FITNESS

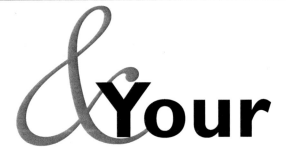

&Your

HEALTH

David C. Nieman

Appalachian State University

Fifth Edition

Kendall Hunt

publishing company

Cover Images Credits:
Skiier image (c) Shutterstock, Inc.
Images of scale and food © PhotoDisc
images of dumb bells, arm lifting weight, man holding weight, and backbone © 2009, JupiterImages, Inc.

Kendall Hunt
publishing company

www.kendallhunt.com
Send all inquiries to:
4050 Westmark Drive
Dubuque, IA 52004–1840

ISBN 978-0-7575-8398-8

Printed in the United States of America
10 9 8 7 6 5 4 3 2 1

To my loving wife, Cathy,
for her wisdom, strength,
and support,
and my two children,
Jonathan and Jennifer,
who fill my life with joy.

Contents

Preface

I have taught collegiate-level fitness and health courses for over 30 years, and it has been a most rewarding and informative experience. Drawing from this background, I have pulled together all the important fitness and health concepts that have proven useful and appealing to young adults.

- What is the meaning of health?
- What does it mean to be physically fit?
- How can one measure health and fitness?
- What is a healthy body fat percentage and how can it be estimated?
- What diet is recommended for healthy and fit individuals?
- What type of lifestyle is recommended to prevent heart disease or avoid obesity?
- What is an optimal blood cholesterol and blood pressure?
- Can the aging process be retarded?
- Can stress be managed in this modern era?

These are the sorts of issues that are emphasized in this book.

About This Book

In many colleges and universities across the United States, the general education requirement for physical education (e.g., 1 or 2 semester hours of badminton, tennis, basketball, etc.) is being supplemented or substituted with the option that students can take a class that focuses on fitness and health issues. *Fitness and Your Health* has been written to meet this need. Specifically, this book uses a physical fitness approach to educate the student on the most important health issues of our time. I have found this approach to be much more stimulating and interesting to collegiate-level students than the most traditional health class (which tends to be more theoretical than practical).

Organization

The eleven chapters of *Fitness and Your Health* are grouped into four parts:

Part 1: An Introduction to Health and Fitness. Chapter 1 reviews the meaning of health and the modern-day fitness and health movement. Chapter 2 outlines the important concepts behind physical fitness.

Part 2: Testing for Physical Fitness. Chapter 3 summarizes the important issues involved in determining whether one is ready to safely start an exercise program. Chapters 4 through 6 describe a wide variety of tests that estimate cardiorespiratory fitness, body composition, and musculoskeletal fitness.

Part 3: Conditioning for Physical Fitness. Chapter 7 outlines five important elements in a comprehensive physical fitness program, while Chapter 8 reviews important nutrition issues for both active and inactive individuals.

Part 4: Physical Activity, Health, and Disease Prevention. Chapters 9 through 11 deal with heart disease prevention, prevention and treatment of obesity, and psychological health. The issues are reviewed in detail, with an emphasis on exercise and nutrition relationships.

Features

Illustrations and Tables

The numerous figures and tables will help reinforce the fitness and health information presented in the text. All information is up-to-date, and is depicted in an easy-to-understand format and style.

Health and Fitness Insight

Each chapter contains a *Health and Fitness Insight* that focuses on a particular topic of current interest.

Summary

A summary at the end of each chapter highlights all the important chapter information, allowing students to gain a final overview prior to quizzes and exams.

Health and Fitness Activities

Each chapter ends with self-assessment questionnaires, surveys, testing activities, or other practical assignments to help the student apply and understand various health and fitness concepts. This is one of the strongest features of the book, and students are encouraged to complete each one.

Chapter Quizzes

A list of quiz questions (and answers) is given at the end of each chapter to help the student prepare for class exams.

Appendices

Two appendices are included with this book, including a pictorial outline of recommended exercise calisthenics, human anatomical charts, and an extensive glossary.

Supplementary Materials

Supplementary materials accompanying this text are designed to help instructors plan coursework, presentations, and exams. These supplementary materials include:

Instructor PowerPoint Presentations

Each chapter has been outlined and prepared as a PowerPoint presentation to guide the instructor during lectures.

TestPak

More than 200 questions have been prepared and put onto a computer diskette for instructor use in preparing quizzes and exams.

PART ONE

An Introduction to Health and Fitness

chapter one

Health and Exercise in America

"The increasing costs associated with health care will compel public policy to emphasize measures such as physical fitness to enhance health." —U.S. Public Health Service

The Meaning of Health

The most notable, and undoubtedly still the most influential definition of health is that of the World Health Organization (WHO), which appeared in the preamble of their constitution during the late 1940s:

"Health is a state of complete physical, mental, and social well-being, and not merely the absence of disease and infirmity."

This definition was built on the conviction of the organizers of WHO that the security of future world peace would lie in the improvement of physical, mental, and social health. Basically it suggests that health involves more than the absence of disease, and extends to how one feels and functions physically, mentally, and socially.

Physical health is defined as the absence of disease and disability, together with sufficient energy and vitality to accomplish daily tasks and active recreational pursuits without undue fatigue. We will discuss this in detail in Chapter 2.

Social health refers to the ability to interact effectively with other people and the social environment, enjoying satisfying personal relationships. There is good evidence that people who have many social ties to other people experience less disease and greater feelings of well-being (see Chapter 11).

Mental or psychological health refers to both the absence of mental disorders and the ability to meet the daily challenges and social interactions of life without undue mental, emotional, or behavioral problems. Later in this book we will review the mounting evidence that psychological well-being has much to do with one's physical health (see Chapter 11).

The *American Journal of Health Promotion* has proposed an updated definition of health because of its belief that spiritual health is an important and separate component. They have defined optimal health as "a balance of physical, emotional, social, spiritual, and intellectual health." [*Am J Health Promotion* 3(3):5, 1989].

FIGURE 1.1
The Health Continuum shows
that between optimal health
and death lies disease, which
is preceded by a prolonged
period of negative lifestyle
habits.

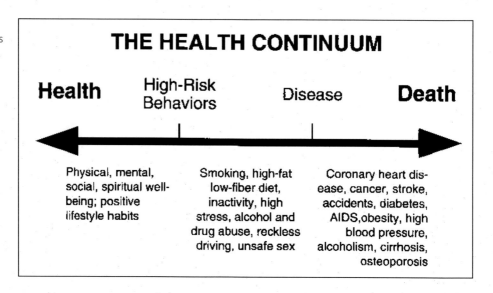

Several articles on **spiritual health** have been published by this journal, and the following definition proposed:

> "Optimal spiritual health is defined as the ability to develop one's spiritual nature to its fullest potential. This includes our ability: to discover, articulate and act on our own basic purpose in life; to learn how to give and receive love, joy and peace; to pursue a fulfilling life; and to contribute to the improvement of the spiritual health of others." [*Am J Health Promotion* 1(2):12–17, 1987.]

This definition represents the position that humankind does have a spiritual dimension, and that health professionals should address it in their day-to-day contacts with patients and clients, while at the same time avoiding "religious proselytizing, singular theism, or dogmatism. . . ." This journal concludes that " . . . we may have limited our theories of human possibility through the exclusion of spirituality." [*Am J Health Promotion* 5(4):273–281, 1991].

Figure 1.1 depicts and summarizes this discussion on the definition of health. The absence of health is death, but before death comes disease (or an accident), and before disease most people go through a sustained period of undesirable habits of living. Health represents a dynamic state of positive well-being, where positive habits are practiced, making the risk of premature disease and death less likely.

The Healthy People Initiative

Healthy People is the prevention agenda for the nation, a road map to better health for all. Since 1980, the U.S. Department of Health and Human Services has used health promotion and disease prevention objectives to improve our health.

It all started in 1979 with the release of *Healthy People: The Surgeon General's Report on Health Promotion and Disease Prevention*. Noting that the nation's first public health revolution against infectious diseases had been very successful, the Surgeon General issued a challenge to begin a second public health revolution—this time against chronic disease or the lifestyle-related diseases such as heart disease, cancer, stroke, and diabetes, which together accounted for two-thirds of all death (see figure 1.2).

The Surgeon General's call for action was followed up with the first set of national health objectives, *Promoting Health/Preventing Disease: Objectives for the Nation*, which were published in 1980. It set out 226 health objectives for 1990, emphasizing 15 focus areas for health improvement. This was the first time that health promotion received

FIGURE 1.2

Leading causes of death in 1900 and current.

Source: Centers for Disease Control and Prevention.

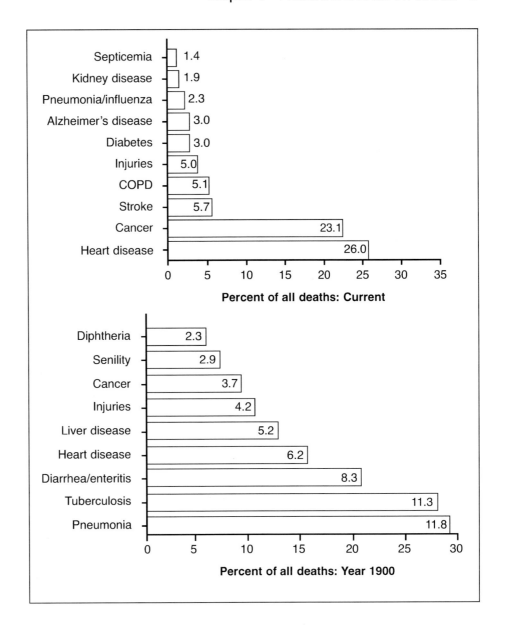

attention by the nation's highest health official, and was defined as the science and art of helping people change their lifestyle to move toward a state of optimal health.

In 1990, another set of objectives was published to improve the health of the nation. The 310 health objectives were divided into 22 focus areas, with three overarching goals: to increase years of healthy life, reduce disparities in health among different population groups, and achieve access to preventive health services for all. This framework provided good direction for individuals to change personal health behaviors, and for health organizations to support good health through health promotion policies.

National health objectives for the year 2010 were published in 2000. *Healthy People 2010* was the United States' contribution to the World Health Organization's "Health for All" strategy. *Healthy People 2010* had two major goals:

Goal #1: Increase quality and years of healthy life. A healthy life translates to a full range of function from infancy through old age, allowing one to enter into satisfying relationships with other people, and to work and play. The average baby born can expect to live 78 years, but only 64 of these years will be healthy.

Goal #2: Eliminate health disparities. There are many barriers to good health, but it is unfortunate that in America race, income, education, and age often interfere with access to quality health care and opportunities to practice good health habits. Healthy People

2020 was published in 2010, and has a vision for a society in which all people live long, healthy lives. The goals for Healthy People 2020 are similar in scope to those of 2010:

- Attain high quality, longer lives free of preventable disease, disability, injury, and premature death.
- Achieve health equity, eliminate disparities, and improve the health of all groups.
- Create social and physical environments that promote good health for all.
- Promote quality of life, healthy development and healthy behaviors across all life stages.

The Problem of Inactivity in This Country

A Brief Historical Review

Early Concepts of Exercise During the Late 1800s

As America experienced increasing urbanization and industrialization, the health of Americans became a growing concern to many leaders. Social reformers such as Dr. Oliver Wendell Holmes, Catharine Beecher, and Dr. Dioclesian Lewis were leaders in encouraging Americans to exercise more.

In the schools, several progressive colleges hired medical doctors to teach students health, light gymnastics with dumbbells, European gymnastics, and anthropometric measurements. Most of the programs were based upon German and Swedish gymnastic programs, which consisted of marching, free exercises with rings and clubs, and apparatus work on balance board, rings, and vaulting box.

The emphasis of these programs was on the health-related value of proper physical exercise. Muscle strength and size were seen as most important. Sports and play and cardiorespiratory exercise were not generally included.

Around the turn of the century, however, public interest and participation in sports grew strongly. This interest was mirrored in the schools as leadership shifted from medical doctors to "physical educators" who promoted sports and games as the best way to develop intellectual awareness and moral and social behavior, along with physical fitness. The promotion of exercise for physical fitness, however, became secondary to the development of game and sport skills (motor fitness), and the attainment of psychosocial goals.

This was the beginning of a furious debate that has continued to this day—should physical education emphasize health-related physical activities (exercises that develop the heart, lungs, and musculoskeletal system), or should it emphasize motor-fitness-related activities (exercises that develop coordination, balance, agility, speed, and power)? (See the discussion of terms in Chapter 2.)

Several major events of the 1940s and 1950s prompted Americans to take a closer look at both school physical education programs and adult fitness.

The Fitness Awakening

Statistics on draftees during World War II spurred the media to report that school sports programs were not adequately developing students' physical fitness. Out of nine million registrants examined for the armed services in early 1943, almost three million were rejected for physical or mental reasons. The chief of Athletics and Recreation for the Army responded by recommending at the 1943 War Fitness Conference that "physical education through play must be discarded and a more rugged program substituted."

After World War II, heart disease reached epidemic proportions. Obesity became a major public health problem, and healthcare costs skyrocketed. In the midst of these health problems, however, the public was still focusing on such men as Charles Atlas and Jack La Lanne, who emphasized muscular strength and muscle size.

The first evidence of national fitness awareness concerned the young. The shocking results of the Kraus-Weber tests of minimum muscular fitness of school children were released in 1953. The tests consisted of six simple movements of key muscle groups. Of U.S. children, 59 percent failed, while only 8.7 percent of European' children failed. When President Eisenhower learned of this study, he immediately called for a special White House Conference, which was finally held in June 1956. As a result, the President's Council on Youth Fitness and a President's Citizens Advisory Committee on the Fitness of American Youth were formed.

A surge in public concern about adult fitness took place in the late 1960s. In 1967, Oregon track coach Bill Bowerman toured New Zealand and discovered "jogging." He returned to America and wrote *Jogging,* igniting the first running boom in the United States, with the book selling over 300,000 copies.

In 1968, Dr. Kenneth H. Cooper, a medical doctor for the Air Force, published his book *Aerobics,* followed two years later by *The New Aerobics.* In these books, Cooper challenged Americans to take personal charge of their lifestyles, and to counter the epidemics of heart disease, obesity, and rising health care costs by engaging in regular exercise. Cooper emphasized, however, that the best exercise for stimulating the heart, lungs, and blood vessels is aerobic:

> I'll state my position early. The best exercises are running, swimming, cycling, walking, stationary running, handball, basketball, and squash, and in just about that order. . . . Isometrics (static muscle contractions against immovable objects), weight lifting and calisthenics, though good as far as they go, don't even make the list, despite the fact that most exercise books are *based* on one of these three, especially calisthenics.

These two books provided the necessary theoretical fuel for an adult fitness revolution that soon gripped the country. Millions took up the "aerobic challenge" and began jogging, cycling, walking, and swimming programs. Ken Cooper's wife, Mildred Cooper, joined her husband in 1972, writing *Aerobics for Women.* Within nine years, these three books on aerobics sold over six million copies and were translated into 15 foreign languages, and into Braille.

In 1972, Frank Shorter won the Olympic marathon gold medal in Munich. The extensive television coverage of both this marathon, and later of Shorter's silver medal effort in 1976 (Montreal), helped to spawn the road racing movement that has since become so popular (see figure 1.3).

FIGURE 1.3

Running has become a symbol of the modern fitness revolution.

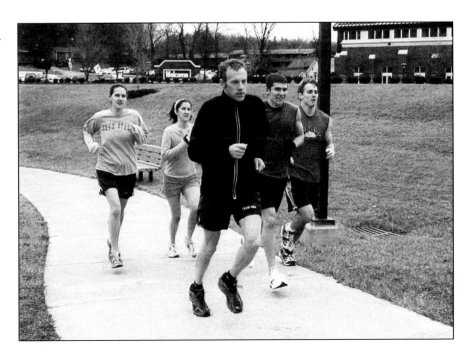

Running, which quickly became a symbol of the American exercise movement, was promoted by a spate of successful books by Joe Henderson, Joan Ullyot, George Sheehan, and others, climaxed by *The Complete Book of Running* by Jim Fixx. Fixx's book topped the bestseller lists for nearly two years, second in history at that time only to *Games People Play.* In the space of one year, 1977 to 1978, the magazine *Runner's World* tripled its circulation from 85,000 to 270,000.

Another popular form of adult exercise, aerobic dance, started at about the same time as the running movement. Aerobic dancing, in making exercise fun and socially oriented, has attracted millions who might otherwise not have joined the fitness movement. It is probably the most popular organized fitness activity for women in the United States, with approximately 25 million participants.

Aerobic dance traces its origins to Jacki Sorenson, the wife of a naval pilot, who began conducting exercise classes at a U.S. Navy base in Puerto Rico in 1969. Its growth has been stimulated more recently by the popularity of videotaped dance exercise programs.

The original aerobic dance programs consisted of a combination of various dance forms, including ballet, modern jazz, disco, and folk, as well as calisthenic-type exercises. More recent innovations include water aerobics (done in a swimming pool), non-impact or low-impact aerobics (one foot on the ground at all times), specific dance aerobics, step aerobics, and "assisted" aerobics involving weights worn on the wrists and/or ankles.

Current American Physical Activity Patterns

Most of us regard physical activity as important for health, but few are motivated enough by this belief to schedule exercise as a part of the daily routine. As summarized in Figure 1.4, since the late 1990s, 30% to 35% of adults report participation in moderate- or vigorous-intensity activity sufficient to meet existing recommendations, and 35% to 40% report no leisure time activity. About one in five engage in muscle strength and endurance exercises.

FIGURE 1.4
Only about one in three adults engage in regular, moderate, or vigorous physical activity.
Source: U.S. Department of Health and Human Services. *2008 Physical Activity Guidelines for Americans.* www.health.gov/paguidelines.

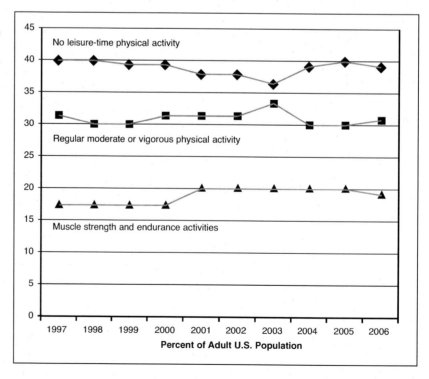

Student Fitness

There is a perceived fitness crisis among American students who are less healthy, active, and fit than is recommended. Key findings include the following:

- An increasing number of American youth are overweight. The prevalence of overweight in children ages 6 to 11 increased from 4.2 percent during the 1960s to a current 17.5 percent; for adolescents ages 12 to 19, the increase was 4.6 percent to 17.0 percent. Nationwide, 20.5 percent of college students are overweight.
- Only 36% adolescents exercise vigorously on a regular basis. Less than four in ten college students participate in aerobic activities that make them sweat and breathe hard for at least 20 minutes on three or more days each week.
- Only one in three students in grades 5 through 12 takes physical education daily, with this proportion falling to 28 percent among high school students. Even among students taking physical education, many students do not participate in moderate to vigorous physical activity.
- Young people aged 2 to 18 spend over four hours a day doing sedentary activities such as watching television, playing video games, or using a computer.
- Upper-body strength is poor for many children and youths. Half of high school male and two-thirds of female students do not engage in strengthening exercises on a regular basis.
- Many young people have disease risk factors. Nearly two in three adolescents have two or more of five major risk factors for chronic disease. Chronic disease is a long-term process that begins with the indiscretions of childhood and youth, so there is much concern about the future health and fitness of the next generation. One in five college students is overweight, less than four in ten exercise vigorously on a regular basis, and significant proportions smoke, have poor diets, and possess disease risk factors (see figure 1.5).

FIGURE 1.5

National surveys on the fitness status of American children and youth have aroused much public concern.

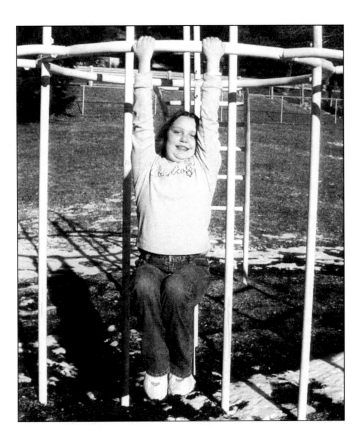

HEALTH AND FITNESS INSIGHT
The Wellness Revolution

As this chapter indicates, a growing number of Americans are entering the fitness movement. The fitness movement, however, is only one part of a much larger "wellness revolution" that is sweeping the United States. Let's consider some trends about this wellness revolution.

Health/Fitness Success Stories

Since 1979 when the *Healthy People* process began, many positive changes in the health of Americans have been measured. A major goal of this book is to help you follow the *Healthy People* road map to health and fitness. Health and fitness highlights of the past quarter-century include the following successes:

- **Life expectancy,** or the number of years one is expected to live at birth, has increased from about 47 years in 1900 to a current 78 years, the highest ever in U.S. history (see Figure 1.6). Most of this increase is attributable to widespread vaccination, control of infectious diseases from cleaner water and improved sanitation, safer and healthier foods, safer workplaces and motor vehicles, a decline in deaths from coronary heart disease and stroke, improvements in personal behavior and lifestyles, and a recognition of tobacco use as a health hazard.
- Stroke and coronary heart disease deaths rates reached epidemic levels about 50 years ago, but have been falling ever since. Since 1950, the American death rate for stroke decreased 74 percent, and for heart disease, 64 percent. This is one of the greatest health success stories of the past half-century, and is due to improvements in American health habits and medical care.
- Cancer death rates decreased during the 1990s after decades of concern over increases. As with heart disease, much of the decrease is because of improvements in lifestyles (especially better diets and less smoking), and an emphasis on early screening for cancer.
- Cigarette consumption has decreased. In 1965, 52 percent of men and 33 percent of women smoked. Now only 20 percent of all Americans smoke.
- Diets have improved. Fat intake has decreased from over 40 percent of total calories in the 1960s to a current 33 percent of calories. Americans are consuming more poultry, fish, and low-fat dairy products, and less beef, pork, eggs, and whole milk.
- Alcohol consumption has fallen. Since the 1980s, alcohol intake has decreased due in part to the public's increasing awareness of alcohol's associated dangers.
- Prevalence of high blood pressure, a major risk factor for stroke and coronary heart disease, has fallen from 39 percent in the 1960s to a current 31 percent of Americans.
- Prevalence of high blood cholesterol, another risk factor for heart disease, has fallen from 32 percent in the 1960s to a current 17 percent.

Key Health/Fitness Challenges for the Future

Despite the successes, some important health-related areas still need improvement:

- Too many Americans adults, about 66 percent, are overweight and obese. Despite a nationwide obsession with ideal body weight, government studies over the past 40 years have shown that Americans are losing the war, especially among the poor and minority groups. Among our youth, the prevalence of overweight is rising strongly.

- Too few American young people and adults exercise regularly. As emphasized in this chapter, about 40% of adults are physically inactive, despite the common knowledge that inactivity is related to heart disease, certain types of cancer, obesity, osteoporosis, and frailty in old age.
- Disease risk factors are still too widely prevalent among both adults and adolescents. One in five Americans smokes, three in ten has high blood pressure, and one in five has high blood cholesterol. About two in three adolescents have two or more of five major risk factors for chronic disease, and these often remain into adulthood.
- Mental stress levels are high. About six in ten American adults report that they experience moderate to high levels of stress, posing one of the greatest health challenges for the next century.

Summary

1. Health and health promotion were defined and discussed. According to the World Health Organization, health is a state of complete physical, mental, and social well-being, not merely the absence of disease and infirmity.
2. A brief historical review of the problem of inactivity in this country was given. A turning point in adult fitness awareness took place in 1968 with the publication of Dr. Kenneth Cooper's first book, *Aerobics*.
3. Many surveys have been conducted trying to evaluate the magnitude of the present fitness revolution. Only one out of four Americans is exercising appropriately; these proportions are even worse among those with less education and income, the elderly, and females.
4. American children and youth have low fitness levels. Of particular concern are test results showing low upper-body strength and cardiorespiratory fitness status in many children and youth. The prevalence of overweight has risen sharply since the 1960s.
5. The wellness revolution, of which the fitness movement is a part, was reviewed in the *Health and Fitness Insight*. While there have been enheartening improvements in American health, there is still much room for progress.

FIGURE 1.6

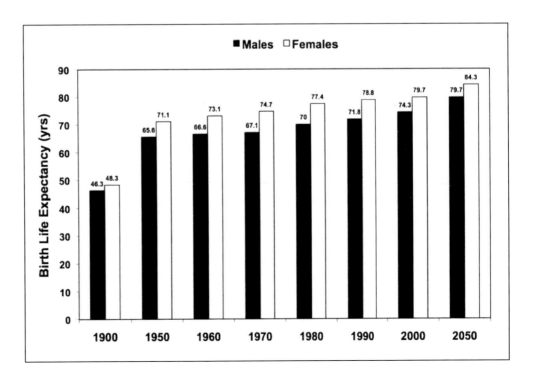

HEALTH AND FITNESS ACTIVITY 1.1
What Is Your Personal Exercise Program?

In this chapter, the exercise habits of Americans were fully described. The National Health Interview Survey (NHIS) by the National Center for Health Statistics is presently one of the best data sources for this type of information. Data from NHIS have been collected continuously since 1957.

In this *Physical Fitness Activity*, you will be answering questions on exercise taken directly from the NHIS Health Promotion and Disease Prevention Survey. Fill in the blanks in Table 1.1 on the next page, and then summarize your exercise program by answering the questions listed below.

Physical Fitness Activity Questions

1. Summarize your answers to the NHIS questionnaire by filling in the following:

    A. What was your average *frequency per week* of exercise during the last 2 weeks? *Note:* Count only the sessions where intensity was high or moderate.

    _____ average frequency/week

    Note: Total the number of times in past 2 weeks and divide by 2. For example, if you jogged 2 times in the past 2 weeks, biked 2 times, and played soccer once, your average frequency would be 5 divided by 2, or 2.5 times/week.

    B. What was your average *duration per exercise session in minutes?* (from "A")

    _____ average duration per exercise session (in minutes)

    Note: Total the number of minutes spent in exercise during past 2 weeks and divide by number of exercise sessions. For example, if the jogging sessions lasted 15 minutes each, the biking sessions 30 minutes each, and soccer 40 minutes, the average duration per exercise session in minutes would be 130 min/5 = 26 minutes per session.

    How do you compare with American College of Sports Medicine standards?

    Yes   No
    ___ ___   3 or more times per week?
    ___ ___   20 or more minutes per session?
    ___ ___   Moderate or high heart rate/breathing levels for each session?

The American College of Sports Medicine recommends that people exercise at least three times per week, for at least 20 to 30 minutes, at moderate-to-hard intensity levels (at least 50 percent maximal oxygen capacity). (See Chapter 7.)

Source: National Health Interview Survey, Health Promotion and Disease Prevention. National Center for Health Statistics, T. Stephens and Schoenborn. 1988. Adult Health Practices in the United States and Canada. Vital and Health Statistics. Series 5, No. 3. DHHS Pub. No. (PHS) 88–1479. Public Health Service. Washington, D.C.: U.S. Government Printing Office.

TABLE 1.2   National Health Interview Survey

A	B	C	D			
In the past 2 weeks, have you engaged in any of the following exercises, sports, or physically active hobbies?	How many times in the past 2 weeks did you play/go/do (activity in A)?	On the average, about how many minutes did you actually spend on (activity in A) on each occasion?	What usually happened to your heart rate or breathing when you undertook (activity in A)? Did you have a small, moderate, or large increase, or no increase at all in your heart rate or breathing?			
	Yes	No	Times	Minutes	Small	Moderate	Large	None

A			B	C	D			
	Yes	No	Times	Minutes	Small	Moderate	Large	None
1. Walking for exercise	—	—	—	—	—	—	—	—
2. Jogging or running	—	—	—	—	—	—	—	—
3. Hiking	—	—	—	—	—	—	—	—
4. Gardening/yard work	—	—	—	—	—	—	—	—
5. Aerobic dancing	—	—	—	—	—	—	—	—
6. Other dancing	—	—	—	—	—	—	—	—
7. Calisthenics	—	—	—	—	—	—	—	—
8. Golf	—	—	—	—	—	—	—	—
9. Tennis	—	—	—	—	—	—	—	—
10. Bowling	—	—	—	—	—	—	—	—
11. Biking	—	—	—	—	—	—	—	—
12. Swimming	—	—	—	—	—	—	—	—
13. Yoga	—	—	—	—	—	—	—	—
14. Weight lifting	—	—	—	—	—	—	—	—
15. Basketball	—	—	—	—	—	—	—	—
16. Baseball	—	—	—	—	—	—	—	—
17. Football	—	—	—	—	—	—	—	—
18. Soccer	—	—	—	—	—	—	—	—
19. Volleyball	—	—	—	—	—	—	—	—
20. Handball/racquetball	—	—	—	—	—	—	—	—
21. Skating	—	—	—	—	—	—	—	—
22. Skiing	—	—	—	—	—	—	—	—
23. Any other type of exercise not mentioned here	—	—	—	—	—	—	—	—
List here _____	—	—	—	—	—	—	—	—

Source: Health Promotion and Disease Prevention Supplement, Section R: Exercise (adapted).

HEALTH AND FITNESS ACTIVITY 1.2
Health/Fitness Check

Name: _____   Today's Date: _____

Mailing Address: _____

City: _____   State: _____   Zip: _____

Your age? _____ years:

Sex: ❏ Male   ❏ Female

How tall are you (without shoes)? _____ feet _____ inches

How much do you weigh (minimal clothing and without shoes)? _____ pounds

Points for Body Weight
2   Too lean, have eating disorder
0   Lean, underweight
0   I am at desirable weight
2   10–20 pounds overweight
3   21–50 pounds overweight
4   more than 50 pounds overweight

Please check the appropriate box for each question.

Yes   No

4   0 Points
❏   ❏   1. Has your father or brother had a heart attack or died suddenly of heart disease before age 55 years; has your mother or sister experienced these heart problems before age 65 years?

4   0
❏   ❏   2. Has a doctor told you that you have high blood pressure (more than 140/90 mm Hg), or are you on medication to control your blood pressure?

4   0
❏   ❏   3. Is your total blood cholesterol greater than 240 mg/dl, or has a doctor told you that your cholesterol is at a high risk level?

4   0
❏   ❏   4. Do you have diabetes?

3   0
❏   ❏   5. During the past year, would you say that you experienced enough stress, strain, and pressure to have a significant effect on your health?

4   0

❏   ❏   6. Do you eat foods nearly *every day* that are high in fat and cholesterol, such as fatty meats, cheese, fried foods, butter, whole milk, ice cream, or eggs?

---

7. In general, compared to other persons your age, rate how healthy you are:

❏ 1   ❏ 2   ❏ 3   ❏ 4   ❏ 5   ❏ 6   ❏ 7   ❏ 8   ❏ 9   ❏ 10

Not at all   Somewhat   Extremely
healthy   healthy   healthy

Scoring: [if you checked 1 or 2 = 3 points]
[if you checked 3 or 4 = 2 points]
[if you checked 5, 6, or 7 = 1 point]

8. Outside of your normal work or daily responsibilities, how often do you engage in exercise that at least moderately increases your breathing and heart rate, and makes you sweat, for at least 20 minutes (such as brisk walking, cycling, swimming, jogging, aerobic dance, stair climbing, rowing, basketball, racquetball, vigorous yard work, etc.).
   0 ❏ 5 or more times per week   **3** ❏ Less than 1 time per week
   1 ❏ 3 to 4 times per week   **4** ❏ Seldom or never
   2 ❏ 1 to 2 times per week

9. On average, how many servings of fruit and vegetables do you eat per day? (One serving = 1 medium fruit, 1/2 cup of chopped, cooked, or canned fruit/vegetable, 3/4 cup of fruit or vegetable juice).
   4 ❏ none   **3** ❏ 1–2   **2** ❏ 3–4   **1** ❏ 5–6   **0** ❏ 7–8   **0** ❏ 9 or more

10. On average, how many servings of bread, cereal, rice, or pasta do you eat per day? (One serving = 1 slice of bread, 1 ounce of ready-to-eat cereal, 1/2 cup of cooked cereal, rice, or pasta).
   3 ❏ none   **3** ❏ 1–2   **2** ❏ 3–5   **1** ❏ 6–8   **0** ❏ 9–11   **0** ❏ 12 or more

11. How have you been feeling in general during the past month?
   0 ❏ In excellent spirits   **1** ❏ In good spirits mostly   **2** ❏ In low spirits mostly
   0 ❏ In very good spirits   **1** ❏ I've been up and   **3** ❏ In very low spirits
                                        down in spirits a lot

12. On average, how many hours of sleep do you get in a 24-hour period?
   2 ❏ Less than 5   **1** ❏ 5 to 6.9   **0** ❏ 7 to 9   **0** ❏ More than 9

13. How would you describe your cigarette smoking habits?
   0 ❏ Never smoked
   0 ❏ Used to smoke
   How many years has it been since you smoked? (Check appropriate box)
            3 ❏ less than 1 year   **1** ❏ 6–15
            2 ❏ 1–5   **0** ❏ More than 15

❏ Still smoke

How many cigarettes a day do you smoke on average?

3 ❏ 1–10   **4** ❏ 21–30   **5** ❏ More than 40
3 ❏ 11–20   **4** ❏ 31–40

14. How many alcoholic drinks do you consume? (A "drink" is a glass of wine, a wine cooler, a bottle/can of beer, a shot glass of liquor, or a mixed drink).

0 ❏ Never use alcohol   **0** ❏ Less than 1 per week   **0** ❏ 1 to 6 per week
0 ❏ 1 per day   **3** ❏ 2 to 3 per day   **4** ❏ More than 3 per day

15. When driving or riding in a car, do you wear a seat belt:

0 ❏ All or most of the time   **2** ❏ Once in a while
1 ❏ Some of the time   **3** ❏ Rarely or never

Norms:

Total Points:	Classification:
0–7	Excellent health habits
8–15	Good, but some improvement needed
16–24	Fair, improvement needed
25 or more	Poor, at high risk for disease

CHAPTER 1 QUIZ
Health and Exercise in America

Note: Answers are given at the end of the quiz.

1. Regarding exercise in America:
   A. A minority of Americans are exercising appropriately.
   B. A greater percentage lift weights versus aerobics.
   C. Three in four are physically inactive.
   D. Nearly all adults have an exercise program.

2. _____ is the leading cause of death in the U.S. today, followed by _____ .
   A. COPD/heart disease
   B. heart disease/accidents
   C. cancer/liver disease
   D. heart disease/cancer
   E. cancer/heart disease

3. _____ is physical, mental, and social well-being, and not merely the absence of disease and infirmity.
   A. Exercise
   B. Physical fitness
   C. Health
   D. Cardiovascular endurance
   E. Energy

4. Regarding the fitness of American youth:
   A. They have become fatter since the 1960s.
   B. A majority take daily P.E.
   C. Nearly all obtain enough exercise in P.E. classes.
   D. Upper-body strength is unusually high.

5. Who wrote the book entitled *Aerobics*, which helped to fuel the fitness revolution during the 1970s?
   A. Jim Fixx
   B. Dr. Kenneth H. Cooper
   C. Frank Shorter
   D. Bill Bowerman

6. About _____ % of adults smoke.
    A. 5
    B. 10
    C. 20
    D. 30
    E. 50

7. T   F   Heart disease death rates are increasing.

chapter two

The Meaning of Physical Fitness

"Over the years, I have come to look upon physical fitness as the trunk of a tree that supports the many branches which represent all the activities that make life worth living: intellectual life, spiritual life, occupation, love life and social activities."

—Thomas Kirk Cureton, Jr.

Introduction

There is a connection between fitness and health. Exercise, a good diet, and other lifestyle habits together are a powerful medicine, quite unlike any pill available. If claims were made for a magical elixir that lengthened the span and quality of life, decreased risk of heart disease and cancer, alleviated anxiety and depression, improved muscle tone and heart function, and lowered blood pressure, would not everyone try it? This book will describe these powerful benefits of a healthy, active lifestyle, and provide you with the tools to help get you there.

Your Body Is Designed for Action

Your body is designed to move. Your muscles, tendons, and ligaments empower your arms, legs, and trunk to engage in many different types of physical movements, work activities, and sport. Centers in your brain devoted to muscular motion coordinate the delivery of blood and oxygen from the heart and lungs to your working muscles. The energy your body needs comes from fuel stores that are burned using nutrients supplied from the stomach and intestines. All of the systems of the body communicate with each other through a complex set of chemical and nerve pathways. The more all of these systems are used, the easier and more enjoyable physical activity becomes, enhancing health and the quality of life at the same time.

Benefits of Physical Activity

Physical activity is defined as any bodily movement produced by your muscles, resulting in expenditure of calories. Physical activity includes everything from walking to your class to taking the stairs instead of the elevator to tossing and turning while you sleep.

Exercise is a type of physical activity that is planned for purposes of becoming physically fit. Examples include lifting weights in the weight room or swimming laps in the pool. In other words, physical activity is general muscular movement that encompasses all activities of daily living, while exercise is done on purpose to increase fitness. All types of physical activities burn calories, and if you repeat them on a regular basis, they will not only make you physically fit, but they will also produce healthful changes in your body.

Prevention of Chronic Diseases

Every year, chronic diseases claim the lives of more than one and a half million Americans. Chronic diseases are diseases that develop slowly and are caused by many factors including multiple poor lifestyle habits. Diseases such as heart disease, cancer, diabetes, and others related to lifestyle account for seven of every ten deaths in the United States, and for more than 60 percent of total medical care expenditures. The prolonged illness and disability from chronic diseases result in a low quality of life for millions of Americans. Each of the leading killers are strongly related to lifestyle habits such as inactivity, smoking, poor eating habits, and excessive alcohol consumption.

One of the most important lifestyle habits that you can adopt for disease prevention and quality of life is regular physical activity. Inactivity is a strong factor in causing many diseases, and is to be avoided at all costs. Regular physical activity also helps you feel more energetic, allowing you to function successfully physically, mentally, and socially. Here is a list of the chief benefits of regular physical activity:

- Reduces the risk of dying prematurely (i.e., improves life expectancy).
- Reduces the risk of dying from coronary heart disease, the nation's leading cause of death.
- Reduces the risk of developing diabetes, especially the type that is associated with obesity after turning 40 years of age (called Type 2 diabetes mellitus).
- Helps prevent and treat high blood pressure, a risk factor for heart disease that afflicts over 50 million Americans.
- Reduces the risk of developing colon cancer, the third most common form of cancer death in the United States.
- Reduces feelings of depression and anxiety, while improving mood state and self-esteem.
- Helps control body weight and prevent obesity, which is prevalent in more than one-third of all Americans.
- Helps build and maintain healthy bones and muscles, and improve heart and lung fitness.
- Improves the life quality of older adults, patients with disease, and people of all ages.
- Decreases blood fat levels and increases the "good" cholesterol, called HDL-cholesterol.

You will be receiving more information on the benefits of regular physical activity in Chapters 9 through 11. To review what physical activity benefits are most important for you, visit *Health and Fitness Activity 2.2.* Also search the Internet on current research findings on the health benefits of regular aerobic exercise, using the information provided in *Health and Fitness Activity 2.3.*

How Much Physical Activity Is Enough?

To avoid the health pitfalls of inactivity, every child, teenager, and adult should accumulate 150 minutes or more of moderate-intensity physical activity each week. The physical activity can be spread throughout the week. In Chapter 7, intensity will be defined in detail, but in general, a moderate-intensity activity is similar to a brisk walk. Examples include morning and evening 15 to 30 minute brisk walks, recreational sports play, or a combination of stair climbing and walking bouts each time you have a break in the daily schedule. The good news is that an active lifestyle linked to good health does not require a regimented, vigorous exercise program.

Can you gain additional health and fitness benefits by exercising for more than 150 minutes per week? In other words, if you put in 300 minutes per week of swimming laps, running, training for sports, cycling, or rowing, can you expect greater benefits than walking 30 minutes 5 days a week? The answer is "yes," according to the landmark *2008 Physical Activity Guidelines for Americans*. Additional health and fitness benefits of physical activity can be achieved by adding more time in moderate-intensity activity, or by substituting more vigorous activity (and, of course, by doing both). See Box 2.1 for more information from this report. These recommendations will be covered in greater detail in Chapter 7.

BOX 2.1

Major Findings from the *2008 Physical Activity Guidelines for Americans*

In 2008, the U.S. Department of Health and Human Services (DHHS) released the *Physical Activity Guidelines for Americans*. The *2008 Physical Activity Guidelines* define "low activity" as fewer than 150 minutes of moderate-intensity physical activity a week or 75 minutes of vigorous-intensity activity, "medium activity" as 150 to 300 minutes of moderate-intensity activity a week or 75 to 150 minutes of vigorous-intensity physical activity a week, and "high activity" as more than 300 minutes of moderate-intensity or 150 minutes of vigorous-intensity physical activity a week.

The 2008 Physical Activity Guidelines for adults include the following:

- All adults should avoid inactivity. Some physical activity is better than none, and adults who participate in any amount of physical activity gain some health benefits.
- For substantial health benefits, adults should do at least 150 minutes a week of moderate-intensity, or 75 minutes a week of vigorous-intensity aerobic physical activity, or an equivalent combination of moderate- and vigorous-intensity aerobic activity. Aerobic activity should be performed in episodes of at least 10 minutes, and preferably, it should be spread throughout the week.
- For additional and more extensive health benefits, adults should increase their aerobic physical activity to 300 minutes a week of moderate-intensity, or 150 minutes a week of vigorous-intensity aerobic physical activity, or an equivalent combination of moderate- and vigorous-intensity activity. Additional health benefits are gained by engaging in physical activity beyond this amount.
- Adults should also do muscle-strengthening activities that are moderate or high intensity and involve all major muscle groups on 2 or more days a week, as these activities provide additional health benefits.

Source: U.S. Department of Health and Human Services. *2008 Physical Activity Guidelines for Americans.* www.health.gov/paguidelines.

Aerobic exercise like walking, cycling, swimming, and running is most important for health benefits, but keeping the muscles toned and strong improves life quality and the ability to accomplish the common tasks of everyday life, especially in old age. In other words, a comprehensive physical activity program includes both aerobic and muscular strength components, and is continued for a lifetime.

Physical Fitness

Physical fitness is a set of attributes that people have or achieve that relates to the ability to perform physical activity. The World Health Organization has defined physical fitness as "the ability to perform muscular work satisfactorily." The American College of Sports Medicine has proposed that "fitness is the ability to perform moderate to vigorous levels of physical activity without undue fatigue and the capability of maintaining such ability throughout life."

The President's Council on Physical Fitness and Sports has offered one of the more widely used definitions, describing physical fitness as the "ability to carry out daily tasks with vigor and alertness, without undue fatigue and with ample energy to enjoy leisure-time pursuits and to meet unforeseen emergencies."

Because modern-day tasks require so little energy expenditure, and because of the human tendency to equate leisure time with inactivity, some researchers would add three other reasons (in addition to providing energy for work, leisure, and emergency) for being physically fit:

1. To help avoid diseases associated with too little activity (such as heart disease, hypertension, diabetes, osteoporosis, and others). (See Part 4 of this book.)
2. To make the most of mental capacities. (See Chapter 11.)
3. To feel good, energetic, buoyant.

In other words, a good level of physical fitness may no longer be needed to work in our technologically dominated world, but it is needed to make the most of mental potentialities, to avoid many of the chronic diseases that plague Americans today, to feel good and energetic, and to make the most of what life has to offer. The focus of fitness is not to have just minimal amounts of energy to barely make it through the day, but more to live an integrated, meaningful, joyous, and satisfying, "self-actuated" life.

Rene Dubos spoke of health as a mirage. You can reach for it but never fully grasp it. Physical fitness is similar. Fitness is not so much a possession as a procession; not so much something to have as a way to be. One can never say, "I am physically fit." Instead, one is always within the process, seeking to come as close as possible to a goal that in itself is unattainable.

One can subjectively measure physical fitness by determining how much energy one has for doing what is enjoyable in life, and experiencing all the natural adventure possible. From snow skiing to mountain climbing, country cycling to weekend backpacking, those who are physically fit have the energy to maximize their enjoyment of all the natural resources of their environment.

Physical fitness has also been described as the ability to last, to bear up, to withstand stress, and to persevere under difficult circumstances where an unfit person would give up. Physical fitness is the opposite from being fatigued from ordinary efforts, from lacking the energy to enter zestfully into life's activities, and from becoming exhausted from unexpected, demanding physical exertion. It is a positive quality, extending on a scale from death to "abundant life."

How to obtain this energy and zest for life is the subject of Part 3 of this book. Basically, when the heart, lungs, blood vessels, and muscles are regularly stimulated through physical activity, in time, every physical movement throughout the day seems easier. This means that more energy is available for active leisure-time as well as emergencies, along with both physiological and psychological benefits.

The following definition of physical fitness summarizes these thoughts:

Physical fitness is a dynamic state of energy and vitality that enables one to carry out daily tasks, to engage in active leisure-time pursuits, and to meet unforeseen emergencies without undue fatigue. In addition, those who are physically fit have a reduced risk of inactivity-related diseases, and are better able to function at the peak of their intellectual capacity, while enjoying "joie de vivre."

The Measurable Elements of Physical Fitness

The above definition of physical fitness is philosophical. Variables such as vigor, alertness, fatigue, and enjoyment are not easily measured. To clarify the meaning of physical fitness, it is important to identify separately the components that can actually be measured and defined and developed. Although in the past there has been misunderstanding and confusion regarding the measurable elements of physical fitness, there is now a growing consensus on this important matter.

The most frequently cited components fall into two groups: one related to health and the other related to skills that pertain more to athletic ability in sports. Figure 2.1 summarizes the components of *health-related fitness* and *skill-related fitness* with examples of the continuum of physical activities that covers the entire range of sports.

THE MEASUREABLE ELEMENTS OF PHYSICAL FITNESS

SKILL-RELATED FITNESS	HEALTH-RELATED FITNESS

1. AGILITY
2. BALANCE
3. COORDINATION
4. SPEED
5. POWER
6. REACTION TIME
	1. CARDIORESPIRATORY ENDURANCE
	2. BODY COMPOSITION
	3. MUSCULOSKELETAL
	   a. flexibility
	   b. muscular strength
	   c. muscular endurance

THE SPORTS CONTINUUM

SKILL-RELATED FITNESS	BOTH	HEALTH-RELATED FITNESS
ARCHERY BOWLING FENCING GOLF TABLE TENNIS VOLLEYBALL BADMINTON BASEBALL DOWNHILL SKIING FOOTBALL TENNIS	BASKETBALL HANDBALL ICE SKATING RACQUETBALL ROLLER SKATING SOCCER SQUASH	AEROBIC DANCING CALISTHENICS CROSS-COUNTRY SKIING ROPE JUMPING ROWING SNOWSHOEING BACKPACKING BICYCLING RUNNING STAIR CLIMBING SWIMMING WALKING WEIGHT LIFTING

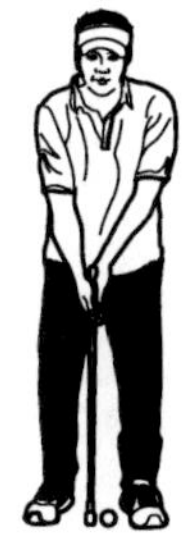

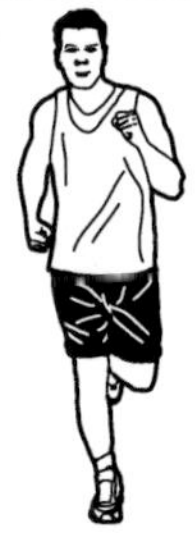

FIGURE 2.1

Most physical activities exist on a continuum between health- or skill-related fitness.

Notice that these activities demand these components in varying degrees. While some physical activities such as archery, bowling, and table tennis demand and develop mainly skill-related attributes, others such as walking, running, and stair climbing are almost entirely health-related. Some activities such as soccer, handball, basketball, and skating require high levels of both components.

While the elements of skill-related fitness are important for participation in various dual and team sports, they have little significance for the day-to-day tasks of Americans or for their general health. Thus, people with poor athletic skills should understand that they can still be healthy, through the development of the health-related components of physical fitness. Just as importantly, the person who excels in throwing a ball or swinging a golf club should understand that the related, athletic activity may leave the core elements of health-related physical fitness underdeveloped. The trend today in public policy recommendations is to emphasize the development of the health-related fitness elements, and to push for their prominence in school, worksite, and community programs.

The Elements of Skill-Related Fitness Defined

The elements of skill-related fitness are:

Agility—The ability to rapidly change the position of the entire body in space, with speed and accuracy.

Balance—Maintenance of equilibrium while stationary or moving.

Coordination—The ability to use the senses, such as sight and hearing, together with body parts in performing motor tasks smoothly and accurately.

Speed—Ability to perform a movement within a short period of time.

Power—Rate at which one can perform work (strength over time).

Reaction Time—The time elapsed between stimulation and the beginning of the reaction to it.

The Elements of Health-Related Fitness Defined

Each of the components of health-related physical fitness can be measured separately from the others, with specific exercises applied to the development of each. The levels of the health-related components of physical fitness need not vary together; for example, a person may be strong but lack flexibility, or a person may have good heart and lung endurance, but lack muscular strength. To develop "total" physical fitness for health, each of the five components discussed below must be included within the exercise prescription (see Chapter 7).

Cardiorespiratory Endurance

Cardiorespiratory endurance can be defined as the ability to continue or persist in strenuous tasks involving large muscle groups for extended periods of time. It is the ability of the circulatory and respiratory systems to adjust to and recover from the effects of whole-body exercise or work.

For many people, being in good shape means having good cardiorespiratory endurance, exemplified by such feats as being able to run, cycle, and swim for prolonged periods of time (see figure 2.2). To most fitness leaders, cardiorespiratory endurance is the most important of the health-related physical fitness components.

High levels of cardiorespiratory endurance indicate a high physical work capacity, which is the ability to release relatively high amounts of energy over an extended period of time. As will be explained in Part 4, there are many benefits associated with cardiorespiratory endurance. Testing for cardiorespiratory endurance will be the subject of Chapter 4; conditioning for cardiorespiratory endurance will be covered in Part 3.

FIGURE 2.2
Cardiorespiratory endurance can be defined as the ability to continue or persist in strenuous tasks involving large muscle groups for extended periods of time. Jogging and running are two examples.

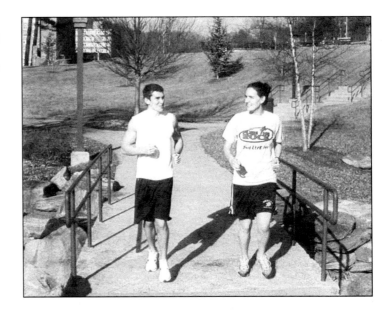

FIGURE 2.3
Body composition is the body's relative amounts of fat and lean body tissue, or fat-free mass (muscle, bone, water).

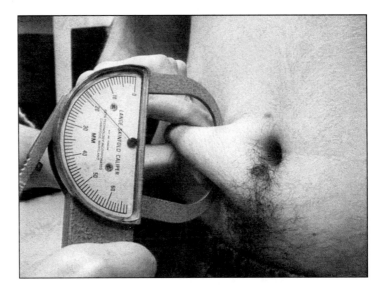

Dr. Kenneth H. Cooper, who coined the term **aerobics,** which is merely another term for cardiorespiratory endurance, gives this definition:

> Aerobics refers to a variety of exercises that stimulate heart and lung activity for a time period sufficiently long to produce beneficial changes in the body. Running, swimming, cycling, and jogging—these are typical aerobic exercises. There are many others. . . . They have one thing in common: by making you work hard, they demand plenty of oxygen. That's the basic idea. That's what makes them aerobic.

Body Composition

Body composition refers to the body's relative amounts of lean body tissue, or fat-free mass for example, muscle, bone, water (see figure 2.3). Body weight can be subdivided simply into two components: fat weight (the weight of fat tissue) and fat-free weight (the weight of the remaining lean tissue). Obesity is defined as an excessive accumulation of fat weight.

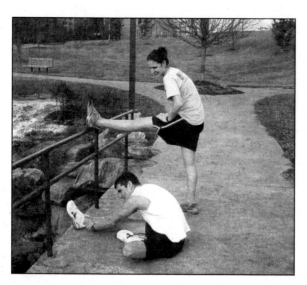

FIGURE 2.4

Flexibility is defined as the functional capacity of the joints to move through a full range of movement.

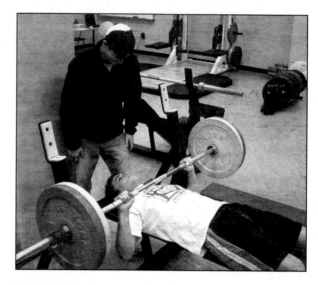

FIGURE 2.5

Strenth is the maximal one-effort force that can be exerted against a resistance.

Percent body fat, the percent of total weight represented by fat weight, is the preferred index for evaluating a person's body composition. The optimal body fat level for men is 15 percent or less; they are considered obese when their body fat percentage is 25 percent and higher. The optimal body fat level for women is 22 percent or less, and they are considered obese when their body fat percentage is 32 percent or higher.

Chapters 5 and 10 will describe how to measure body fat accurately, theories of obesity, the impact of obesity on health, and how to treat obesity.

Musculoskeletal Fitness

Musculoskeletal fitness is comprised of three components: flexibility, muscular strength, and muscular endurance.

1. **Flexibility** is defined as the functional capacity of the joints to move through a full range of movement (see figure 2.4). Flexibility is specific to each joint of the body. Muscles, ligaments, and tendons largely determine the amount of movement possible at each joint. Common flexibility exercises include touching the floor with the hands while the legs are nearly straight, or spreading the legs far out to the side while sitting.

   Chapter 6 will explain how to test for flexibility, and explore the benefits. Chapter 7 will discuss the principles of flexibility exercise.

2. **Muscular strength** the maximal one-effort force that can be exerted against a resistance (see figure 2.5). It is the absolute maximum amount of force that one can generate in an isolated movement of a single muscle group. The stronger the individual, the greater the amount of force that he or she can generate. Common muscular strength exercises include weight lifting with heavy weights.

   Chapters 6 and 7 will discuss how to test and develop muscular strength.

3. **Muscular endurance** is defined as the ability of the muscles to apply a submaximal force repeatedly or to sustain a muscular contraction for a certain period of time (see figure 2.6). Common muscle endurance exercises are sit-ups, push-ups, chin-ups, or repetitions of lifting weights. Chapters 6 and 7 will describe how to test and develop muscular endurance.

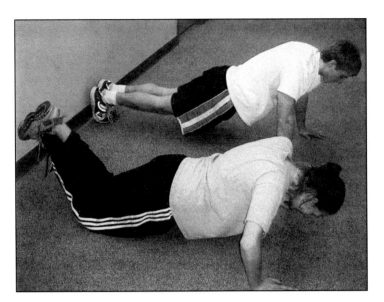

FIGURE 2.6
Muscular endurance is defined as the ability of the muscles to apply a submaximal force repeatedly or to sustain a muscular contraction for a certain period of time.

HEALTH AND FITNESS INSIGHT
What Is Health Promotion?

Health promotion is the science and art of helping people change their lifestyles to move toward a state of optimal health. The focus is on behaviors that result in improved lifestyle, because only when people take action, only when their behaviors change, do they improve their health.

Health promotion programs have three levels: awareness, behavior [lifestyle] change, and supportive environments. Awareness programs increase the participants' understanding of or interest in health-related topics. Lifestyle change programs are designed to help participants change physical and emotional health-related behaviors (starting to exercise, quitting smoking, learning to manage stress, etc.).

Lifestyle change programs have a greater chance of success if they take place over time, involve a multi-step process, and include a combination of educational, behavior modification and experiential components.

The third level, supportive environments, concerns the importance of the environment in determining behavior. Families, friends, organizational cultures, community laws, and other forces shape these environments. If environments can be created that encourage a healthy lifestyle, there is a greater chance of helping people sustain long-term lifestyle change.

Self-responsibility is a central theme in health promotion. A health promotion program will be most successful when it provides the skills and environment necessary for the participant to take responsibility for making choices that are consistent with good health habits.

Summary

1. "Physical activity," "exercise, and "physical fitness" are terms that describe different concepts. Physical activity is defined as any bodily movement produced by skeletal muscles that results in energy expenditure.
2. Exercise is a subcategory of physical activity which is planned, structured, repetitive, and purposive in the sense that improvement or maintenance of physical fitness is an objective.
3. A comprehensive definition of physical fitness is: Physical fitness is a dynamic state of energy and vitality that enables one to carry out daily tasks, to engage in active leisure-time pursuits, and to meet unforeseen emergencies without undue fatigue. In addition, physically fit individuals have a decreased risk of hypokinetic diseases (diseases associated with inactive lifestyles), and are better able to function at their peak intellectual capacity while experiencing a sense of "joie de vivre."
4. The measurable elements of physical fitness fall into two groups, "skill-related fitness" and "health-related fitness." The former include agility, balance, coordination, speed, power, and reaction time. The latter include cardiorespiratory endurance, body composition, and musculoskeletal fitness, which includes flexibility, muscular strength, and muscular endurance.

HEALTH AND FITNESS ACTIVITY 2.1
Ranking Activities by Health-Related Value

As discussed in this chapter, there are five measurable elements of health-related fitness:

The Measurable Elements of Health-Related Physical Fitness

Cardiorespiratory Endurance
Body Composition
Musculoskeletal Fitness
    Flexibility
    Muscular Endurance
    Muscular Strength

Sports and other forms of physical activity vary in their capacity to develop each component. In this physical fitness activity, you will be ranking different sports and exercises in terms of their capacity to promote such development, using a five-point scale for each of the five health-related fitness components. Answer the questions to the best of your ability, and then *compare your answers in a group session with your teacher or your local fitness expert.*

Rate each physical activity or sport in terms of its capacity to develop each of the five health-related components: 1 = not at all; 2 = somewhat or just a little bit; 3 = moderately; 4 = strongly; 5 = very strongly. Then answer the following question:

1. What five activities received the highest total score (add the five component scores for each activity)?

    #1 Activity _____

    #2 Activity _____

    #3 Activity _____

    #4 Activity _____

    #5 Activity _____

Physical Activity	Cardio-respiratory	Body Composition	Flexibility	Muscular Endurance	Muscular Strength	Total
Archery						
Backpacking						
Badminton						
Basketball						
non-game						
gameplay						
Bicycling						
pleasure						
15 mph						

Physical Activity	Cardio-respiratory	Body Composition	Flexibility	Muscular Endurance	Muscular Strength	Total
Bowling						
Canoeing, Rowing, Kayaking						
Calisthenics						
Dancing						
social and square						
aerobic						
Fencing						
Fishing						
bank, boat, or ice						
stream, wading						
Football (touch)						
Golf						
power cart						
walking, with bag						
Handball						
Hiking, Cross-Country						
Horseback Riding						
Paddleball, Racquetball						
Rope Jumping						
Running						
12 min per mile						
6 min per mile						
Sailing						
Scuba Diving						
Skating						
ice						
roller						
Skiing, Snow						
downhill						
cross-country						
Skiing, Water						
Sledding, Tobagganing						
Snowshoeing						
Squash						
Soccer						
Stair Climbing						
Swimming						

Physical Activity	Cardio-respiratory	Body Composition	Flexibility	Muscular Endurance	Muscular Strength	Total
Table Tennis						
Tennis						
Volleyball						
Walking, Briskly						
Weight Training, Circuit						
Brick Laying, Plastering						
Shoveling Light Earth						
Splitting Wood						
Digging Ditches						

HEALTH AND FITNESS ACTIVITY 2.2
Rating the Benefits of Physical Activity

As reviewed in this chapter, major benefits of regular exercise training include the following:

1. Improved heart and lung fitness.
2. Stronger, larger, and firmer muscles.
3. Stronger and denser bones.
4. Reduced body fat and better long-term control of body weight.
5. Reduced risk of high blood pressure.
6. Improved blood lipid profile.
7. Reduced risk of dying prematurely (i.e., improves life expectancy).
8. Reduced risk of dying from coronary heart disease.
9. Reduced risk of developing diabetes.
10. Reduced risk of developing colon cancer.
11. Reduced feelings of depression and anxiety, with improvement of mental mood state and self-esteem.
12. Improvement in life quality of older adults, patients with disease, and people of all ages.

Review this list carefully, and then, drawing on your own experience and that of your immediate family, list three benefits that you personally feel are most valuable. List the benefits, and explain why you chose it. List the benefits in order of importance.

#1 benefit:

Your reasons:

#2 benefit:

Your reasons:

#3 benefit:

Your reasons:

HEALTH AND FITNESS ACTIVITY 2.3

Internet Activity: Current Research on the Health Benefits of Exercise

Search the health and fitness Internet site of the Medline Plus: http://www.nlm.nih.gov/medlineplus/exerciseandphysicalfitness.html. Study the research findings listed at this site, and list two major current findings regarding the health benefits of exercise.

Exercise Health Benefit Finding #1

_____

_____

_____

_____

_____

_____

Exercise Health Benefit Finding #2

_____

_____

_____

_____

_____

_____

HEALTH AND FITNESS ACTIVITY 2.4
What Does Physical Fitness Mean to You?

As reviewed in the text, physical fitness places an emphasis on having vigor and energy to perform physical work, sports, and exercise, and is related to a low risk of chronic disease. The most frequently cited measurable components of physical fitness fall into two groups, one related to health and the other related to athletic skills. Skill-related fitness includes such components as agility, balance, coordination, power, reaction time, and speed. These are integral to success in sports such as tennis, football, baseball, volleyball, golf, and basketball. Individuals who engage in regular physical activity and sports to develop cardiorespiratory endurance, musculoskeletal fitness, and optimal body fat levels improve their basic energy levels, and place themselves at lower risk for the common chronic diseases.

What does physical fitness mean to you? What elements of physical fitness are most important for you? Review the text and then write two paragraphs below summarizing your personal feelings on what physical fitness means to you personally.

_____

_____

_____

_____

_____

_____

_____

_____

_____

_____

_____

_____

_____

CHAPTER 2 QUIZ
The Meaning of Physical Fitness

Note: Answers are given at the end of the quiz.

1. Which activity listed below scores highest in the development of all five of the measurable elements of health-related physical fitness?
   A. badminton
   B. running
   C. bowling
   D. rowing
   E. baseball

2. _____ is physical activity that is planned for purposes of improving health.
   A. Physical fitness
   B. Exercise
   C. Work
   D. Aerobics

3. Musculoskeletal fitness has three components, including _____ , muscular strength, and muscular endurance.
   A. cardiovascular endurance
   B. flexibility
   C. agility
   D. coordination
   E. speed

4. Aerobics is another term for:
   A. flexibility.
   B. cardiorespiratory endurance.
   C. muscular endurance.
   D. power.
   E. body composition.

5. Which one of the following is *not* a measureable element of health-related physical fitness?
   A. flexibility
   B. cardiorespiratory endurance
   C. muscular endurance
   D. agility
   E. body composition

Answers: 1. D   2. B   3. B   4. B   5. D

PART TWO

Testing for Physical Fitness

chapter three

Before You
Start Exercising

"Obviously, there is no precise and completely reliable way of gauging a person's phyical fitness. The real test is intuitive, and the truly fit person can know that he is truly fit only by sensing that he is deriving the most possible satisfaction from living."

—*Thomas K. Cureton*

Pre-Exercise Precautions

Much has been learned about physical activity and health since 1968 when the modern fitness movement began. In general, aerobic exercise has been found to be both safe and beneficial for most people. However, there are some individuals who can suffer ill health from exercise. There's probably not a single fitness enthusiast in America who has not read the reports of famous athletes dying on basketball courts, runners found dead with their running shoes on, executives discovered slumped over their treadmills, or middle-aged men suffering heart attacks while shoveling snow.

Whether exercise is beneficial or hazardous to the heart depends on the individual. For most, regular aerobic exercise reduces the risk of heart disease by about one-half, compared to those who are physically inactive. However, for those who are at high risk for heart disease to begin with, vigorous exercise bouts can trigger fatal heart attacks. About 75,000 Americans suffer a heart attack during or after exercise each year. These victims tend to be men who were sedentary, over age 35 years, already had heart disease or were at high risk for it, and then exercised too hard for their fitness levels.

Also of concern is congenital heart disease, now the major cause of athletic death in high school and college. In one study of 158 athletes who died young (average age 17) and in their prime, 134 of them had heart or blood vessel defects that were present at birth. Most common was an abnormal thickening of the heart's main pumping muscle. In other words, when a young athlete dies during or shortly after exercise, it is most often due to a birth defect of the heart and blood vessel system.

Health screening is a vital process in first identifying individuals at high risk for exercise-induced heart problems, and then referring them to appropriate medical care. A brief, self-administered medical questionnaire called the **Physical Activity Readiness Questionnaire (PAR-Q)** has been used very successfully (see Box 3.1). You should fill this in before starting an exercise program, to ensure your safety and health.

BOX 3.1

Physical Activity Readiness Questionnaire (PAR-Q)

Regular physical activity is fun and healthy, and increasingly more people are starting to become more active every day. Being more active is very safe for most people. However, some people should check with their doctor before they start becoming much more physically active.

If you are planning to become much more physically active than you are now, start by answering the seven questions in the box below. If you are between the ages of 15 and 69, the PAR-Q will tell you if you should check with your doctor before you start. If you are over 69 years of age, and you are not used to being very active, check with your doctor.

Common sense is your best guide when you answer these questions. Please read the questions carefully and answer each one honestly:

Check YES or NO. Checking YES to any answer will require you to get a physicians clearance before starting an exercise program.

Yes	No	
❏	❏	1. Has your doctor ever said that you have a heart condition and that you should only do physical activity recommended by a doctor?
❏	❏	2. Do you feel pain in your chest when you do physical activity?
❏	❏	3. In the past month, have you had chest pain when you were not doing physical activity?
❏	❏	4. Do you lose balance because of dizziness or do you ever lose consciousness?
❏	❏	5. Do you have a bone or joint problem that could be made worse by a change in your physical activity?
❏	❏	6. Is your doctor currently prescribing drugs (for example, water pills) for your blood pressure or heart condition?
❏	❏	7. Do you know of any other reason why you should not do physical activity?

If "yes", please describe reason:

_____

_____

_____

In general, most individuals, except for those with known serious disease, can begin a moderate exercise program, such as walking, without an evaluation from a medical doctor. Whenever you are in doubt about your own personal health and safety while exercising, a medical evaluation is recommended.

American College of Sports Medicine Guidelines

The American College of Sports Medicine (ACSM) recommends that all individuals interested in participating in organized exercise programs be evaluated for heart disease risk factors, using guidelines from the National Cholesterol Education Program. Box 3.2 summarizes ACSM guidelines for risk and symptom analysis prior to exercise. These include the following eight risk factors (which should not be viewed as an all-inclusive list, but which are used by ACSM for counting risk factors prior to risk stratification):

- *Age* Men 45 and older; women 55 and older.
- *Family history* (major heart disease or death before 55 years of age in father or brother, or before 65 years of age in mother or sister).
- *Cigarette smoking* (current cigarette smoker or those who quit within the previous 6 months).
- *High blood pressure* (systolic blood pressure of 140 mm Hg and higher, or diastolic blood pressure of 90 mm Hg and higher, confirmed by measurements on at least two separate occasions, or on medication to control high blood pressure).
- *High blood cholesterol* (total serum cholesterol of 200 mg/dl and higher or high-density lipoprotein cholesterol of less than 40 mg/dl, or on lipid-lowering medication).
- *Borderline high glucose level* (fasting blood glucose of 100 mg/dl and higher, confirmed by measurements on at least two separate occasions).
- *Obesity* (body mass index of 30 kg/m^2 and higher, or waist circumference of 40 inches and higher for males, and 35 inches and higher for females).
- *Sedentary lifestyle* (persons not participating in a regular exercise program or meeting the minimal physical activity recommendations.

ACSM also recommends that people with these major signs or symptoms suggestive of heart and lung disease see a doctor before exercising:

- Pain in the chest, neck, jaw, arms, or other areas from potential heart disease.
- Shortness of breath at rest, when sleeping, or when exercising moderately.
- Dizziness or lightheadedness.
- Swollen ankles.
- Irregular heart beats or an unusually fast heart rate of over 100 beats per minute at rest.
- Pain in the leg muscles when walking.
- Unusual fatigue or shortness of breath with usual activities.

ACSM Risk Levels

Prior to starting an exercise program, adults can be ranked by health/fitness professionals into one of three ACSM risk levels:

- *Low risk* (individuals who have no symptoms and no more than one risk factor threshold).
- *Moderate risk* (individuals who have no symptoms and have two or more risk factors).
- *High risk* (individuals with one or more signs/symptoms or known heart/lung disease or diabetes).

BOX 3.2

Screening Questionnaire
Assess your health needs by marking all **true** statements.

History
You have had:
- ❏ a heart attack
- ❏ heart surgery
- ❏ cardiac catheterization
- ❏ coronary angioplasty (PTCA)
- ❏ pacemaker/implantable cardiac
- ❏ defibrillator/rhythm disturbance
- ❏ heart valve disease
- ❏ heart failure
- ❏ heart transplantation
- ❏ congenital heart disease

Other health issues:
- ❏ You have musculoskeletal problems.
- ❏ You have concerns about the safety of exercise.
- ❏ You take prescription medication(s).
- ❏ You are pregnant.

Symptoms
- ❏ You experience chest discomfort with exertion.
- ❏ You experience unreasonable breathlessness.
- ❏ You experience dizziness, fainting, blackouts.
- ❏ You take heart medications.

Recommendations
*If you marked any of the statements in this section, consult your healthcare provider before engaging in exercise. You may need to use a facility with a **medically qualified staff.***

- ❏ You have diabetes
- ❏ You have asthma or other lung disease
- ❏ You have burning or cramping in lower legs when walking

Cardiovascular risk factors
- ❏ You are a man older than 45 years.
- ❏ You are a woman older than 55 years or you have had a hysterectomy or you are postmenopausal.
- ❏ You smoke.
- ❏ Your blood pressure is greater than 140/90 mm Hg.
- ❏ You don't know your blood pressure.
- ❏ You take blood pressure medication.
- ❏ Your blood cholesterol level is >200 mg/dl.
- ❏ You don't know your cholesterol level.
- ❏ You have a blood relative who had a heart attack before age 55 (father/brother) or 65 (mother/sister).
- ❏ You are diabetic or take medicine to control your blood sugar.
- ❏ You are physically inactive (i.e., you get less than 30 minutes of physical activity on at least 3 d/wk).
- ❏ You are more than 20 pounds overweight.

Recommendations
*If you marked two or more of the statements in this section, you should consult your healthcare provider before engaging in exercise. You might benefit by using a facility with a **professionally qualified staff** to guide your exercise program.*

- ❏ **None of the above is true.**

You should be able to exercise safely without consulting your healthcare provider.

FIGURE 3.1
For people of all ages, information from the maximal graded exercise test is valuable in establishing an effective and safe exercise prescription.

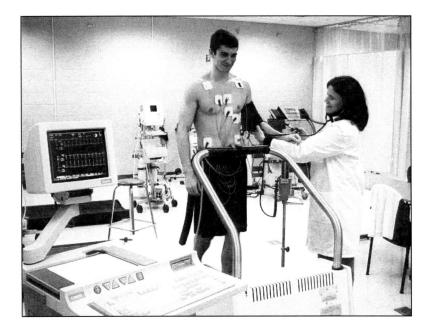

Medical examination and exercise testing is not necessary for low risk individuals or those at moderate risk desiring to initiate a moderate exercise program (e.g., brisk walking, but are recommended for high risk individuals and those at moderate risk desiring to initiate a vigorous exercise program (e.g., running) (see figure 3.1).

Concepts and Purposes for Physical Fitness Testing

There are many health clubs and fitness centers that offer physical fitness tests before one signs up as a member or starts an exercise program. The YMCA, for example, measures resting heart rate and blood pressure, body fat percentage through skinfolds, heart and lung fitness with a submaximal bicycle test, flexibility with the sit-and-reach test, and muscular strength and endurance with the bench press test and one-minute timed sit-up test.

In Canada, a sample of the population is tested periodically through the Canada Fitness Survey, which includes a step test for determination of cardiorespiratory fitness, skinfold measurements for body fat percentage, the sit-and-reach test for flexibility, the hand-grip dynamometer test (both hands) for muscular strength, one-minute timed sit-ups for abdominal muscular endurance, and push-ups for upper body muscular strength and endurance.

Reduced to its simplest terms, the function of measurement is to determine physical fitness status, which should be assessed before giving individualized exercise counseling. The information from the physical fitness testing is used, along with any medical test information, to tailor the program to the individuals needs.

Several important test criteria should be considered before you allow an organization or fitness club to test you;

1. **Are their tests valid?** This refers to the degree to which the test measures what it was designed to measure. A valid test is one that measures accurately what it is used to measure.
2. **Are their tests reliable?** This deals with how consistently a certain element is measured by the particular test. It is concerned with the repeatability of the test—if you are measured two separate times by two different people, the results should be consistent.
3. **Are norms for the tests available?** Norms represent the achievement level of a particular group to which the measured scores can be compared. Norms provide a useful basis for interpretation and evaluation of test results.

4. Are the tests basic and economical? This refers to ease of administration, the use of inexpensive equipment, the limitation of time needed to administer the test, and the simplicity of the test so that you can easily understand the purpose and results.

So in other words, a good physical fitness test measures what it is supposed to, accurately; it can be consistently used by different people; it produces results that can be compared to a data set; and is relatively inexpensive, simple, and easy to administer.

In a complete physical fitness program, testing of participants before, during, and after participation is important for several reasons:

1. To assess current fitness levels
2. To identify special needs for individualized counseling
3. To evaluate progress
4. To motivate

Test results are a means to an end. They should not be considered as an end in themselves. Expensive, elaborate, and lengthy testing is seldom needed, and can detract from the exercise program itself. Scores on the various items of simple and inexpensive test batteries are adequate to identify the strengths and weaknesses of participants, so that special attention can be given within individualized programs. If anything, it is better to undertest than overtest, so that more time and attention can be given to counseling and guiding each participant through the exercise program.

It is important to emphasize that the testing process should never be allowed to become a separate entity. The testing process is merely the stepping stone in the progress toward better understanding, attitudes, and practices in health and fitness.

Summary

1. In general, most individuals, except for those with known serious disease, can begin a moderate exercise program, such as walking, without an evaluation from a medical doctor. Whenever you are in doubt about your own personal health and safety while exercising, a medical evaluation is recommended.
2. Health screening is a vital process in first identifying individuals at high risk for exercise-induced heart problems, and then referring them to appropriate medical care. A brief, self-administered medical questionnaire called the *Physical Activity Readiness Questionnaire (PAR-Q)* has been used very successfully.
3. The American College of Sports Medicine (ACSM) recommends that all individuals interested in participating in organized exercise programs be evaluated for heart disease risk factors and signs or symptoms suggestive of heart disease or other medical problems.
4. Physical fitness testing is recommended prior to the start of an exercise program, to help determine current fitness levels, to identify special needs for counseling by fitness leaders, to provide a base for evaluation of progress, and for motivation. There is little need for sophisticated and expensive testing. Many valid, reliable, and economical testing packages with excellent norms have been established, including those from the YMCA and the Canadian Fitness Survey.

Name _____   Date _____

HEALTH AND FITNESS ACTIVITY 3.1
Are You Ready To Exercise?

As described in this chapter, health screening is a vital process in first identifying individuals at high risk for exercise-induced heart problems, and then referring them to appropriate medical care. A brief, self-administered medical questionnaire called the *Physical Activity Readiness Questionnaire (PAR-Q)* has been used very successfully. You should fill this in before starting an exercise program to ensure your safety and health. Go to Box 3.1 and answer the seven questions. According to your answers and the recommendations given in the PAR-Q, what should you do next? Comment below:

_____

_____

_____

_____

_____

_____

_____

_____

_____

_____

_____

_____

_____

_____

_____

_____

CHAPTER 3 QUIZ
Before You Start Exercising

Note: Answers are given at the end of the quiz.

1. Health screening is a vital process in first identifying individuals at high risk for exercise-induced heart problems, and then referring them to appropriate medical care. A brief, self-administered medical questionnaire called the _____ has been used very successfully.
   A. PAR-Q
   B. ACSM
   C. NCEP
   D. AHA
   E. ACS

2. _____ is now the major cause of athletic death in high school and college.
   A. Cancer
   B. Injury
   C. Congenital heart disease
   D. Stroke
   E. COPD

3. About 75,000 Americans suffer a heart attack during or after exercise each year. These victims tend to be men who were sedentary, over age ____ years, who already had heart disease or were at high risk for it, and then exercised too hard for their fitness levels.
   A. 75
   B. 25
   C. 50
   D. 35
   E. 65

4. T   F   In general, most individuals, except for those with known serious disease, can begin a moderate exercise program, such as walking, without an evaluation from a medical doctor.

5. How many risk factors does a 40-year-old male have, according to ACSM, if he has no family history, does not smoke, has a blood pressure of 134/84 mm Hg, a serum cholesterol of 244 mg/dl, a sedentary lifestyle, and a body mass index of 32 kg/m².

   A. 1
   B. 2
   C. 3
   D. 4
   E. 5

6. Individuals at "moderate risk," according to the American College of Sports Medicine, are those with _____ or more major coronary risk factors.

   A. 1
   B. 2
   C. 3
   D. 4
   E. 5

7. Which risk factor listed below is NOT on the American College of Sports Medicine's list for classifying individuals prior to exercise?

   A. serum cholesterol >200 mg/dl
   B. HDL-cholesterol ≤ 45 mg/dl
   C. body mass index ≥ 30 kg/m²
   D. systolic BP ≥140 or diastolic BP ≥ 90 mm Hg
   E. family history of heart disease in parents or siblings prior to age 55 for males, age 65 for females

chapter four

Assessment of Cardiorespiratory Fitness

"The key to endurance training is oxygen consumption. The body needs it to produce energy. It can't store it, so it must bring it in constantly and deliver it to the organ or tissue where the energy is needed. The amount that ther body can bring in and deliver—your maximum oxygen consumption—is the best measure of your fitness."
— Dr. Kenneth H. Cooper

Aerobic Fitness: The Basics

Your heart and lung system is an incredible machine. Often called the **cardiorespiratory system,** the heart and lungs are designed to deliver oxygen and nutrients to your body during both rest and exercise.

The lungs take in air and pass oxygen to the blood through 300 million tiny "air sacs" known as **alveoli.** The enormous number of these alveoli provides a surface area equal to that of a tennis court, allowing oxygen to diffuse rapidly into the blood.

Your heart, about the size of the human fist, pumps about 60 to 80 times per minute, delivering five liters of blood and one-fourth liter of oxygen through 60,000 miles of blood vessels each minute at rest. During exercise, your heart and lungs are capable of greatly increasing the amount of blood and oxygen delivered to working muscles.

In Chapter 2, aerobic fitness was defined as the ability to continue or persist in strenuous tasks involving large muscle groups for extended periods of time. Also called cardiorespiratory fitness, it is the ability of the heart and lungs to adjust to and recover from the effects of such activities as brisk walking, running, swimming, cycling, and other moderate-to-vigorous activities.

Aerobic fitness is enhanced when the body is involved in continuous and rhythmic muscular activity for at least three to five exercise sessions a week, 20 to 60 minutes a session (see Chapter 7). Typical aerobic activities include running, swimming, cycling, brisk walking, and various vigorous sports. In this chapter, emphasis will be placed on how to measure aerobic or cardiorespiratory fitness.

Aerobic fitness improves your quality of life, making you feel more energetic. Those who avoid aerobic exercise have a markedly increased risk of heart disease and other health problems. This point will be reviewed in greater detail in Part 4 of this book.

The Concept of $\dot{V}O_{2max}$

Maximal Oxygen Uptake ($\dot{V}O_{2max}$) is defined as the greatest rate at which oxygen can be consumed during exercise. "$\dot{V}$" is the volume of oxygen used per minute, "O_2" is oxygen, "max" represents maximal exercise conditions, and the dot over the "$\dot{V}$" means "per minute." The maximal rate of oxygen uptake is the maximal rate at which oxygen can be taken up, distributed, and used by the body during physical activity.

$\dot{V}O_{2max}$ is usually expressed in terms of oxygen consumed per kilogram of body weight per minute. With this adjustment for body weight, the $\dot{V}O_{2max}$ of individuals of varying size and in different environments can be compared with one another. $\dot{V}O_{2max}$ can also be expressed as liters per minute, representing the oxygen consumption of the entire body.

Figure 4.1 shows that at rest, a 70-kilogram male consumes about one fourth of a liter of oxygen each minute to keep alive. This represents 3.5 milliliters of oxygen per kilogram of body weight per minute (or 1 MET—a shorthand method that exercise physiologists use to represent resting oxygen consumption). Notice that as a 70-kg male starts walking, then running, and finally "maxing out," the oxygen consumption increases to provide the working muscles with enough oxygen to fuel the movement.

The highest $\dot{V}O_{2max}$ value ever recorded in any athlete (in milliliters of oxygen per kilogram of body weight per minute) was 94, for a high-altitude runner from Colorado (who has been very successful in the Pike's Peak Marathon). A $\dot{V}O_{2max}$ of 93 has been reported

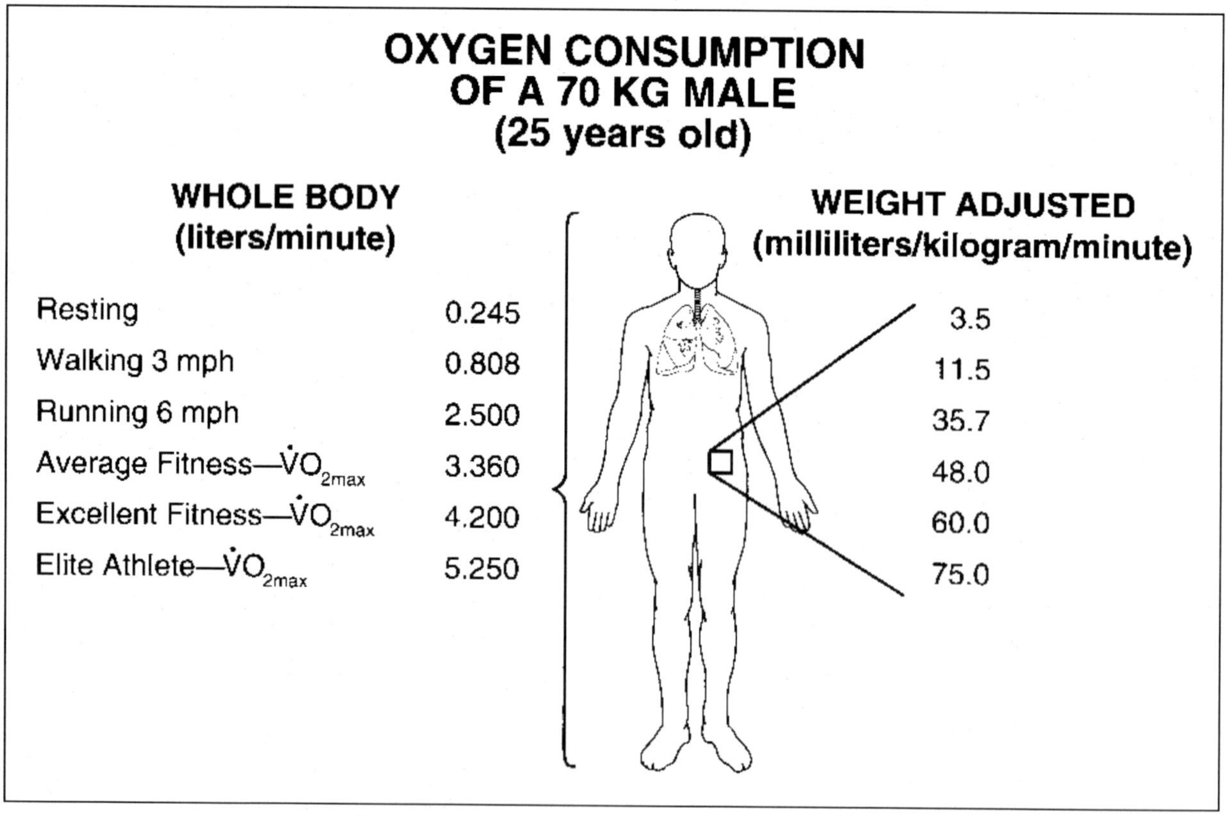

OXYGEN CONSUMPTION OF A 70 KG MALE (25 years old)

	WHOLE BODY (liters/minute)	WEIGHT ADJUSTED (milliliters/kilogram/minute)
Resting	0.245	3.5
Walking 3 mph	0.808	11.5
Running 6 mph	2.500	35.7
Average Fitness—$\dot{V}O_{2max}$	3.360	48.0
Excellent Fitness—$\dot{V}O_{2max}$	4.200	60.0
Elite Athlete—$\dot{V}O_{2max}$	5.250	75.0

FIGURE 4.1

The oxygen consumption ($\dot{V}O_{2max}$) can be expressed in units of liters per minute for the entire body, or in units of milliliters per kilogram of body weight per minute, to represent the oxygen consumption for each kilogram of body weight.

for a Scandinavian cross-country skier. In contrast, $\dot{V}O_{2max}$ values measured for untrained but healthy young adult males are usually between 44 and 51, and for young adult females, between 35 and 43. The highest value ever recorded for a female was 78 for Joan Benoit Samuelson, winner of the 1984 Los Angeles Olympic marathon.

Table 4.1 summarizes the $\dot{V}O_{2max}$ values for various age groups. As one ages, $\dot{V}O_{2max}$ falls about 9 percent per decade after the age of 25. Females have lower $\dot{V}O_{2max}$ values than do males, in part because women tend to have higher body fat content, smaller muscle mass, and less hemoglobin to carry oxygen in the blood. In the general population, $\dot{V}O_{2max}$ varies widely because of many factors, including age, gender, and degree of training. Researchers from Canada have determined that 40 percent of the variance is due to genetic differences. In other words, some people can train hard but not increase their $\dot{V}O_{2max}$ as much as others who have genetic capacities for high $\dot{V}O_{2max}$ levels.

Although important, $\dot{V}O_{2max}$ is only one of several factors that determines success in running. There is a large variation in performance between runners of equal $\dot{V}O_{2max}$. Some top-class marathon runners have had relatively low $\dot{V}O_{2max}$ values. Derek Clayton, former world record holder in the Marathon had a $\dot{V}O_{2max}$ of only 66.8. Joan Benoit Samuelson's is much higher than Clayton's, yet her Marathon time is much slower. Obviously, other factors play an important role in cardiorespiratory endurance performance.

Exercise Oxygen Economy is the oxygen cost of exercise, usually expressed in terms of oxygen usage ($\dot{V}O_{2max}$), at a certain running or exercise pace. This rate can vary considerably between individuals. While it is not possible to explain this variation precisely, biomechanical, physiological, psychological, and biochemical factors probably all play a part. In other words, some runners, cyclists and swimmers use oxygen more efficiently than others, and even though they may not have high $\dot{V}O_{2max}$ values, they use less oxygen at any given workload.

The Assessment of $\dot{V}O_{2max}$

The laboratory test generally regarded as the best measure of heart and lung endurance is the direct measurement of oxygen uptake during maximal graded exercise. The exercise is usually performed using a bicycle ergometer or treadmill, which allows the tester to progressively increase the workload from light to exhaustive (maximal) exercise. The amount of oxygen consumed during the test can be measured by a variety of methods (see figure 4.2).

TABLE 4.1 $\dot{V}O_{2max}$ **Norms (in milliliters of oxygen per kilogram of body weight per minute)**

Age	Low	Fair	Average	Good	High	Athletic	Olympic
Women							
20–29	<28	29–34	35–43	44–48	49–53	54–59	60+
30–39	<27	28–33	34–41	42–47	48–52	53–58	59+
40–49	<25	26–31	32–40	41–45	46–50	51–56	57+
50–65	<21	22–28	29–36	37–41	42–45	46–49	50+
Men							
20–29	<38	39–43	44–51	52–56	57–62	63–69	70+
30–39	<34	35–39	40–47	48–51	52–57	58–64	65+
40–49	<30	31–35	36–43	44–47	48–53	54–60	61+
50–59	<25	26–31	32–39	40–43	44–48	49–55	56+
60–69	<21	22–26	27–35	36–39	40–44	45–49	50+

Source: Adapted from Astrand *ACTA Physiol Scand 49* (Suppl): 169, 1960.

FIGURE 4.2
$\dot{V}O_{2max}$ is best measured in the laboratory during a maximal exercise test in which the oxygen consumed is measured by a computerized matabolic cart.

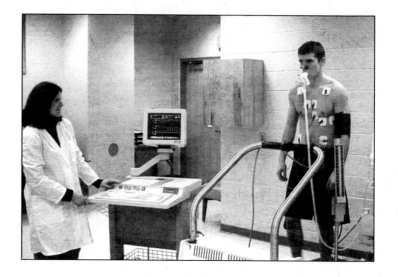

A high level of $\dot{V}O_{2max}$ depends upon the proper functioning of three important systems in the body:

1. the respiratory system, which takes up oxygen from the air in the lungs and transports it into the blood;
2. the cardiovascular system, which pumps and distributes the oxygen-laden blood throughout the body; and
3. the musculoskeletal system, which uses the oxygen to convert stored carbohydrates and fats into an energy source for muscle contraction and heat production.

As a person exercises vigorously week after week, his or her $\dot{V}O_{2max}$ increases (up to that person's maximum potential), as various changes take place in the body. The lungs can take in more air and diffuse more oxygen to the blood, the heart gets bigger and can pump out more blood with each beat, the amount of blood in the body increases, the number of capillaries around muscle fibers increases, and the muscles' supply of important energy-producing enzymes increases, allowing fuels to be burned better.

During graded exercise testing, the active muscle tissue needs more and more oxygen to burn the carbohydrate and fats needed for energy production. For every liter of oxygen that the body consumes during exercise, approximately 5 Calories of energy are produced. Figure 4.3 demonstrates that as the workload increases (faster speed and increasing grade), oxygen consumption increases up to the last stage of exercise. At this point, $\dot{V}O_2$ plateaus, and the person has reached his or her $\dot{V}O_{2max}$. If the person is willing to push hard enough, a small decrease in oxygen volume can be obtained just prior to exhaustion, as demonstrated in Figure 4.3.

Laboratory measurement of $\dot{V}O_{2max}$ is expensive, time-consuming, requires highly-trained personnel, and therefore, is not practical for mass testing situations. Various field tests that can be easily administered to large numbers of people have been developed, including the one-mile run, one-mile walk, 12-minute run, or cycling. Various equations are used to estimate the $\dot{V}O_{2max}$, based on performance in these field tests.

As indicated above, where they are practical, the best laboratory tests for estimating $\dot{V}O_{2max}$ are maximal graded treadmill and bicycle tests. These will be discussed in detail later in this chapter. Basically, the tests require that the individual exercise for as long as possible on a treadmill or bicycle, for which the workload is adjusted every three minutes according to a set protocol. Based on the length of time or the workload achieved when the subject becomes "maxed out," equations are used to estimate $\dot{V}O_{2max}$.

Some of the more important of these exercise tests will be discussed in this chapter. It is assumed that the preliminary considerations outlined in the previous chapter have been addressed before these tests are conducted, with a medical screening of those with disease or at high risk.

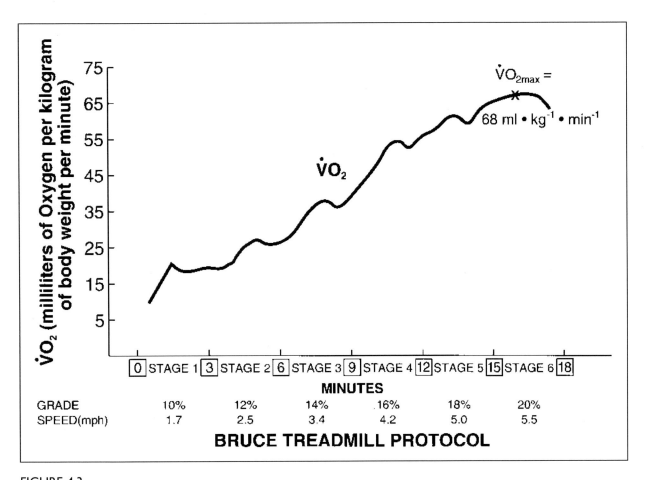

FIGURE 4.3

With increasing workload, oxygen consumption increases up to the last stage of exercise. At this point, oxygen volume plateaus, at what is called the $\dot{V}O_{2max}$.

Resting and Exercise Blood Pressure and Heart Rate Determination

Resting Blood Pressure

Blood pressure is the force of blood against the walls of the arteries and veins created by the heart as it pumps blood to every part of the body. **Hypertension** is simply a condition in which the blood pressure is chronically elevated above optimal levels. The Joint National Committee on Detection, Evaluation, and Treatment of High Blood Pressure has established blood pressure classifications (see Table 4.2).

Hypertension is diagnosed for adults when the average of two or more a **diastolic** measurements (blood pressure when the heart is resting) on at least two separate visits is 90mm Hg or higher. If the **diastolic** blood pressure is below 90 mm Hg, **systolic** hypertension is diagnosed when the average of multiple systolic blood pressure (pressure when heart is pumping) measurements on two or more separate visits are consistently greater than 140 mm Hg.

Nearly one in three Americans have elevated systolic blood pressure of 140 mm Hg or greater and/or diastolic blood pressure of 90 mm Hg or greater, or are taking antihypertensive medication. Table 4.3 summarizes important lifestyle changes that decrease systolic blood pressure in people with hypertension. Prevalence increases with age, and is higher among blacks than whites. Healthcare professionals are urged to measure blood pressure at each patient visit.

TABLE 4.2   Classification of Blood Pressure

	Systolic BP, mm Hg	Diastolic BP, mm Hg
Normal	<120	and <80
Prehypertension	120–139	or 80–89
Stage 1 hypertension	140–159	or 90–99
Stage 2 hypertension	>160	or >100

TABLE 4.3   Lifestyle Changes Help Lower High Blood Pressure

Lifestyle Change	Approximate Decrease in Systolic Blood Pressure
Weight loss of 20–25 pounds	5–20 mm Hg
Adopt healthy eating plan	8–14 mm Hg
Reduce dietary sodium	2–8 mm Hg
Regular physical activity	4–9 mm Hg
Keep alcohol intake moderate	2–5 mm Hg

FIGURE 4.4

Blood pressure is taken with a stethoscope (A) and sphygmomanometer, which consists of an inflatable cuff (B) connected by rubber tubes to a manometer, which measures pressure in millimeters at mercury (C), and a rubber bulb that regulates air during the measurements (D). Blood pressure is the force of blood against the walls of the arteries and veins created by the heart (E) as it pumps. The blood pressure cuff fits over the brachial artery (F). The upper circle (G) represents the common carotid artery, and the lower circle (H) the radial artery, for sensing the heart rate.

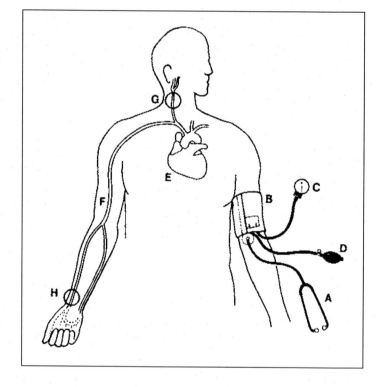

To take the resting blood pressure, a sphygmomanometer and a stethoscope are needed. The **sphygmomanometer** consists of an inflatable compression bag enclosed in an unyielding covering called the cuff, plus an inflating bulb, a manometer from which the pressure is read, and a controlled exhaust valve to deflate the system. The *stethoscope* is made of rubber tubing attached to a device that amplifies the sounds of blood passing through the blood vessels (see figure 4.4). This equipment can be obtained in most drug stores for under $30, though more expensive blood pressure equipment is available.

Those taking blood pressure should be trained by qualified instructors. A single blood pressure reading does not provide an accurate measure. Blood pressure should be measured two or three times until consistency is achieved. If the initial readings are high, several blood pressure readings by different observers, or on different occasions by the same observer, are recommended (see Health and Fitness Activity 4.2).

For best results in taking blood pressure:

- Measurements should be taken with a mercury sphygmomanometer, a recently calibrated aneroid manometer, or a validated electronic device.
- Two or more readings should be averaged. If the first two readings differ by more than 5 mm Hg, additional readings should be obtained.
- Take the measurement in a quiet room with the temperature approximately 70 to 74 degrees Fahrenheit (21 to 23 degrees C).
- Having the upper arm bare makes it easier to adjust the cuff.
- With older people, because of potential arterial obstructions, it is best to take readings on both arms.
- Use the proper size cuff. The rubber bladder should encircle at least two thirds of the arm. The three most frequently used cuff sizes are child (13 to 20 cm), adult (17 to 26 cm) and large adult (32 to 42 cm). If the person's arm is large, the normal size cuff will be too small, resulting in an inaccurately high reading (and vice versa).
- Allow at least 30 to 60 seconds between readings for normal circulation to return to the arm.
- The person being checked should be comfortably seated, with the arm straight (just slightly flexed), palm up, and the whole forearm supported at heart level on a smooth surface.
- Anxiety, emotional turmoil, food in the stomach, bladder distension, climate variation, exertion, and pain all may influence blood pressure, and when possible, should be controlled or avoided. Heavy exercise or eating shortly before the examination should be avoided, and the individual being tested should sit quietly for at least five minutes before the test. One should also avoid smoking or ingesting caffeine for at least 30 minutes prior to measurement.
- Place the cuff (deflated) with the lower margin about 1 inch above the inner elbow crease. The rubber bag should be over the brachial artery (inner part of upper arm).
- The stethoscope should be applied lightly. It has been determined recently that excessive pressure on the stethoscope head can erroneously lower diastolic readings. The stethoscope should not touch clothing, the cuff, or the cuff tubing (to avoid unnecessary rubbing sounds).
- With the stethoscope in place, as the cuff bladder is inflated, the pressure will close off the blood flow in the brachial artery, causing the pulse sound to stop. The pressure should be raised 20 to 30 mm Hg above the point at which the pulse sound disappears (listen carefully through the stethoscope).
- The pressure should be slowly released at a rate of 2 to 3 mm Hg/second. Do not go more slowly than this, because it can cause pain, and also raise blood pressure.
- As the pressure is released, the blood pressure sounds (the **Korotkoff's sounds**) become audible and pass through several phases.

Systolic blood pressure readings

Phase One (the systolic pressure) is marked by the appearance of faint, clear tapping sounds, which gradually increase in intensity. This represents the blood pressure when the heart is contracting.

A true systolic blood pressure cannot be obtained unless the Korotkoff's sounds are relatively sharp. Korotkoff's sounds can be made louder by having the person being tested open and clench his fist about 10 times during cuff inflation, inflating the cuff quickly, and elevating the arm before inflating the cuff.

Diastolic blood pressure readings

At rest—diastolic blood pressure equals the disappearance of the pulse sound (also called the fifth sound).

During exercise testing—sometimes the disappearance of sound drops all the way to zero. Therefore, the point at which there is an abrupt muffling sound (fourth phase) should be used for the diastolic blood pressure.

Blood pressures taken during exercise are difficult to measure, and only experienced or certified exercise testing personnel should make these measurements (figure 4.5).

As figure 4.6 shows, during exercise of increasing intensity, the systolic blood pressure rises while the diastolic stays the same. Some people's blood pressure rises to an abnormally high level during testing, indicating a potential problem with hypertension at rest.

FIGURE 4.5

Blood pressure determination during exercise is a difficult skill, and requires considerable experience. Korotkoff sounds are easier to hear it the tubes are not allowed to rub or bump the subject or the treadmill. The stethoscope head should be attached to the subject's arm. The manometer should be at the level of the subject's heart.

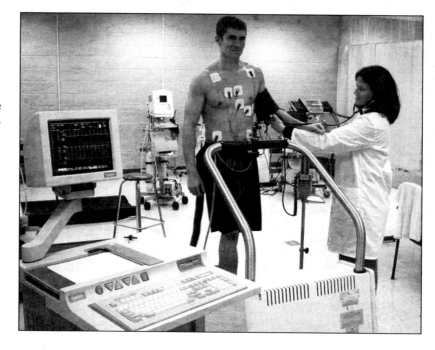

FIGURE 4.6

Pattern of systolic and diastolic blood pressures during graded exercise testing.

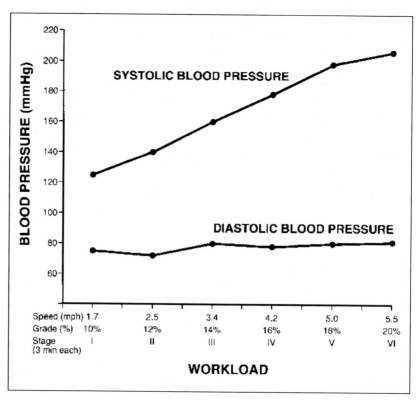

Resting Heart Rate

The resting heart rate can be obtained through a stethoscope, feeling the pulse with your fingers, or EKG recordings.

The pulse rate is best determined during rest at the radial artery (lateral aspect of the palm side of the wrist in line with the base of the thumb) (see figure 4.4). The tip of the middle and index fingers should be used (not the thumb, which has a pulse of its own). Start the stopwatch simultaneously with the pulse beat. Count the first beat a zero. Continue counting for 30 seconds and then multiply by two to get total heart beats per minute.

During exercise, the carotid artery (in the neck just lateral to the larynx) is easier to measure by, because it is bigger than the radial artery (see figure 4.4). Heavy pressure should not be applied when measuring the carotid artery, because pressure receptors (baroreceptors) in that artery can detect the pressure and cause a reflex slowing of the heart rate.

The heart rate fluctuates widely and easily due to the same factors that influence blood pressure. Resting heart rate is best determined upon awakening, averaged from measurements taken on at least three separate mornings. Lower heart rates are usually (but not always) indicative of a heart conditioned by exercise training, a heart able to push out more blood with each beat (having a larger stroke volume) and therefore needing fewer beats. Accordingly, the resting heart rate usually drops with regular exercise, decreasing approximately one beat every one or two weeks for the first 10 to 20 weeks of the program. Some of the best endurance athletes in the world have resting heart rates as low as 35 to 45 beats per minute, whereas sedentary adults may have rates between 75 and 85 beats per minute. See Table 4.4 for YMCA resting heart rate norms. Also see Health and Fitness Activity 4.1. We will discuss measurement of heart rate during exercise in Chapter 7.

Figure 4.7 shows that the heart rate rises with increase in workload (just like oxygen consumption). At the point of exhaustion, the heart is beating as fast as it can. This is called the **maximal heart rate (Max HR),** which can be estimated by subtracting one's age from the number 220. (220 – AGE = Max HR.)

For example, a 25-year-old individual would have a maximal heart rate of 195 (220 – 25 = 195), while a 60-year-old's would be estimated to be 160.

Estimating Your Aerobic Fitness or $\dot{V}O_{2max}$

As emphasized earlier, direct measurement of $\dot{V}O_{2max}$ with computerized metabolic carts is the "gold standard" method. It is very expensive and difficult, however, to measure $\dot{V}O_{2max}$ this way. Many simpler methods have been developed, and will be reviewed in the following sections of this chapter.

TABLE 4.4 YMCA Norms for Resting Heart Rate (beats per minute)

Age (yrs.) Gender	18–25 M	F	26–35 M	F	36–45 M	F	46–55 M	F	56–65 M	F	Over 65 M	F
Excellent	49–55	54–60	49–54	54–59	50–56	54–59	50–57	54–60	51–56	54–59	50–55	54–59
Good	57–61	61–65	57–61	60–64	60–62	62–64	59–63	61–65	59–61	61–64	58–61	60–64
Above Average	63–65	66–69	62–65	66–68	64–66	66–69	64–67	66–69	64–67	67–69	62–65	66–68
Average	67–69	70–73	66–70	69–71	68–70	70–72	68–71	70–73	68–71	71–73	66–69	70–72
Below	71–73	74–78	72–74	72–76	73–76	74–78	73–76	74–77	72–75	75–77	70–73	73–76
Poor	76–81	60–84	77–81	78–82	77–82	79–82	79–83	78–84	76–81	79–81	75–79	79–84
Very Poor	84–95	86–100	84–94	84–94	86–96	84–92	85–97	85–96	84–94	85–96	83–98	88–96

Source: Adapted from YMCA. *The Y's Way to Fitness.* 3rd edition. Champaign, IL: Human Kinetics Publishers, Inc., 1989.

FIGURE 4.7

Heart rate results during the graded exercise test of a 20-year-old before and after exercise training. Notice that his pre-test exercise heart rate is much higher than his true resting heart rate. The exercise heart rate increases in a linear (fashion with increase in workload until the maximal heart rate is reached, when it plateaus.

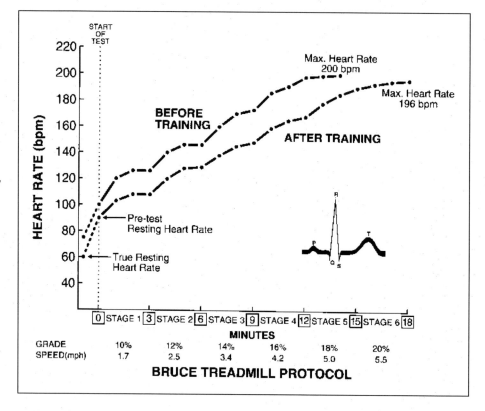

The easiest of all methods is the use of an equation to predict $\dot{V}O_{2max}$ using personal factors such as age, gender, body weight and height, and amount of physical activity. Although these prediction equations are not as accurate as laboratory testing of $\dot{V}O_{2max}$, people can be broadly classified as having poor, average, or good cardiorespiratory fitness.

Go to Health and Fitness Activity 4.3, and estimate your $\dot{V}O_{2max}$ using an equation, and then use Table 4.1 to classify your result. You will need a calculator and some patience to work through this equation.

Field Tests for Cardiorespiratory Fitness

As was mentioned earlier, a number of performance tests such as maximal endurance runs on a track have been devised for testing large groups in field situations. These tests are practical, inexpensive, less time-consuming than laboratory tests, easy to administer for large groups, and quite accurate when properly conducted.

Endurance runs should be a mile or longer to test the aerobic system. For ease of administration, the one-mile and 1.5-mile runs are most commonly used. See Health and Fitness Activity 4.4. Various set-timed runs such as the 9-minute run are hard to administer because exact distance determination is difficult.

With the one-mile or 1.5-mile runs, those being tested simply run the set distance around a track (or other precisely measured course) while their time is measured. The objective is to cover the distance in the shortest possible time. The effort should be maximal, and is appropriate only for those properly motivated and experienced in running. Updated norms for the 1.5-mile run test are set out in Table 4.5.

TABLE 4.5   Norms for the 1.5 Mile Run Test (for people between the ages of 17 and 35

Fitness Category	Time: Age 17–25	Time: Age 26–35
Superior		
Males	less than 8:30	less than 9:30
Females	less than 10:30	less than 11:30
Excellent		
Males	8:30–9:29	9:30–10:29
Females	10:30–11:49	11:30–12:49
Good		
Males	9:30–10:29	10:30–11:29
Females	11:50–13:09	12:50–14:09
Moderate		
Males	10:30–11:29	11:30–12:29
Females	13:10–14:29	14:10–15:29
Fair		
Males	11:30–12:29	12:30–13:29
Females	14:30–15:49	15:30–16:49
Poor		
Males	more than 12:29	more than 13:29
Females	more than 15:49	more than 16:49

Note: Before taking this running test, it is highly recommended that the student or individual be "moderately fit." Sedentary people should first start an exercise program, and slowly build up to 20 minutes of running, 3 days per week, before taking this test.

Source: Draper DO, Jones GL. The 1.5 Mile Run Revitited—An Update in Women's Times. *JOPERD,* September 1990:78–80.

The one-mile run is used in both the AAHPERD college student health-related physical fitness test, and also the Public Health Service National Children and Youth Fitness test (see Activity 4.4).

Recently, equations have been developed to predict $\dot{V}O_{2max}$ from one's ability to run various distances at maximal speed.

Table 4.6 summarizes the relationships between $\dot{V}O_{2max}$ and running performance for races ranging from 1.5 km to 42.195 km (marathon). Notice, for example, that running a mile in 6:01 demands the same $\dot{V}O_{2max}$ as running the 5 km in 21:23, the 10 km in 46:17, or the marathon in 3:49:28.

The maximal endurance run tests are only for the healthy (ACSM "apparently healthy" category). Dr. Kenneth Cooper suggests that the 1.5-mile run test should not be taken unless one can already jog nonstop for fifteen minutes. In addition, there always should be a proper warm-up of slow jogging and calisthenics. After the test, there should be an adequate "warm-down" or "cool-down," with several minutes of walking, followed by flexibility exercises.

A one-mile walk test was developed recently by a team of researchers at the University of Massachusetts. Walking is safer than running and more easily performed by most Americans. In this study, 343 males and females, 30 to 69 years of age, were tested using a one-mile walk test. They walked a mile as fast as possible, performing the test a minimum of two times, with heart rates monitored. They then were given a treadmill $\dot{V}O_{2max}$ test, and the one-mile walk results correlated very highly with actual measured $\dot{V}O_2$ (see Health and Activity 4.5).

Table 4.6 **Equivalent Peformances for Various Distances**

VO$_{2max}$	Performance Times (hours:minutes:seconds)				
(ml • kg^{-1} • min^{-1})	1.5 km	Mile	5 km	10 km	Marathon
28	13:30	14:46	56:49	2:39:14	31:41:25
31.5	11:27	12:29	47:04	2:02:00	16:35:05
35	9:56	10:49	40:10	1:38:53	11:13:52
38.5	8:46	9:33	35:02	1:23:08	8:29:26
42	7:51	8:33	31:04	1:11:43	6:49:30
45.5	7:07	7:44	27:54	1:03:03	5:42:21
49	6:30	7:03	25:20	0:56:15	4:54:07
52.5	5:59	6:29	23:11	0:50:47	4:17:48
56	5:32	6:01	21:23	0:46:17	3:49:28
59.5	5:09	5:36	19:50	0:42:30	3:26:44
63	4:50	5:14	18:30	0:39:33	3:08:06
66.5	4:32	4:55	17:20	0:36:33	2:52:34
70	4:17	4:38	16:18	0:34:10	2:39:23
73.5	4:03	4:23	15:23	0:32:12	2:28:05
77	3:50	4:09	14:34	0:30:12	2:18:41
80.5	3:39	3:57	13:50	0:28:33	2:09:41
84	3:29	3:46	13:10	0:27:04	2:02:06
87.5	3:20	3:36	12:34	0:25:44	1:55:21

Source: Tokmakidis S.P., Leger L., Mercier D., Peronnet F., Thibault G. New approaches to predict $\dot{V}O_{2max}$ and endurance from running performance. *J Sports Med* 27:401–409, 1987.

FIGURE 4.8
The step test for college students.

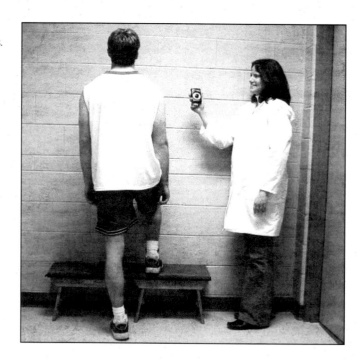

A Step Test for College Students

A step test has been developed for college students to predict $\dot{V}O_{2max}$ (figure 4.8). This step test is easy to take, and requires only a stopwatch, metronome, and a stepping bench. Health and Fitness Activity 4.6 provides a recording form for the test data. The heart rate is taken for 15 seconds after stepping up and down on a 16.25 inch bench for three minutes at a rate of 24 steps per minute for men, and 22 for women, and then applied to equations to determine $\dot{V}O_{2max}$. Overweight individuals and those with medical problems or leg injuries should not take this test.

The YMCA Three-Minute Step Test

The YMCA uses the three-minute step test for mass testing of participants.

The equipment involved includes a 12-inch-high, sturdy bench; a metronome set at 96 bpm (24 up-down cycles—four clicks of the metronome equals one cycle, up 1, 2, down 3, 4), which should be properly calibrated with a wrist watch; a timing clock for the 3-minute stepping exercise and 1-minute recovery; and preferably a stethoscope to count the pulse rate.

It is important to first practice the stepping technique before being tested (four counts—right foot up onto the bench on 1, left foot up on 2, right foot down to the floor on 3, and left foot down on 4). The exerciser should have some preliminary practice, and should be well rested, with no prior exercise of any kind.

The test involves stepping up and down at the 24-steps-per-minute rate for 3 minutes, then immediately sitting down. Within 5 seconds the person giving the test should be counting the pulse with the stethoscope, *continuing for one full minute.* The exerciser can take his own pulse at the same time by monitoring the radial artery, providing a means of verifying the tester's count. (The one-minute count limit reflects the heart's ability to recover quickly.)

The total number of heart beats for the one minute provides the score for the test, and should be recorded. It can he affected by many factors other than fitness, such as emotion, tiredness, prior exercise, resting, and maximum heart rates that differ from population averages, and miscounting. See Table 4.7 for the YMCA norms.

A Treadmill Test for College Students

Many colleges and universities have fitness centers with good treadmills. If you have access to a good treadmill that provides an accurate output of both grade and speed, then a treadmill test is highly recommended, because it provides a much better estimate of your

Table 4.7 YMCA 3-Minute Step Test
Post Exercise 1-Minute Heart Rate (beats/mm)

Age (yrs.) Gender	18–25 M	F	26–35 M	F	36–45 M	F
Excellent	70–75	72–83	73–79	72–86	72–81	74–87
Good	82–88	88–97	83–88	91–97	86–94	93–101
Above Average	91–97	100–106	91–97	103–110	98–102	104–109
Average	101–104	110–116	101–106	112–118	105–111	111–117
Below Average	107–114	118–124	109–116	121–127	113–118	120–127
Poor	118–126	128–137	119–126	129–135	120–128	130–138
Very Poor	131–164	142–155	130–164	141–154	132–168	143–152

Age (yrs.) Gender	46–55 M	F	56–65 M	F	over 65 M	F
Excellent	78–84	76–93	72–82	74–92	72–86	73–86
Good	89–96	96–102	89–97	97–103	89–95	93–100
Above Average	99–103	106–113	98–101	106–111	97–102	104–114
Average	109–115	117–120	105–111	113–117	104–113	117–121
Below Average	118–121	121–126	113–118	119–127	114–119	123–127
Poor	124–130	127–133	122–128	129–136	122–128	129–134
Very Poor	135–158	138–152	131–150	142–151	133–152	135–151

Note: Pulse is to be counted for one full minute following 3 minutes of stepping at 24-steps cycles/min on a 12-inch bench.

Source: Adapted from YMCA. *Y'S Way to Fitness,* 3rd edition. Champaign, IL: Human Kinetics Publishers, Inc., 1989.

fitness than does a running or walking test. College students in good health and without underlying medical problems can take this test. Your class instructor should be present to help monitor the test.

A maximal treadmill graded exercise test for college students has been developed by researchers at Arizona State University that allows the participant to select a comfortable walking-jogging speed. The test protocol is described in Health and Fitness Activity 4.7. After a six-minute warm-up at a self-selected speed, the treadmill grade is increased 1.5 percent each minute until you can no longer continue because of fatigue. The ending speed in miles per hour (mph) and the final treadmill percent grade that you were able to sustain for close to one minute is entered into a formula to estimate $\dot{V}O_{2max}$ in $ml \cdot kg^{-1} \cdot min^{-1}$.

Maximal Graded Exercise Treadmill Test Protocols

Figures 4.9 and 4.10 describe the most commonly used maximal treadmill protocols. Of the treadmill protocols, the Bruce is by far the most commonly used, followed by the Balke. The Bruce has relatively large, abrupt increases in work load every three minutes, and some have criticized the test for this. Nonetheless, excellent maximal data can be obtained, and because the test is so widely used, there are an abundance of comparative data.

FIGURE 4.9

The Bruce maximal graded exercise test protocol. Every 3 minutes, the speed and grade of the treadmill are increased until the subject can no longer exercise due to exhaustion.

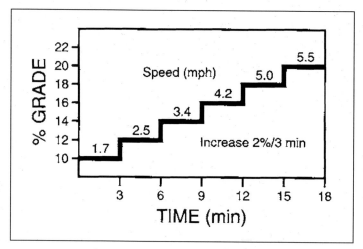

FIGURE 4.10

The Balke maximal graded exercise test protocol. Every minute, the grade is increased one percent while the speed is kept at 3.3 mph. If the subject is still able to exercise when the treadmill is at the 25 percent grade, the speed is increased 0.2 mph each minute.

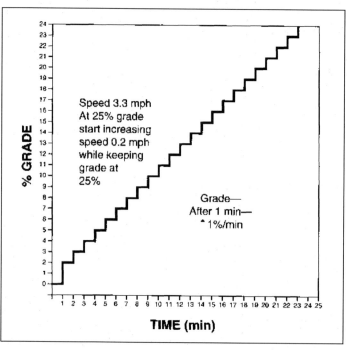

The main criticism of the Balke test is its length (nearly twice as long as the Bruce), which is prohibitive for testing large numbers of people. Ken Cooper uses the Balke protocol in his Cooper Institute for Aerobic Research in Dallas because he feels the Balke allows for a more gradual warm-up and is therefore safer. The Balke is basically an uphill walking test, while the Bruce starts out as an uphill walking test, and then in Stage 4 becomes an uphill running test.

The basis of these tests is that $\dot{V}O_{2max}$ can be estimated accurately from length of time to exhaustion following treadmill protocols, if the person being tested is taken to a "true max," which means:

- The person is allowed to practice one time before the maximal test to become "habituated" to the treadmill.
- He is *urged* to exercise until exhaustion is reached.
- When he is "maxed-out," there is no additional increase in heart rate despite an increase in workload, he shows signs of exertional intolerance (fatigue, staggering, inability to keep up with the workload, facial pallor), or the subject refuses to continue despite urging.
- During the test, he is not allowed to hang onto the treadmill bar in any way.

To ensure valid and reliable $\dot{V}O_{2max}$ values, the test should utilize the type of exercise the person is accustomed to. The temperature in the laboratory should be 20–23°C, with 50 percent humidity. If follow-up testing is conducted, tests should be repeated at the same time of the day, using the same procedures.

Table 4.8 shows the relationship between length of time on the treadmill and $\dot{V}O_{2max}$.

Table 4.8 $\dot{V}O_{2max}$ Estimation from Treadmill Test
From length of time in minutes on treadmill until exhaustion

VO_{2max}	Bruce (min:sec)	Balke (min:sec)
14.0	2:30	2:00
15.7	4:00	3:00
20.2	6:00	6:00
24.2	7:20	8:00
27.7	8:20	9:45
31.1	9:15	12:00
34.8	10:10	14:30
38.2	11:00	17:00
42.5	12:00	19:00
45.7	12:45	21:30
49.6	13:40	24:15
53.0	14:30	26:15
56.1	15:15	27:45
59.7	16:10	29:00
62.7	17:00	30:00
66.1	18:00	31:15
70.0	19:20	32:00
73.6	21:00	33:45
75.4	22:30	35:45

Note: $\dot{V}O_{2max}$ is in milliliters of oxygen per kilogram of body weight per minute.

Sources. Estimated $\dot{V}O_{2max}$ for Bruce's treadmill protocol based on the equation: $\dot{V}O_{2max}$ ml • kg⁻¹ • min⁻¹ = 14.8 − 1.379(TIME) + 0.451(TIME²) − 0.012(TIME³), *Note:* TIME = total time to exhaustion during the Bruce maximal graded treadmill exercise test. Foster C, Jackson AS, Pollock ML, et al. Generalized Equations for Predicting Functional Capacity From Treadmill Performance. *Am Heart J* 108:1229–1234, 1984. Estimated $\dot{V}O_{2max}$ for Balke protocol taken from table adapted from Pollock M. L. Wilmore J. H. and Fox S.M.: *Health and Fitness Through Physical Activity.* New York: Macmillan, 1978.

Summary

1. While the direct measurement of $\dot{V}O_{2max}$ is the best measure of heart and lung endurance, for various practical reasons other tests have been developed as substitutes. These include field tests (mainly running tests), step tests (YMCA 3-minute step test), submaximal laboratory tests, and maximal laboratory tests (both bicycle and treadmill).
2. Resting and exercise blood pressure and heart rate determination are reviewed.
3. Principles for taking blood pressure measurements are listed. At rest, diastolic blood pressure equals the disappearance of the pulse sound (fifth Korotkoff's sound).
4. A number of performance tests, such as maximal endurance runs on a track, have been devised for testing large groups in field situations. Equations for predicting $\dot{V}O_{2max}$ from one's ability to run various distances at maximal speed have been developed. Recently, a one-mile walk test was developed to more safely test American adults.
5. Both maximal and submaximal step tests have been developed for predicting $\dot{V}O_{2max}$.

HEALTH AND FITNESS ACTIVITY 4.1
Measurement of Your Resting Heart Rate

As emphasized in the test, a low resting heart rate usually indicates a heart conditioned by regular aerobic exercise. Some people have a low resting heart rate due to various genetic factors, but even they can lower their resting heart rates through exercise training.

Many factors can increase the resting heart rate to levels that are higher than normal (see the text). To rule out these factors, the resting heart rate is best measured a few minutes after awakening when seated on the edge of the bed. In this Health and Fitness Activity, you will take your resting heart rate, using the artery in your wrist or neck, three mornings in a row after getting out of bed. Record these values in the blanks below, average them, and then using Table 4.4, classify your resting heart rate from the YMCA norms. If you have never counted your pulse, it is best to have your instructor explain the procedure using Figure 4.4. Put three fingers at the base of your thumb on the bottom of your wrist to count the heart beats for one full minute using the radial artery, or three fingers on either side of your voice box on the neck (carotid artery). Do not press too hard.

Resting heart rate measurements:

First morning: _____ beats per minute

Second morning: _____ beats per minute

Third morning: _____ beats per minute

Average resting heart rate: _____ beats per minute

Classification (Table 4.4) _____

HEALTH AND FITNESS ACTIVITY 4.2
Measurement of Your Resting Blood Pressure

As emphasized in the text, the person taking the blood pressure should be trained and skilled in the procedure (e.g., a nurse or other health professional). Have your instructor organize a class session for blood pressure measurement by a visiting health professional.

You should sit quietly for at least five minutes before having your blood pressure measured. Be totally relaxed. The same factors that raise the resting heart rate can elevate the blood pressure (stress and anxiety, food in the stomach, a full bladder, pain, extreme hot or cold, tobacco use, caffeine, and certain kinds of medications). Ideally, two measurements should be taken on two separate days. If this is not practical, have your blood pressure measured twice during the class session, and then average. Use Table 4.2 to classify your blood pressure.

Resting blood pressure measurements:

First reading: _____ mm Hg

Second reading: _____ mm Hg

Average resting blood pressure: _____ mm Hg

Classification (Table 4.2)   _____

HEALTH AND FITNESS ACTIVITY 4.3
Estimation of $\dot{V}O_{2max}$ Using an Equation

Low levels of cardiorespiratory fitness have been linked to most of the leading causes of death, including heart disease, stroke, cancer, and diabetes. Direct measurement of cardiorespiratory fitness or $\dot{V}O_{2max}$ is expensive, and requires trained technicians and medical supervision. There has been much interest in developing simple methods of estimating $\dot{V}O_{2max}$, especially for large groups of people. One method gaining widespread acceptance is the use of an estimating equation that factors in several personal characteristics including age, gender, height, weight, and physical activity habits.

Use the equation below to estimate your $\dot{V}O_{2max}$. You will need a calculator. Calculate your body mass index (BMI) from figure 5.6. It should be emphasized that this equation provides a "ballpark" estimate of your $\dot{V}O_{2max}$, and that other methods, especially running and walking tests, are preferred. Once you estimate your $\dot{V}O_{2max}$, use Table 4.1 to obtain your classification.

Equation for Estimating $\dot{V}O_{2max}$

$\dot{V}O_{2max}$ ml · kg^{-1} · min^{-1} = _____   _____

Classification (Table 4.1)

56.363 – (_____ × 0.381)
               age

– (_____ × 0.754)
   Body mass index

+ (_____ × 1.921)
        physical activity rating, 0 to 7*

+ 10.987 (if you are a male) or 0 (if you are a female)

Example: Calculate $\dot{V}O_{2max}$ in ml $\cdot$ kg^{-1} $\cdot$ min^{-1} for a 20-year-old female college student who is 5 foot, 5 inches tall (65 inches), weighs 130 pounds, and swims laps 45 minutes each week.

$\dot{V}O_{2max}$ ml $\cdot$ kg^{-1} $\cdot$ min^{-1} = ____42.0____   _____Average_____
                                              Classification (Table 4.1)

56.363 – (____20____ × 0.381)
              age

– (____21.7____ × 0.754)
   Body mass index

+ (_____5_____ × 1.921)
     physical activity rating, 0 to 7*

+ 0 (female)

* Pick a physical activity rating that best fits your typical habits:

- I. Does not participate regularly in programmed recreation sport or physical activity.

     0 points: Avoids walking or exertion (e.g., always uses elevator, drives whenever possible instead of walking).

     1 point: Walks for pleasure, routinely uses stairs, occasionally exercises sufficiently to cause heavy breathing or perspiration.

- II. Participates regularly in recreation or work requiring modest physical activity, such as golf, horseback riding, calisthenics, gymnastics, table tennis, bowling, weight lifting, or yard work:

     2 points: 10 to 60 minutes per week.

     3 points: Over one hour per week.

- III. Participates regularly in heavy physical exercise (such as running or jogging, swimming, cycling, rowing, skipping rope, running in place) or engages in vigorous aerobic type activity (such as tennis, basketball, or handball).

     4 points: Runs less than one mile per week or spends less than 30 minutes per week in comparable physical activity.

     5 points: Runs one to five miles per week or spends 30 to 60 minutes per week in comparable physical activity.

     6 points: Runs 5 to 10 miles per week or spends one to three hours per week in comparable physical activity.

     7 points: Runs over 10 miles per week or spends over three hours per week in comparable physical activity.

HEALTH AND FITNESS ACTIVITY 4.4
Estimation of $\dot{V}O_{2max}$ by Running One or 1.5 Miles

As described in the text, running tests can provide a fairly accurate estimate of your $\dot{V}O_{2max}$ if the following criteria are met:

1. The distance in accurately measured on a track.
2. The time is measured accurately with a stopwatch by a friend or instructor.
3. The distance (one or 1.5 miles) is run in the shortest possible time, with a maximal effort.
4. You are properly motivated and experienced in running (especially pacing).
5. Participants include those who are healthy and fit, with no underlying medical condition.
6. First engage in a proper warm-up of at least 5–10 minutes (enough to work up a light sweat). Afterwards, be sure to cool-down and stretch.

One-Mile Run Test: Follow the criteria listed above, run one mile as fast as possible, and then insert your time and other personal characteristics in the equation listed below. This equation is for males and females between the ages of 8 and 25 years. You will need Figure 5.6 from the next chapter to calculate your BMI or body mass index.

$\dot{V}O_{2max}$ ml · kg^{-1} · min^{-1} = _____   _____

Classification (Table 4.1)

108.94 – (_____ × 0.8.41) + (_____ × 0.34)
        mile time   mile time^2

+ (0.21 × _____ × _____) – (0.84 × _____)
        age   sex   BMI

Note: Mile time should be in minutes (using a decimal for seconds); sex = 1 for males, 0 for females; BMI = body mass index, which can be obtained using height and weight from figure 5.6.

For example, if a 20-year-old male can run a mile in 7.0 minutes and has a BMI of 21:

$\dot{V}O_{2max}$ ml · kg^{-1} · min^{-1} = _____53.3_____   _____Good_____
Classification (Table 4.1)

108.94 – (___7___ × 8.41) + (___49___ × 0.34)
        mile time   mile time^2

+ (0.21 × ___20___ × ___1___) – (0.84 × ___21___)
        age   sex   BMI

1.5-Mile Run Test: Follow the criteria listed above; run 1.5 miles as fast as possible, and then insert your time and other personal characteristics in the equation listed below.

$\dot{V}O_{2max}$ ml · kg^{-1} · min^{-1} = _____   _____

Classification (Table 4.1)

88.02 – (_____ × 2.767)
     1.5 mile time

+ (3.716 × _____)
          sex

– (0.0753 × _____)
          body weight in pounds

Note: 1.5 mile time should be in minutes (using a decimal for seconds); sex = 1 for males, 0 for females.

For example, if a 20-year-old female can run 1.5 miles in 13.0 minutes and weighs 130 pounds:

$\dot{V}O_{2max}$ ml · kg^{-1} · min^{-1} = _____ 42.3 _____   _____ Average _____

Classification (Table 4.1)

88.02 – (___ 13 ___ × 2.767)
     1.5 mile time

+ (3.716 × ___ 0 ___)
          sex

– (0.0753 × ___ 130 ___)
          body weight in pounds

HEALTH AND FITNESS ACTIVITY 4.5
The One-Mile Walk Test

Would you rather walk than run to determine your cardiorespiratory fitness level? Then the one-mile walk test is for you.

To take the test, walk a mile around a track or measured course as fast as possible, measure the total walking time, and then take the heart rate just after finishing.

This equation is recommended for college students:

$\dot{V}O_{2max}$ ml · kg^{-1} · min^{-1} = 88.768 + (8.892 × _____

(gender with M = 1, F = 0)

− (0.0957 × _____

(weight in pounds)

− (1.4537 × _____

(walk time in minutes in decimal format)

− (0.1194 × _____

(ending exercise heart rate)

For example, a college female weighing 128 pounds and able to walk one mile in 13 minutes with an ending heart rate of 133 beats per minute would have this estimated $\dot{V}O_{2max}$: 88.768 + (8.892 × 0) − (0.0957 × 128) − (1.4537 × 13.0) − (0.1194 × 133) = 41.7 ml · kg^{-1} · min^{-1}.

One-mile walking time: _____ minutes

Ending heart rate: _____ beats per minute

Fitness rating (from Table 4.1) _____

HEALTH AND FITNESS ACTIVITY 4.6
A Step Test For College Students

As explained in the text, in this step test, the heart rate is taken for 15 seconds after stepping up and down on a 16.25 inch bench for three minutes at a rate of 24 steps per minute for men, and 22 for women, and then applied to the equations listed below to determine $\dot{V}O_{2max}$. Overweight individuals and those with medical problems or leg injuries should not take this test.

1. The step test requires the following equipment: stopwatch, metronome, and stepping bench (16.25 inches high, typical of most gymnasium bleachers). The metronome should be set at 96 beats per minute for men, and 88 beats per minute for women. Practice stepping to a four-step cadence (up with the right foot, up with the left foot, down with the right foot, down with the left foot) to ensure 24 complete step-ups per minute for men, and 22 step-ups per minute for women.
2. Begin the test and perform the step-ups for exactly three minutes.
3. After stepping, remain standing, wait 5 seconds, and then count the heart rate at the wrist or neck for 15 seconds.
4. Convert the 15-second pulse count into beats per minute by multiplying by four.
5. Use these equations and to estimate $\dot{V}O_{2max}$, and Table 4.1 to classify your fitness status.

MALES: Predicted $\dot{V}O_{2max}$ = 111.33 – (0.42 × heart rate in bpm)

FEMALES: Predicted $\dot{V}O_{2max}$ = 65.81 – (0.1847 × heart rate in bpm)

15-second pulse count after stepping: _____   beats

Convert heart rate to beats per minute   _____   beats/minute

Estimated $\dot{V}O_{2max}$ from equations   _____ $ml \cdot kg^{-1} \cdot min^{-1}$

$\dot{V}O_{2max}$ classification from Table 4.1   _____

HEALTH AND FITNESS ACTIVITY 4.7
A Treadmill Test For College Students

A maximal treadmill graded exercise test has been developed that allows you to select a comfortable walking-jogging speed. After a six-minute warm-up at a self-selected speed, the treadmill grade is increased 1.5 percent each minute until you can no longer continue because of fatigue. The ending speed in miles per hour (mph) and the final treadmill percent grade that you were able to sustain for close to one minute are entered into a formula to estimate $\dot{V}O_{2max}$ in ml · kg^{-1} · min^{-1}. Only healthy individuals without underlying medical conditions should take this test. It is highly recommended that your class instructor supervise this test.

Follow these stages:

- Warm-up: Walk or jog up a 5% grade on the treadmill at a self-selected pace for six minutes.
- Test: Increase treadmill grade by 1.5% each minute while keeping the speed constant until you are unable to continue despite verbal encouragement from your instructor. Note the ending speed in miles per hour (mph) and the final treadmill percent grade that you were able to sustain for close to one minute.

$\dot{V}O_{2max}$ in ml · kg^{-1} · min^{-1} is estimated from this formula:

$\dot{V}O_{2max}$ **ml · kg^{-1} · min^{-1}** = _____

Classification (Table 4.1)

4.702 – (0.042 × _____)

                         weight in pounds

+ (6.191 × _____) + (1.311 × _____)

               treadmill mph   ending treadmill % grade

+ (2.674 × 1 (for males) or 0 (for females)

For example, if a 154-pound college male chooses a jogging speed of 5.4 mph, and is "maxed out" after the treadmill grade reaches 11%, the estimated $\dot{V}O_{2max}$ is:

$\dot{V}O_{2max}$ **ml · kg^{-1} · min^{-1}** = _____48.8_____   ____Average____

Classification (Table 4.1)

4.702 – (0.042 × _____154_____)

                         weight in pounds

+ (6.191 × _____5.4_____) + (1.311 × _____11_____)

               treadmill mph   ending treadmill % grade

+ (2.674 × 1) (for males)

CHAPTER 4 QUIZ
Assessment of Cardiorespiratory Fitness

Note: Answers are given at the end of the quiz.

1. The pressure in the artery when the heart is resting and is between beats is called the:

   A. systolic.

   B. diastolic.

2. $\dot{V}O_{2max}$ is defined as the greatest rate at which oxygen can be consumed during maximal exercise conditions, and is usually expressed in terms of:

   A. ml/kg/min.

   B. mg/min.

   C. kg/min.

   D. g/kg.

   E. none of the above.

3. During a graded exercise test on a treadmill, the systolic blood pressure:

   A. increases.

   B. stays the same.

   C. decrease.

4. The resting oxygen consumption for the average human is _____ ml/kg/min.

   A. 11.5

   B. 3.5

   C. 50

   D. 245

   E. 75

5. When the diastolic blood pressure is greater than _____ mm Hg, this is an indication of high blood pressure (when based on two or more readings).

   A. 60

   B. 70

   C. 80

   D. 90

6. Which fitness test uses a one-minute recovery heart rate to determine fitness classification?

   A. College Treadmill Test

   B. YMCA 3-minute step test

   C. 1.5-mile run test

   D. Bruce treadmill test

7. A high level of $\dot{V}O_{2max}$ depends on the proper functioning of three important systems of the body. Which one listed below is *not* included?

   A. respiratory system
   B. cardiovascular system
   C. gastrointestinal system
   D. musculoskeletal system

chapter five

Body Composition Measurement

"Whether your weight is 'healthy' depends on how much of your weight is fat, where in your body the fat is located, and whether you have weight-related medical problems, such as high blood pressure, or a family history of such problems."

—U.S. Department of Health and Human Services

The Best "Weigh"

How much should you weigh? This is a challenging question! We come in all shapes and sizes. Some of us are of slight build, with little muscle, bone, or fat. Athletes are often angular, with plenty of muscle and bone, but little fat, to accomplish feats of strength and endurance.

An increasing number of college students and adults in America carry too much body fat, placing themselves at increased risk for most of the common diseases of this era (see Chapter 10). At the other end of the spectrum, some are quite dissatisfied with their body weight and build, leading to heightened anxiety and the potential for eating disorders.

In this chapter, you will learn more about body weight, body fat, and ideal body weight, and how these can be measured. In Chapter 2, *body composition* was defined as the relative amount of body fat and fat-free mass. There are many techniques for measuring body composition and determining ideal body weight. These range from simple height-weight tables to sophisticated and expensive procedures used for research. You will learn several practical methods in this chapter that you can use throughout your lifetime.

Body Composition: The Basics

Body weight can be divided into fat mass and fat-free mass. The fat mass is the weight of your body that is fat. The fat-free mass is the weight of your body that is not fat—primarily water, protein (mostly in muscle tissue), and bone. **Body composition** is often defined as the ratio of fat to fat-free weight, with **obesity** specified as an excessive accumulation of fat weight. **Percent body fat** or **relative body fat,** the percent of total weight represented by fat weight, is the preferred index used to evaluate a person's body composition.

To illustrate, let's say you have a friend who weighs 200 pounds, and was measured at 25 percent body fat. One fourth of his body weight is fat (i.e., 50 pounds), while three fourths is fat-free mass (i.e., 150 pounds). About two thirds of the fat-free mass is water, with muscle and bone accounting for another third.

Reasons for Measuring Body Composition

Interest in measurement of body composition has grown tremendously since the early 1970s when the modern-day fitness movement began. Elite athletes, people involved with weight management programs, and patients in hospitals have all benefitted from the increased popularity and accuracy of body composition measurement.

There are several important reasons for measuring body composition:

- *To assess the decrease in body fat weight that occurs in response to a weight management program.* About 150 million American adults are overweight, with the highest rates found among the poor and minority groups (see Chapter 10). Body composition measurement throughout the entire weight-loss process helps people make informed decisions about their diet and exercise programs.
- *To help athletes determine the best body composition for performance.* Most athletes are very concerned with body composition. In some sports such as wrestling, gymnastics, ballet dancing, bodybuilding, and distance running, athletes attempt to reach the lowest body fat levels possible. In other sports such as weight lifting, football, baseball, and rowing, a large fat-free mass is paramount. Accurate body composition measurement is critical to guide athletes as they seek the optimal level of fat and fat-free mass associated with their sport.
- *To monitor fat and fat-free weight in patients with disease.* High body fat is an important risk factor for some diseases (e.g., heart disease, certain types of cancer, diabetes, and high blood pressure). Low muscle and bone mass predicts future development of osteoporosis. Thus, body composition measurement serves an important role in the prevention of chronic disease.
- *To track long-term changes that occur in body fat and fat-free mass with aging.* Body fat doubles between the ages of 20 and 65 years. Often, during middle-age, extra fat is gained around the stomach and trunk areas, which is especially harmful to long-term health. Muscular strength in most people is maintained to about 45 years of age, but then falls by about 5 to 10 percent per decade thereafter. In older people, muscle weakness may decrease the ability to accomplish the common activities of daily living, leading to dependency on others. Body composition measurement throughout the life-cycle helps people prepare for the changes that occur late in life.

Methods for Measuring Body Composition

Figure 5.1 shows that weight measurement alone cannot always accurately determine the body fat status of a person. Weight measurement does not differentiate between fat-free mass and fat mass. People genetically endowed with unusually high or low amounts of fat-free mass can be misclassified with respect to obesity if the only measure is total weight.

In other words, some people with **mesomorphic** or athletic, muscular body types (such as football players) can have normal or low body fat even though they are overweight according to standard charts. Some people who are **ectomorphic** (or lean, thin, and linear) with low amounts of fat-free mass can be underweight according to the weight charts, but be overly fat when their fat tissue is measured.

FIGURE 5.1

There are five ways of classifying people, in terms of their over-all weight and the fat-lean composition of their bodies. Obesity exists only in cases where the fat percentage is high, and is not directly related to weight.

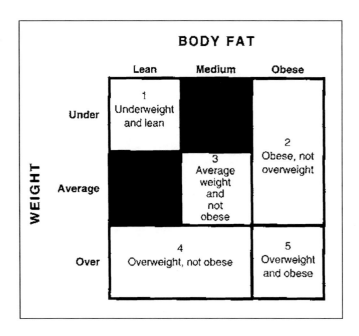

Height-Weight Tables and Indexes

During the last century, many different methods for determining body fat percentage were developed. The most basic of all methods is use of height-weight tables and indexes. Height-weight tables provide weight ranges that are recommended for a certain height. Height-weight indexes attempt to classify groups of individuals into various body composition categories (e.g., overweight, mild-, moderate-, and severe-obesity) by using mathematical formulas based on height and weight. Height-weight tables and indexes are quick and easy to use, and provide a fairly accurate classification.

The greatest problem with height and weight tables and indexes is that we vary widely in their fat-free mass. If you are muscular and athletic, you will usually be defined as "overweight" despite having low amounts of body fat. At the same time, if you have a slight build with little muscle and bone, you may be designated as "underweight" when your body fat may be normal or even slightly high. For these reasons, it is recommended that you have your body fat measured by a trained fitness professional (e.g., your instructor) to gain a true picture of your body fat percent and ideal body weight. Measurement of height and weight is an important beginning, but don't stop there if you want to know the real truth about your body composition.

Measurement of Body Weight

Your body weight should be measured using an electronic scale or a physician balance-beam scale. Scales should be placed on a flat, hard surface that will allow them to sit securely without rocking or tipping. Stand still in the middle of the scale's platform without touching anything and with the body weight equally distributed on both feet (see Figure 5.2). Ideally, you should be weighed with minimal clothing, no shoes, and after going to the bathroom.

Measurement of Height

The measurement of your height requires a vertical ruler with a horizontal headboard or right-angle measuring block that can be brought into contact with the highest point on the head. The headboard and ruler taken together are called a stadiometer.

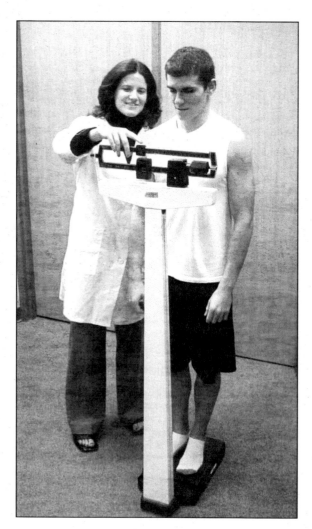

FIGURE 5.2
Body weight should be measured on a physician's balance beam scale, with minimal clothing.

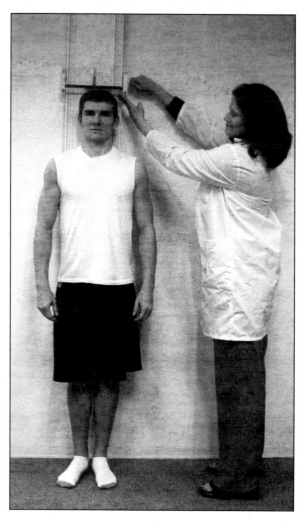

FIGURE 5.3
Height should be measured while standing erect, heels, buttocks, back of shoulders, and head touching the vertical ruler. A right-angle object should be brought into contact with the highest point on the head after a deep inhalation and holding of breath.

To accurately measure your height, stand without shoes, heels together, back as straight as possible, heels, buttocks, shoulders and head touching the wall, and looking straight ahead. Your weight should be distributed evenly on both feet, arms hanging freely by the sides of your body. Just before measurement, inhale deeply, and hold your breath, while the headboard is brought onto the highest point of your head, with sufficient pressure to compress the hair (see Figure 5.3).

Body Mass Index

Your height and weight measurements can be mathematically adjusted to provide an indirect estimate of obesity. The most common height-weight index is the **body mass index (BMI),** defined as your weight in kilograms divided by your height in meters squared (kg/m^2). Use of the BMI is simple, quick, and inexpensive, and is fairly accurate in classifying you as underweight, normal weight, overweight, or obese. As with any use of height and weight, however, BMI can classify you as overweight if you are very muscular, and underweight if you have little muscle even though your body fat is normal.

FIGURE 5.4
The Body Mass Index (kg/m^2) is calculated from this nomogram by reading the central scale after a straight edge is placed between height and body weight.

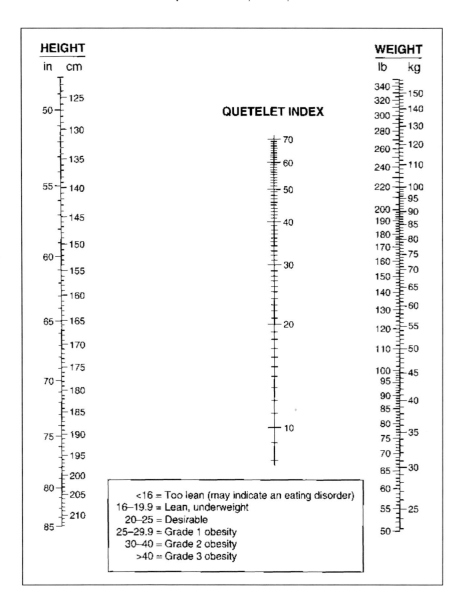

Figure 5.4 and Table 5.1 provide easy methods for calculating the BMI. If you desire to calculate the BMI mathematically, the following example can be used. A man weighing 154 pounds or 70 kilograms (one pound=0.4536 kg), standing 68 inches tall or 1.727 meters (one inch = 2.54 cm = 0.0254 m) has a BMI of 23.5 (kg/m^2) (70/1.727^2). To estimate BMI from pounds and inches, use this formula: (pounds/inches^2) x 704.5.

In 1998, the National Heart, Lung, and Blood Institute published updated BMI guidelines for the identification of overweight and obesity in adults. These are summarized in Table 5.2. This table was developed from research data that showed the higher the BMI the higher the disease risk. See Health and Fitness Activity 5.1 to determine your BMI classification.

Body Shape and Waist Circumference

Does body shape affect the link between obesity and disease risk? The answer according to recent evidence is "yes". Disease risk from obesity is high if fat tends to accumulate in the abdominal and trunk areas rather than the hip and thigh areas. This is called upper-body or android obesity in comparison to lower-body or gynoid obesity, which is characterized by body fat accumulation in the hips and thighs. (See Chapter 10 for more information).

TABLE 5.1 Body Mass Index Table

Directions: First find your height (no shoes), next locate your body weight at that height, and then find your BMI (top row).

Height (in)	Healthy Weight						Overweight					Obese											Very Obese													
BMI	19	20	21	22	23	24	25	26	27	28	29	30	31	32	33	34	35	36	37	38	39	40	41	42	43	44	45	46	47	48	49	50	51	52	53	54
												Body Weight (lb)																								
58	91	96	100	105	110	115	119	124	129	134	138	143	148	153	158	162	167	172	177	181	186	191	196	201	205	210	215	220	224	229	234	239	244	248	253	258
59	94	99	104	109	114	119	124	128	133	138	143	148	153	158	163	168	173	178	183	188	193	198	203	208	212	217	222	227	232	237	242	247	252	257	262	267
60	97	102	107	112	118	123	128	133	138	143	148	153	158	163	168	174	179	184	189	194	199	204	209	215	220	225	230	235	240	245	250	255	261	266	271	276
61	100	106	111	116	122	127	132	137	143	148	153	158	164	169	174	180	185	190	195	201	206	211	217	222	227	232	238	243	248	254	259	264	269	275	280	285
62	104	109	115	120	126	131	136	142	147	153	158	164	169	175	180	186	191	196	202	207	213	218	224	229	235	240	246	251	256	262	267	273	278	284	289	295
63	107	113	118	124	130	135	141	146	152	158	163	169	175	180	186	191	197	203	208	214	220	225	231	237	242	248	254	259	265	270	278	282	287	293	299	304
64	110	116	122	128	134	140	145	151	157	163	169	174	180	186	192	197	204	209	215	221	227	232	238	244	250	256	262	267	273	279	285	291	296	302	308	314
65	114	120	126	132	138	144	150	156	162	168	174	180	186	192	198	204	210	216	222	228	234	240	246	252	258	264	270	276	282	288	294	300	306	312	318	324
66	118	124	130	136	142	148	155	161	167	173	179	186	192	198	204	210	216	223	229	235	241	247	253	260	266	272	278	284	291	297	303	309	315	322	328	334
67	121	127	134	140	146	153	159	166	172	178	185	191	198	204	211	217	223	230	236	242	249	255	261	268	274	280	287	293	299	306	312	319	325	331	338	344
68	125	131	138	144	151	158	164	171	177	184	190	197	203	210	216	223	230	236	243	249	256	262	269	276	282	289	295	302	308	315	322	328	335	341	348	354
69	128	135	142	149	155	162	169	176	182	189	196	203	209	216	223	230	236	243	250	257	263	270	277	284	291	297	304	311	318	324	331	338	345	351	358	365
70	132	139	146	153	160	167	174	181	188	195	202	209	216	222	229	236	243	250	257	264	271	278	285	292	299	306	313	320	327	334	341	348	355	362	369	376
71	136	143	150	157	165	172	179	186	193	200	208	215	222	229	236	243	250	257	265	272	279	286	293	301	308	315	322	329	338	343	351	358	365	372	379	386
72	140	147	154	162	169	177	184	191	199	206	213	221	228	235	242	250	258	265	272	279	287	294	302	309	316	324	331	338	346	353	361	368	375	383	390	397
73	144	151	159	166	174	182	189	197	204	212	219	227	235	242	250	257	265	272	280	288	295	302	310	318	325	333	340	348	355	363	371	378	386	393	401	408
74	148	155	163	171	179	186	194	202	210	218	225	233	241	249	256	264	272	280	287	295	303	311	319	326	334	342	350	358	365	373	381	389	396	404	412	420
75	152	160	168	176	184	192	200	208	216	224	232	240	248	256	264	272	279	287	295	303	311	319	327	335	343	351	359	367	375	383	391	399	407	415	423	431
76	156	164	172	180	189	197	205	213	221	230	238	246	254	263	271	279	287	295	304	312	320	328	336	344	353	361	369	377	385	394	402	410	418	426	435	443

Body shape tends to run in the family, and is strongly influenced by genetic factors. The best solution for all body types is to keep body fat at healthy levels. Although android or upper-body obesity is the worst type, all forms of obesity impair health.

Your body shape can be estimated through the waist circumference measurement. The waist or abdominal circumference is defined as the smallest waist circumference below the rib cage and above the belly button, while standing with abdominal muscles relaxed (not pulled in) (see Figure 5.5). Use an inelastic tape that is in a horizontal plane (i.e., parallel to the floor). See Health and Fitness Activity 5.1 to determine and classify your waist circumference.

Using the Waist Circumference to Predict Disease Risk

The National Heart, Lung, and Blood Institute expert panel on overweight and obesity in adults recommends that the waist circumference be used in combination with the BMI to estimate disease risk from obesity. Disease risk climbs strongly if you are a male with a waist circumference greater than 40 inches, or a female measured at greater than 35 inches. Table 5.2 and Box 5.1 summarize the relationship between BMI, waist circumference, and disease risk.

FIGURE 5.5
The waist circumference should be measured below the rib cage and above the belly button. The abdominal muscle should be relaxed and not pulled in. Measure the smallest circumference in this area.

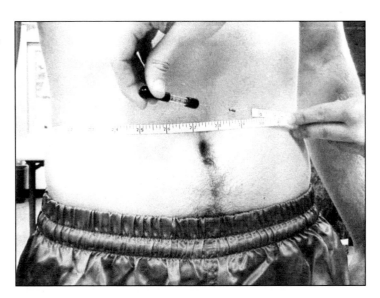

TABLE 5.2   Disease Risk Associated with Body Mass Index and Waist Circumference

Classification	Obesity Class	BMI (kg/m²)	Men ≤40 in / Women ≤35 in	>40 in / >35 in
Underweight		<18.5		
Normal		18.5–24.9		
Overweight		25.0–29.9	Increased	High
Obesity	I	30.0–34.9	High	Very high
	II	35.0–39.9	Very high	Very high
Extreme obesity	III	>40	Extremely high	Extremely high

*Disease risk for type 2 diabetes, hypertension, and cardiovascular disease.

Source: NHLBI Obesity Education Initative Expert Panel (1998). *Clinical Guidelines on the Identification, Evaluation, and Treatment of Overweight and Obesity in Adults.* National Heart, Lung, and Blood Institute: www.nhlbi.nih.gov/nhlbi/.

BOX 5.1

Following the Dietary Guidelines for Americans

How to Evaluate Your Weight (Adults)
1. Weigh yourself and have your height measured. Find your BMI category in the chart. The higher your BMI category, the greater the risk for health problems.
2. Measure around your waist, just above your hip bones, while standing Health risks increase as waist measurement increases, particularly if waist is greater than 35 inches for women or 40 inches for men. Excess abdominal fat may place you at greater risk of health problems, even if your BMI is about right
3. Refer to the list below to find out how many other risk factors you have.

The higher your BMI and waist measurement, and the more risk factors you have, the more you are likely to benefit from weight loss.

Find Out Your Other Risk Factors for Chronic Disease
The more of these risk factors you have, the more you are likely to benefit from weight loss if you are overweight or obese.

- Do you have a personal or family history of heart disease?
- Are you a male older than 45 years, or a postmenopausal female?
- Do you smoke cigarettes?
- Do you have a sedentary lifestyle?
- Has your doctor told you that you have any of the following?
  —High blood pressure
  —Abnormal blood lipids (high LDL cholesterol, low HDL cholesterol, high triglycerides)
  —Diabetes

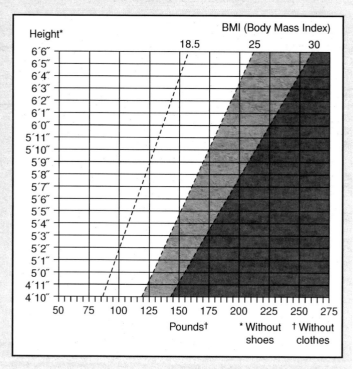

BMI measures weight in relation to height The BMI ranges shown above are for adults. They are not exact ranges of healthy and unhealthy weights. However, they show that health risk increases at higher levels of overweight and obesity. Even within the healthy BMI range, weight gains can carry health risks for adults.

Directions: Find your weight on the bottom of the graph Go straight up from that point until you come to the line that matches your height. Then look to find your weight group.

☐ **Healthy Weight** BMI from 18.5 up to 25 refers to healthy weight.
◻ **Overweight** BMI from 25 up to 30 refers to overweight.
■ **Obese** BMI 30 or higher refers to obesity. Obese persons are also overweight.

Source: Report of the Dietary Guidelines Advisory Committee on the Dietary Guidelines for Americans, 2000.
Note: Weight loss is usually not advisable for pregnant women.

Measurement of Percent Body Fat

Although the BMI and waist circumference provide important information regarding your personal health, they do not measure your percent body fat. The most widely used and practical methods for determining percent body fat are based on bioelectrical impedance analysis (BIA) and skinfold measurements.

Bioelectrical Impedance Analysis

Bioelectrical impedance analysis (BIA) was developed in the 1960s and has become one of the most popular methods for estimating percent body fat. A harmless 50-kHz current is generated by the BIA analyzer and passed through the person being measured (see figure 5.6). The measurement of electrical impedance is detected as the resistance to electrical current, and then translated through equations to percent body fat.

When the appropriate BIA equation is used, and the sources of measurement error are controlled, estimation of percent body fat through the BIA method is about as accurate as the skinfold method. The BIA method, however, may be more preferable in some settings compared to the skinfold method, because it does not require technician skill, and it is more comfortable and less intrusive.

There are several sources of measurement error with the BIA method that need to be controlled as much as possible to improve accuracy and reliability:

Instrumentation: BIA analyzers differ substantially from one company to another, and can be a source of substantial error. To control for this error, the same instrument should be used when monitoring body composition changes in people over time.

Subject and Environmental Factors: The person's state of hydration can greatly affect the BIA process. Factors such as eating, drinking, avoidance of fluids, and exercising can affect hydration state, and therefore introduce error. Cool, ambient temperatures cause a drop in skin temperature that results in an underestimation of fat-free mass. Subject and environmental guidelines prior to BIA measurements include the following:

1. No eating or drinking within four hours of the test.
2. No exercise within 12 hours of the test.

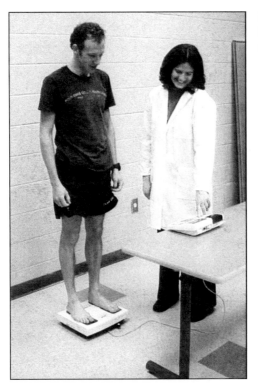

FIGURE 5.6

Bioelectrical impedance analysis is convenient and as accurate as skinfolds in calculating percent body fat.

3. Urinate within 30 minutes of the test.
4. No alcohol consumption within 48 hours of the test.
5. No diuretic medications within 7 days of the test.
6. No testing of female clients who perceive they are retaining water during that stage of their menstrual cycle.
7. BIA measurements should be made in a room with normal ambient temperature.

Technician Skill: Some BIA analyzers require that the person being tested be in a supine position with arms and legs comfortably apart, at about a 45-degree angle to each other. BIA measures are taken on the right side of the body. Electrodes need to be correctly positioned at the wrist and ankle according to manufacturer guidelines. The sensor or proximal electrodes should be placed on the dorsal surface of the wrist, so that the upper border of the electrode bisects the head of the ulna, and the dorsal surface of the ankle, so that the upper border of the electrode bisects the medial and lateral malleoli. The source or distal electrodes should be placed at the base of the second or third metacarpal-phalangeal joints of the hand and foot. There should be at least five centimeters between the proximal and distal electrodes.

A new leg-to-leg bioimpedance analysis system, combined with a digital scale that employs stainless steel pressure-contact foot pad electrodes for standing impedance and body weight measurements, has been developed by the Tanita Corporation (see figure 5.6). This system has been found to perform as well as the conventional arm-to-leg gel electrode BIA system, but is much quicker and easier to use.

Skinfold Measurements

Another widely used method for determining obesity is based on the thickness of skinfolds. *Skinfold measurements* have several advantages:

1. The necessary equipment is inexpensive and takes up little or no space.
2. The measures can be obtained quickly and easily.
3. The measures when performed correctly have a high correlation with body density, providing more accurate estimates of body fat than the various height-weight ratios do.

Seven skinfold sites are described below. To reduce error, skinfold sites should be precisely determined and verified by a *trained* instructor before measurement. The measurements should be made carefully, in a quiet room, and without undue haste.

Figures 5.7 to 5.13 show the correct site marking and method of measurement for the respective sites. *(Appendix B can be of help in finding the various anatomic sites used in skinfold testing.)*

- **Chest** (figure 5.7)—The chest or pectoral skinfold is measured using a skinfold with its long axis directed to the nipple. The skinfold is picked up just next to the anterior axillary fold (front of armpit line). The measurement is taken one-half inch from the fingers. The site is approximately one inch from the anterior axillary line towards the nipple. The measurement is the same for both men and women.
- **Abdomen** (figure 5.8)—A horizontal fold is picked up slightly more than one inch (3 cm) to the side of and one-half inch below the naval.
- **Thigh** (figure 5.9)—A vertical fold on the front of the thigh, midway between the hip (inguinal crease) and the nearest border of the patella or knee cap. The person being tested should first flex his hip to make it easier to locate the inguinal crease. Be sure to pick a spot on the hip crease that is exactly above the midpoint of the front of the thigh. The closest border of the knee cap should be located while the knee is extended. When measuring the thigh skinfold, the body weight should be shifted to the other foot, while the leg on the side of the measurement is relaxed, with the knee slightly flexed and the foot flat on the floor.
- **Triceps** (figure 5.10)—A vertical fold on the rear midline of the upper arm, halfway between the lateral projection of the acromion process of the scapula (bump on back side of shoulder) and the inferior part of the olecranon process (the elbow). The site

FIGURE 5.7
Measurement of the chest or pectoral skinfold.

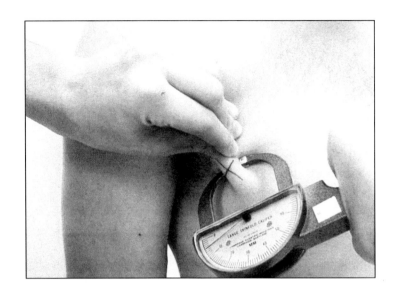

FIGURE 5.8
Measurement of the abdominal skinfold.

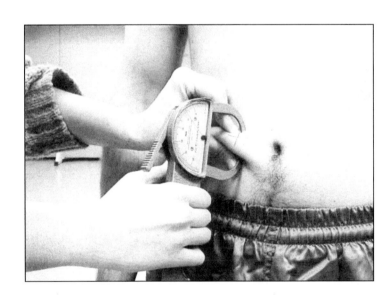

FIGURE 5.9
Measurement of the thigh skinfold.

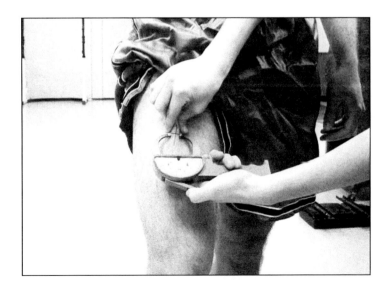

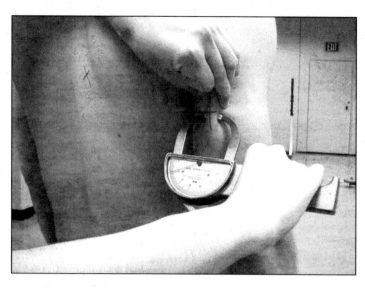 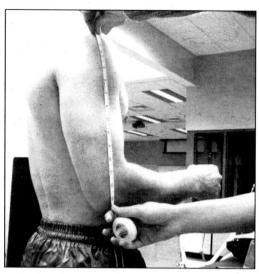

FIGURE 5.10 (A & B)
Measurement of the triceps skinfold.

FIGURE 5.11
Measurement of the suprailiac skinfold.

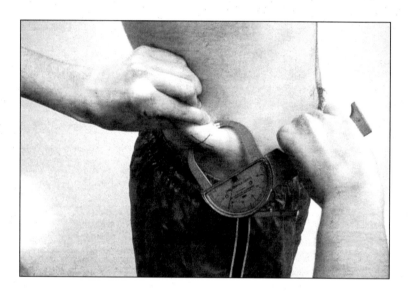

should first be marked by measuring the distance between the lateral projection of the acromial process and the lower border of the olecranon process of the ulna, using a tape measure, with the elbow flexed to 90 degrees. The midpoint is marked on the lateral side of the arm. The skinfold is measured with the arm hanging loosely at the side. The measurer stands behind the person being measured and picks up the skinfold site on the back of the arm, with the thumb and index finger directed down toward the feet. The triceps skinfold is picked up with the left thumb and index finger, approximately one-half inch above the marked level where the tips of the caliper are applied.

- **Suprailiac** (figure 5.11)—A diagonal fold above the crest of the ilium at the spot where an imaginary line would come down from the mid-axillary line. The person being measured should stand erect with feet together. The arms should hang by the sides, but can be moved slightly to improve access to the site. A diagonal fold should be grasped just to the rear of the mid-axillary line, following the natural cleavage lines of the skin. The skinfold caliper jaws should be applied about one-half inch from the fingers.
- **Subscapular** (figure 5.12)—The site is just below the lowest angle of the scapular. A fold is taken on a diagonal line directed at a 45-degree angle toward the right side. To

FIGURE 5.12
Measurement of the subscapular skinfold.

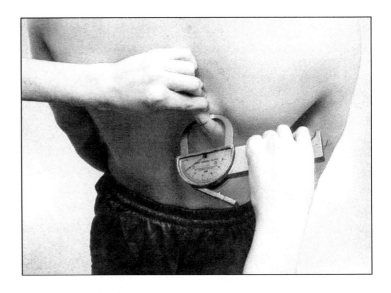

FIGURE 5.13
Measurement of the medial calf skinfold.

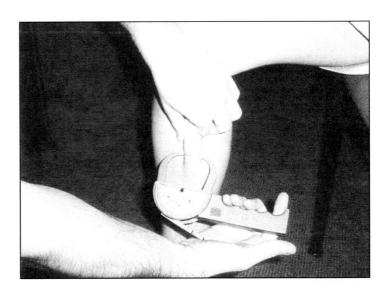

locate the site, the measurer should feel for the bottom of the scapula. In some cases it helps to place the arm of the person being measured behind his back.

- **Medial Calf** (figure 5.13)—For the measurement of the medial calf skinfold, the person being measured sits with his right knee flexed to about 90 degrees, sole of the foot on the floor. The level of the maximum calf circumference is marked on the inside (medial) of the calf. Facing from the front, the measurer raises a vertical skinfold, and measures at the marked site.

Two-Site Skinfold Test for Children, Youth, and Those of College Age

The two-site skinfold test, using the triceps and subscapular sites, has been the most commonly used body composition test for young people age six through college.

The choice of the triceps and subscapular sites over other commonly measured sites (medial calf, abdomen, suprailiac, thigh, etc.) was originally made for several reasons:

- Correlations between these sites and other measures of body fat have been consistently among the highest in many studies.
- These sites are more reliably and objectively measured than most other sites.
- There are available national norms for these sites.

Recently, however, use of the subscapular site has been questioned. Some parents of school-aged children are concerned that the modesty of their children is infringed upon when the physical educator raises the shirt of the child to gain access to the subscapular site. The medial calf skinfold site is more easily accessible, and recent studies have found it to be valid and reliable.

Figures 5.14 and 5.15 outline recently developed skinfold and body fat standards for children and youth, ages 6 to 17.

Teachers are encouraged to attend workshops where training is offered on the skinfold measurement technique. It is recommended that skinfold measurements be taken for all children at least once a year, with records kept to track children from year to year.

FIGURE 5.14

Body fat standards for children and youth (ages 6 to 17) using the triceps and subscapulor skinfolds. Source: The Use of Skinfold to Estimate Body Fatness on Children and Youth. JOPERD, November/December, 1987, pp. 98–102.

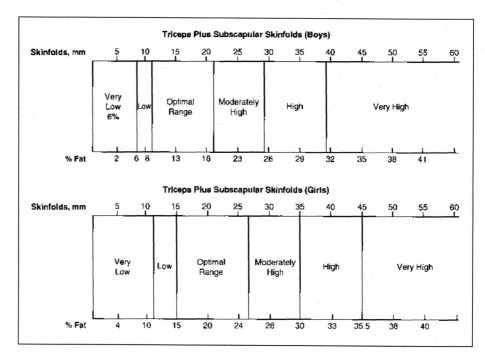

FIGURE 5.15

Body fat standards for children and youth (ages 6 to 17) using the triceps and medial calf skinfolds. Source: The Use of Skinfold to Estimate Body Fatness on Children and Youth. JOPERD, November/December, 1987, pp. 98–702.

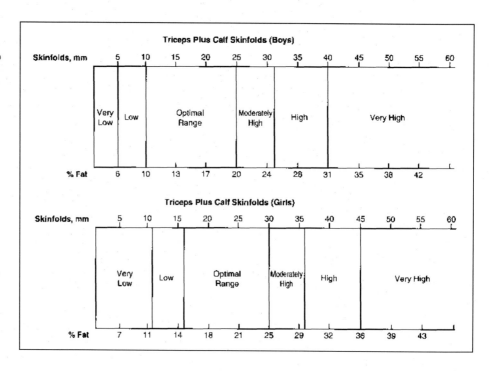

Multiple Skinfold Tests for Adults

To gain an accurate understanding of your percent body fat and ideal body weight, you should have at least three skinfold sites measured by a trained tester.

Since 1951, more than 100 body composition equations (skinfold measurements and circumference and diameter measures) have been published. Most of these equations have been developed for specific types of people (athletes, young men, elderly women, etc.), and are thus limited to the groups for which they were developed.

The more recent trend has been to develop generalized rather than such population-specific equations. These equations have been developed taking into account data from many different research projects. One generalized equation replaces several population-specific equations without a loss in prediction accuracy for a wide range of people. The three-site equations utilizing triceps, suprailiac, and thigh skinfolds for adult females, and chest, abdomen, and thigh skinfolds for adult males have been most widely used.

For ease of determination, a nomogram has been developed to calculate percentage body fat using age and the sum of three skinfolds for both men and women (see figure 5.16). A sample skinfold testing form is outlined in Figure 5.17.

FIGURE 5.16

To use the nomogram, place a straight edge connecting the age and sum of three skinfolds. The percent body fat is read at the point where the straight edge crosses the line representing the gender of the subject.

Source: Baun WB, Baun MR, Raven PB. *Res Quart Exerc Sport* 52:380–384, 1981.

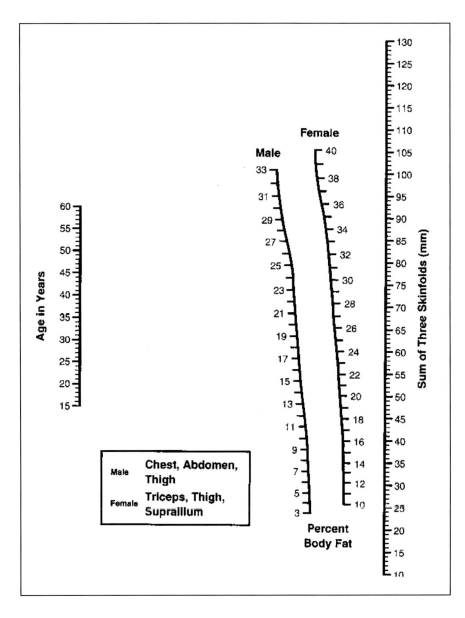

SKINFOLD MEASUREMENTS

NAME _____ DATE _____

AGE _____ SEX _____ HEIGHT _____ WEIGHT _____

MEASUREMENTS (mm)

_____ CHEST   _____ SUPRAILIAC

_____ ABDOMINAL   _____ MID-AXILLARY

_____ THIGH   _____ SUBSCAPULAR

_____ TRICEPS   _____ MEDIAL CALF

CALCULATIONS
(USE APPROPRIATE FORMULA)

_____ BIA
(percent fat)

_____ TOTAL SKINFOLDS (mm)
(skinfolds)

_____ BODY FAT PERCENT
(skinfolds)

_____ POUNDS OF FAT
(Total Wt x Body Fat %)

_____ POUNDS OF LEAN BODY WEIGHT
(Total Wt – Fat Wt)

_____ CLASSIFICATION
(See Norms)

_____ IDEAL BODY WEIGHT
[LBW/(100% – Desired Fat %)]

FIGURE 5.17
Skinfold testing form.

In making the calculations for fat, lean body weight (fat-free mass), and ideal body weight, the following formulas should be used:

pounds of fat = total weight × body fat %

lean body weight = total weight − fat weight

ideal weight = [present lean body weight/(100% − desired fat %)]

For example, if a subject weighs 200 pounds and is 25 percent body fat, and desires to be 15 percent body fat:

body fat = 200 × 0.25 = 50 pounds

lean body weight= 200 − 50 = 150 pounds

ideal weight = 150/0.85 = 176 pounds

Notice that the ideal weight formula assumes that the lean body weight stays the same during weight loss. Excess body weight, however, has been determined to be 75 percent body fat and 25 percent lean body weight (fat-free mass). For some people, therefore, a reduction in lean body weight is actually desirable, and should be represented in the equation by subtracting 25 percent of the excess weight (e.g., 25 percent of 12 excess pounds, or 3 pounds) from the present lean body weight.

Norms for body fat are listed in Table 5.3. Athletes involved in sports where the body weight is supported, such as canoeing, kayaking, and swimming, tend to have higher body fat values than athletes involved in weight-bearing sports such as naming, that are either very anaerobic (sprinting) or very aerobic (marathoning).

HEALTH AND FITNESS INSIGHT
Other Methods for Determining Body Composition

There are many other methods for measuring body fat and fat-free mass. Of these methods, underwater weighing is considered the "gold standard."

Underwater Weighing

Underwater weighing is the most widely used laboratory procedure for measuring body fat. In this procedure, whole body density is calculated from body volume according to Archimedes' principle of displacement, which states that an object submerged in water is buoyed up by the weight of the displaced water.

The protocol requires weighing a person underwater (with their air blown out of their lungs) as well as on land.

The scale and chair can be suspended from a diving board or an overhead beam into a pool, small tank, or hot tub that is four to five feet deep. The water should be warm for comfort (85–92°F), still, and filtered and chlorinated.

Although the underwater weighing method provides a high degree of accuracy, it presents practical problems. First of all, some people have a difficult time blowing their air out of their lungs and then staying underwater for the five to ten seconds it takes for the underwater weight to be measured. Also, the procedure requires special equipment, experience, and significant financial investment. (In particular, sophisticated equipment is needed to measure the residual volume, the air left in the lungs after the exhalation; if it is not measured accurately, the test is no more accurate than skinfold measurement.)

TABLE 5.3   Body Fat Ranges for Ages 18 and Older

Classification	Male	Female
Unhealthy range (too low)	5% and below	8% and below
Acceptable range (lower end)	6–15%	9–23%
Acceptable range (higher end)	16–24%	24–31%
Unhealthy range (too high)	25% and above	32% and above

	Average Body Fat Ranges for Elite Athletes*	
	Male	Females
Endurance athletes	*4–15%*	*12–26%*
Long-distance runners	4–14%	12–20%
Swimmers	5–14%	14–26%
Cross-country skiers	7–14%	15–23%
Canoers/rowers	6–15%	14–24%
Athletes in sports that emphasize leannes	*4–10%*	*10–19%*
Wrestlers	4–10%	
Gymnasts	4–10%	10–19%
Body builders	4–10%	10–17%
Team/dual sport athletes	*7–21%*	*18–27%*
Basketball players	7–11%	18–27%
Baseball players	11–15%	
Football players	9–21%	
Volleyball players	9–15%	20–25%
Tennis players	14–17%	19–22%
Power athletes	*5–20%*	*17–30%*
Shot-putters/discus throwers	15–20%	23–30%
Weight lifters	8–16%	
Sprinters	5–17%	17–21%

*Body fat ranges represent the average for national and international class athletes for a particular sport but do not encompass extreme values sometimes measured.

Sources: Lohman, TG. *Advances in Body Composition Assessment: Current Issues in Exercise Science,* Monograph Number 3. Champaign, IL: Human Kinetics, 1992. Wilmore, JH. Design issues and alternatives in assessing physical fitness among apparently healthy adults in a health examination survey of the general population. In National Center for Health Statistics, Drury, TG (ed.). *Assessing Physical Fitness and Physical Activity in Population-Based Surveys.* DHHS Pub. No. (PHS) 89-1253. Public Health Service. Washington, DC: U.S. Government Printing Office, 1989.

Recently, the whole concept of body density determination has been questioned. While the density of human body fat is relatively constant within and between individuals, and is independent of sex, age, or location within the body, the density of the lean component appears to be quite variable, depending on age, sex, activity, and race. For example, athletes have denser bones and muscles than nonathletes, which leads to an underestimation of body fat. Osteoporosis (thinning of the bones) reduces bone density, and can result in an overestimation of body fat in the elderly.

More research is needed to develop more refined equations for predicting percentage of body fat for humans of all ages. For now, skinfold measurement remains the most practical method for most people. Underwater weighing is best conducted in a research environment.

Summary

1. Body weight can be divided into fat mass and fat-free mass. The fat mass is the weight of your body that is fat. The fat-free mass is the weight of your body that is not fat—primarily water, protein (mostly in muscle tissue), and bone. Body composition is defined as the ratio of fat to fat-free weight, with obesity specified as an excessive accumulation of fat weight. Percent body fat or relative body fat is the percent of total weight represented by fat weight.

2. There are several important reasons for measuring body composition: to assess the decrease in body fat weight that occurs in response to a weight management program; to help athletes determine the best body composition for performance; to monitor fat and fat-free mass in patients with disease; to track long-term changes that occur in body fat and fat-free mass with aging.

3. The most common height-weight index is the Body Mass Index (BMI), defined as your weight in kilograms divided by your height in meters squared (kg/m^2).

4. Height-weight indexes such as the Body Mass Index classify groups of individuals into various body composition categories (e.g., overweight, mild-, moderate-, and severe-obesity) by using mathematical formulas based on height and weight. Height-weight indexes are quick and easy to use, and provide a fairly accurate classification.

5. Body shape affects the link between obesity and disease risk. Disease risk is high if fat tends to accumulate in the abdominal and trunk areas rather than the hip and thigh areas. This is called upper-body or android obesity in comparison to lower-body or gynoid obesity which is characterized by body fat accumulation in the hips and thighs. Your body shape can be estimated through the waist-to-hip ratio (WHR). The waist circumference is easier to use and measure, and by itself can predict disease risk.

6. The most widely used and practical methods for determining percent body fat are based on bioelectrical impedance analysis (BIA) and skinfold measurements. These measurements can be used to estimate your fat mass, fat-free mass, and ideal body weight.

Name _____ Date _____

HEALTH AND FITNESS ACTIVITY 5.1
Classification of Body Mass Index and Waist Circumference

Accurately measure your height, body weight, and waist circumference following the instructions in this chapter, and record them here. Use Figure 5.2 and Table 5.1 to classify body weight and frame size. You will need a good weight scale, stadiometer, and measuring tape, and the guidance of your instructor, to make these measurements.

Measurement   **Classification**

_____ height in inches

_____ weight in pounds

_____ body mass index (BMI) (from Figure 5.4)   _____
(Weight in kilograms/height in meters squared)   (From Table 5.2)

_____ Waist circumference (inches)   _____
                                                       (From Table 5.2)

Review Box 5.1 and Table 5.2, and summarize your disease risk based on your BMI and waist circumference:

_____

_____

_____

_____

_____

_____

_____

_____

HEALTH AND FITNESS ACTIVITY 5.2
BIA and Skinfold Measurements, and Calculation of
Percent Body Fat and Ideal Body Weight

Step 1:
Using the information described in this chapter, have your class instructor measure three skinfolds (chest, abdomen, and thigh for men; triceps, suprailliac, and thigh for women), and record them in the worksheet provided in figure 5.17.

Step 2:
If you have access to a bioelectrical impedance analyzer, take this test (following all of the rules listed in the text) and transfer the percent body fat to the form in figure 5.17 and in the blank below:

Your BIA percent body fat = _____

Step 3:
Total the three skinfolds, and transfer this total to the lower half of the form.

Step 4:
Estimate body fat percent using figure 5.16. Compare this with your BIA measurement and record here:

Your skinfold percent body fat = _____

Step 5:
Use Table 5.3 to classify your body fat percent, and then record this classification on the form and here:

Your percent body fat classification = _____

Step 6:
Calculate fat weight, lean body weight (or fat-free weight), and ideal body weight. The formulas are listed in figure 5.17, with an explanation in the text.

Fat weight =   _____

Fat-free weight =   _____

Ideal body weight =   _____

CHAPTER 5 QUIZ
Body Composition Measurement

Note: Answers are given at the end of the quiz.

A friend of yours weighs 250 pounds, is 70 inches tall, and is measured to be 36% fat. Answer questions 1 to 3 based on this information.

1. What is his fat weight?
   A. 40 pounds
   B. 50
   C. 70
   D. 90

2. What is his lean body weight?
   A. 134
   B. 160
   C. 180
   D. 210

3. If your friend wants to reduce his body fat to 15%, what would his ideal weight be? (Assume lean body weight stays the same.)
   A. 200
   B. 156
   C. 162
   D. 188
   E. 212

4. What is the BMI of a male who weighs 200 pounds at a height of 68 inches?
   A. 30.5
   B. 24.5
   C. 22.3
   D. 34.3
   E. 28.9

5. It a male friend of yours is 10% body fat with a BIA of 30, he probably looks like:
   A. an elite distance runner
   B. a football linebacker
   C. an average college student
   D. a ballet dancer

6. Which body composition technique listed below is the gold standard for estimation of human obesity?

   A. height-weight tables
   B. BIA
   C. underwater weighing
   D. skinfolds
   E. bioelectrical impedance

7. When the waist circumference rises above a threshold of _____ inches in a man, this is an indicaiton of high risk for obesity-related health problems.

   A. 35
   B. 40
   C. 45
   D. 50

8. A BMI above a threshold of _____ is an indication of obesity:

   A. 13
   B. 20
   C. 25
   D. 40

9. Females are considered at "acceptable" levels (low end) when their body fat percentage is 9 to _____ %.

   A. 15
   B. 35
   C. 23
   D. 40

chapter six

Assessment of Musculoskeletal Fitness

"That which is used develops. That which is not used wastes away."
—Hippocrates

"We can learn a lot by observing animals. Watch a cat or a dog. They instinctively know how to stretch. They do so spontaneously, never overstretching, continually and naturally tuning up muscles they will have to use."
—Bob Anderson

Muscular Fitness: The Basics

More than 600 muscles enable you to work, play sports, and accomplish your daily tasks (see Appendix B). Skeletal muscle is the body's most abundant tissue, making up about 23 percent of a female's body weight, and 40 percent of a male's. Millions of tiny protein filaments within the muscle work together to contract and pull on tendons and other tissues to create movement around joints. When your muscles contract, they become shorter—in other words, they pull but cannot push.

Your muscles are very responsive to use and disuse. Those that are forcefully exercised become larger, a phenomenon called muscular hypertrophy. On the other hand, a muscle that is not used will atrophy or decrease in size and strength, and become inflexible. Good muscular fitness depends on the development of three basic components:

- Muscular strength
- Muscular endurance
- Flexibility

Muscular Strength and Endurance

As reviewed in Chapter 2, **muscular strength** is the maximum one-effort force that you can generate against a resistance, while **muscular endurance** is the ability of the muscles to repeat a sub-maximal effort over and over. It takes muscular strength to bench press a heavy weight once or twice before fatigue, but endurance to lift a lighter weight 15 to 20 times.

Strength training builds physical fitness and promotes a high quality of life. The minimum strength training program is performing two sets of 8–12 repetitions of 8 to 10 exercises two to three times per week. The same regimen using 10 to 15 repetitions is recommended for persons over 50 years of age. This is a basic program, however, and greater gains in muscular strength and power can be experienced using higher intensity (fewer repetitions with greater weight) with multiple sets (e.g., 3 sets of 6 reps to fatigue). This will be reviewed in greater detail in Chapter 7.

Flexibility

Exercises to develop flexibility have long been pursued to enhance performance, fitness, and peace of mind. The ancient Greek athletes used flexibility training to enable them to dance, perform acrobatic stunts, and wrestle with greater ease. Stretching positions have been a part of Near Eastern and Far Eastern traditions for thousands of years, and today are practiced by millions in yoga classes to develop equilibrium of body, mind, and spirit. Stretching has long been a vital component of martial arts (e.g., karate and the modern tae kwon do), gymnastics, and ballet.

In the United States, stretching became recognized as an important part of a total fitness program following the publication of the book *Stretching* by Bob Anderson in 1975. This book has since sold more than two million copies in the United States, and has been published in 22 languages for worldwide distribution. In 1998, the American College of Sports Medicine included recommendations on flexibility exercise for the first time in their position stand on exercise "based on growing evidence of its multiple benefits."

The word *flexibility* comes from a Latin term meaning "to bend." In Chapter 2, flexibility was defined as the capacity of the joints to move through a full range of movement. In other words, if you can sit down on the floor with your legs straight and freely reach beyond your toes, you have a flexible hip joint. If you have difficulty reaching your ankles, the hip joint is inflexible. It is important to understand that flexibility is specific to each joint of the body. Some people have flexible shoulder joints, for example, but tight hip joints.

There are three basic types of flexibility:

- **Static flexibility:** Ability to hold a stretched position (e.g., touching the floor with the fingers with legs straight or performing a "leg split").
- **Dynamic flexibility:** Ability to engage in slow, rhythmic movements throughout the full range of joint motion (e.g., the ability of a ballet dancer to raise and hold her leg above the head).
- **Ballistic flexibility:** Ability to engage in bobbing, bouncing, rebounding, and rhythmic motions (e.g., touching one's toes by bobbing up and down). This type of movement is generally not recommended due to injury potential except when included as an inherent part of a sporting endeavor (e.g., certain gymnastic and dance movements).

How can your flexibility in all of the major muscle groups and joints be improved? There are several types of stretching programs, but the most practical one involves static stretching, which involves slowly applying a stretch to a muscle and joint, and then holding it at a position of mild discomfort for 10 to 30 seconds. To develop flexibility, static stretching exercises should be repeated 2 to 4 times for each major muscle group and joint of the body, with a minimum of 2 to 3 sessions per week. As a matter of safety and effectiveness, an active aerobic warm-up should precede vigorous stretching sessions. Muscles that are warm from jogging, cycling, or other aerobic exercise can stretch further and more safely.

Further details on stretching exercises and guidelines will be reviewed in Chapter 7. In this chapter, emphasis will be placed on the benefits of stretching and methods for assessing flexibility.

Factors That Influence Flexibility Why are some people more flexible than others? Each joint is surrounded by ligaments, tendons, and muscles, and these connective tissues determine whether the joint is tight or loose. Ligaments are special tissues that tie bones together, tendons link muscles to bones, and all of these plus other tissues make up the structural or framework connective tissues. Unusual strain to the joint can stretch the ligaments, leading to a loose joint that is then highly susceptible to injury. Stretching exercises help to lengthen the muscles and tendons, increasing the joint range of motion in a healthy way. Gymnasts and ballet dancers, for example, are capable of amazing feats of flexibility due to spending much time each day stretching.

As a person ages, flexibility decreases, although this is thought to be due more to inactivity than the aging process itself. There are good examples of physically active elderly people who have maintained a high degree of flexibility, and studies show that older persons can benefit from flexibility training. In other words, it is never too late in life to perform stretching exercises. But the usual tendency is for people to grow weak and tight as they age. Gender also plays a role, with males tending to have less flexibility than females.

Physically inactive people tend to be less flexible than those who are active. The connective tissues tend to tighten around the joints when the muscles are not used on a regular basis. Warming the joint (either from hot water or aerobic exercise) produces a significant increase in joint range of motion; thus, a good warm-up should precede stretching routines.

The Health Benefits of Muscular Fitness

Development of muscular fitness has several important health-related benefits, including increased bone density (lowering risk of osteoporosis or brittle bones in old age), muscle size, and connective tissue strength, and improved self-esteem. See Box 6.1 on osteoporosis. Between the ages of 30 and 70, muscle size and strength decrease by an average of 30 percent; much of this due to inactivity. This decrease contributes to the weakness and frailty common in old age. According to recent studies, elderly people who train with weights can recapture a good portion of their lost strength, enabling them to better perform the common daily activities of life.

Low back pain has been related to weak spinal and abdominal muscles, and tight lower back muscles. During certain types of lifting or exercise, weak trunk muscles may be unable to support the spine properly, leading to low back pain. Intensive back muscle exercise programs provide excellent therapy for low back pain sufferers, helping to reduce their pain and enabling them to return to work earlier than would otherwise be expected. This benefit will be discussed in the next section of this chapter.

There is little evidence to suggest that weight lifting reduces the risk for heart disease, cancer, diabetes, high blood pressure, or high blood cholesterol. Training with weights does not increase the $\dot{V}O_{2max}$ appreciably, primarily because the heart and lung system is not challenged sufficiently. Thus, weight lifters should supplement their resistance training with aerobic training. Table 6.1 compares the health and fitness benefits of aerobic and strength training.

Flexible Benefits The concept behind stretching is simple: When a muscle is extended slightly beyond its normal length (just short of the pain threshold), it gradually adapts and develops a greater range of motion. That improved range accounts for most of the benefits of stretching.

Many claims have been made for the performance-, fitness , and health related benefits of flexibility. These include:

- more graceful body movements
- enhanced performance of sport skills
- relaxation of mental stress and tension
- muscular relaxation, and relief of muscular cramps and soreness

BOX 6.1

Risk Factors for Osteoporosis, and Prevention Steps

Osteoporosis is a bone disorder where the bones lose density and are more prone to fractures. Osteoporosis afflicts 10 million Americans (80% women) and causing 1.5 million bone fractures each year. Primary osteoporosis has two types: Type I occurs in women when estrogen levels fall after menopause; and Type II is the inevitable loss of bone mass experienced by men and women as they age. Secondary osteoporosis may develop at any age as a consequence of hormonal, digestive, and metabolic disorders and diseases, and also includes loss of bone mineral mass during prolonged bed rest and weightlessness (as in space flight).

During puberty, rapid increases in bone growth and density occur, with peak bone density reached between the ages of 20 and 30 years. About 98% of the adult bone mineral content is deposited by age 20, but this process is affected by both genetic and lifestyle factors. The period between ages 9 and 20 is critical in building up an optimal bone density as a safeguard against losses later in life. Thus the best strategy for preventing osteoporosis is to build strong bones early in life. Many risk factors predict osteoporosis, and people with several of them need to do all they can to reverse the progression. Here is the list of risk factors and prevention steps.*

- Personal history of fracture after age 45
- Current low bone mass
- History of fracture in a first degree relative
- Being female
- Being thin and/or having a small frame
- Advanced age
- A family history of osteoporosis
- Estrogen deficiency as a result of menopause, especially early or surgically induced
- Abnormal absence of menstrual periods (amenorrhea)
- Anorexia nervosa
- Low lifetime calcium intake
- Vitamin D deficiency
- Use of certain medications, such as corticosteroids and anticonvulsants
- Presence of certain chronic medical conditions
- Low testosterone levels in men
- An inactive lifestyle
- Current cigarette smoking
- Excessive use of alcohol
- Being Caucasian or Asian

Prevention

By about age 20, the average woman has acquired 98 percent of her skeletal mass. Building strong bones during childhood and adolescence can be the best defense against developing osteoporosis later. There are four steps, which together can optimize bone health and help prevent osteoporosis. They are:

Step 1: A balanced diet rich in calcium and vitamin D
Step 2: Weight-bearing exercise
Step 3: A healthy lifestyle with no smoking or excessive alcohol intake
Step 4: Bone density testing and medication when appropriate.

*See Health and Fitness Acitivity 6.4

TABLE 6.1 Health and Fitness Benefits of Aerobic Compared to Muscular Fitness

Variable	Aerobic Exercise	Resistance Exercise
Resting blood pressure	↓↓↓	↓
Serum HDL-cholesterol	↑↑	↑
Insulin sensitivity	↑↑	↑↑
Body fat percent	↓↓↓	↓
Bone mineral density	↑	↑↑↑
Strength	↑	↑↑↑
Physical function in old age	↑↑	↑↑↑
VO_{2max}	↑↑↑	↑

One arrow = little benefit; two arrows = moderate benefit; three arrows = strong benefit.

- improved body fitness, posture, symmetry, and self-image
- reduced risk of low-back pain and other spinal aches and pains
- prevention of injury
- rehabilitation/treatment of pain and injury

There is little doubt that flexibility is important for performance by elite athletes in such sports as Olympic weight lifting, ballet dancing, gymnastics, swimming, track and field, and wrestling. Athletes in these sports usually possess an excellent range-of-motion in the applied joints.

Tight lower back and hamstring muscles combined with weak abdominal and trunk muscles allow the pelvis to tilt forward (a condition called **lordosis**), increasing the risk of lower back pain. See Health and Fitness Activity 6.1 to learn how to evaluate your posture.

Is your flexibility important for injury prevention? When questioned, the majority of sports medicine specialists support the use of flexibility training in injury prevention, but also readily admit that there is little scientific support for this practice. Part of the problem is that this is a difficult area to research. For example, U.S. Army studies suggest that both unusually high and low flexibility are associated with increased risk of injury. Most sports medicine specialists still recommend stretching to prevent injuries, because their clinical experience has shown this practice to be beneficial. Flexibility exercises are also advocated in the treatment of many types of injuries to regain range-of-motion and reduce pain symptoms.

Muscular Fitness and Low Back Pain

Low back pain is a common ailment—at some point in their lives, 60 to 80 percent of all Americans will experience a bout of low back pain ranging from a dull, annoying ache to intense and prolonged pain. After headaches, low back pain is the second most common ailment in the United States, and is topped only by colds and flus in time lost from work.

Males and females appear to be affected equally, with most cases of low back pain occurring between the ages of 25 and 60 years, with a peak at about 40 years of age. The first attack often occurs early in life—up to one third of adolescents report they have experienced at least one bout of low back pain.

Fortunately, most low back pain is self-limiting. Without treatment, 60 percent of back pain sufferers go back to work within a week, and nearly 90 percent return within six weeks. Pain remains for a long time in 5 to 10 percent of patients.

The spine is composed of 24 vertebrae, 23 discs, 31 pairs of spinal nerves, and 140 attaching muscles, plus a large number of ligaments and tendons (see Appendix B). Though humans are born with 33 separate vertebrae (the bones that form the spine), by adulthood most have only 24. The nine vertebrae at the base of the spine grow together. The five lumbar vertebrae are most frequently involved in back pain because they carry most of the body's stress.

Risk Factors for Low Back Pain

There are many risk factors for low back pain. (See Health and Fitness Activity 5.2 for a self-quiz to estimate your risk of low back pain.) Most low back pain is due to unusual stresses on the muscles and ligaments that support the spine of people with weak muscles. When the body is in poor shape, weak spinal and abdominal muscles may be unable to support the spine properly during certain types of lifting or physical activities.

But even hardy workers (e.g., firefighters and truck drivers) or athletes who push beyond their limits are susceptible. Rowers, triathletes, professional golfers, tennis players, wrestlers, and gymnasts, for example, have all been reported to have high back injury rates. Any extreme lifting, bending, and twisting can cause low back pain in even the strongest workers and athletes.

Major risk factors for low back pain include:

- heavy lifting with bending and twisting motions, pushing and pulling, slipping, tripping or falling
- long periods of sitting or driving, especially with vibrations
- obesity
- smoking
- poor posture
- mental stress and anxiety
- muscular weakness
- poor joint flexibility

Prevention of Low Back Pain

Prevention of low back pain is based on these recommendations:

- Exercise regularly to strengthen your back and abdominal muscles.
- Lose weight, if necessary, to lessen strain on your back.
- Avoid smoking (which increases degenerative changes in the spine).
- Lift by bending at your knees, rather than the waist, using leg muscles to do most of the work.
- Receive objects from others or platforms near to your body, and avoid twisting or bending at the waist while handling or transferring it.
- Avoid sitting, standing, or working in any one position for too long.
- Maintain a correct posture (sit with your shoulders back and feet flat on the floor, or on a footstool or chair rung. Stand with head and chest high, neck straight, stomach and buttocks held in, and pelvis forward). (See Health and Fitness Activity 6.1).
- Use a comfortable, supportive seat while driving.
- Use a firm mattress, and sleep on your side with knees drawn up or on your back with a pillow under bent knees.
- Try to reduce emotional stress that causes muscle tension.
- Be thoroughly warmed up before engaging in vigorous exercise or sports.
- Undergo a gradual progression when attempting to improve strength or athletic ability.

Treatment of Low Back Pain

Treatment of low back pain has proven to be complex and frustrating. The optimal management of low back pain is still under debate. Many nonsurgical treatments are available for patients with low back pain, but few have been proven effective or clearly superior to others. Physical therapy with exercise is recommended by physicians more than any other nonsurgical treatment for low back pain. Figure 6.1 summarizes exercises used for the treatment and prevention of low back pain.

FIGURE 6.1

Exercise for Treatment and Prevention of Lower Back Pain

Many clinicians agree that one of the best techniques for relieving or preventing back pain is regular conditioning exercise for the muscles that support the back. Four important calisthenics include the following:

A. Hamstring stretch: Lie on your back with one leg straight in front of you and the other bent so that your thigh is resting on your chest. Hold onto the ankle of your bent leg and slowly try to straighten your leg. Keep the lower back on the floor as you straighten your leg. Hold for 10 to 30 seconds, making sure that the stretch does not feel painful. Switch to the other leg, and do the some. Repeat 5 times.

B. Bent-knee sit-ups: Lie on your back as shown, with knees bent and feet and lower back on the floor. Place your arms across your chest with the fingertips of each hand touching the shoulders. Slowly raise your head and shoulders slightly off the ground, using your stomach muscles. Hold for 10 to 15 seconds, then relax. Repeat the sequence 5 to 10 times, increasing the number of repetitions as your fitness level improves.

C. Pelvic tilt: Lie as shown with knees bent and feet flat on the floor. Slowly tighten your stomach and buttocks muscles as you press your lower back onto the floor. Hold for 10 seconds and then relax. Repeat 5 to 10 times.

D. Leg lift: Lie on the floor with one leg straight in front of you and the other bent as shown. Slowly raise your straightened leg as far up as you can. Hold for 10 seconds. Then, slowly lower your leg to the floor. Repeat 5 times. Relax. Switch leg positions and repeat the same sequence with the other leg.

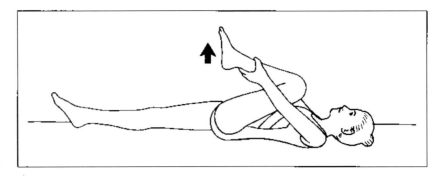

A. Hamstring Stretch

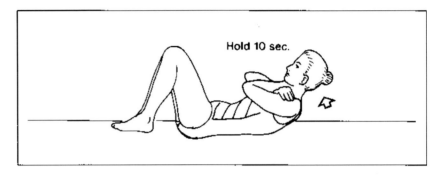

Hold 10 sec.

B. Bent-Knee Sit-Ups

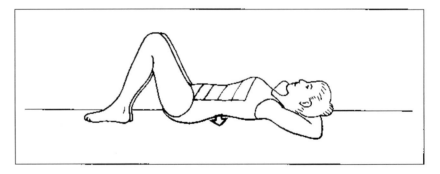

C. Pelvic Tilt

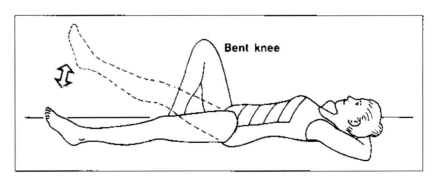

Bent knee

D. Leg Lift

Recommendations to treat low back pain include the following:

- Engage in low-stress activities such as walking, biking or swimming during the first two weeks after symptoms begin, even if the activities make the symptoms a little worse. The most important goal is to return to your normal activities as soon as it is safe.
- Bed rest usually isn't necessary and shouldn't last longer than two to four days. More than four days of rest can weaken muscles and delay recovery.
- Nonprescription pain relievers such as aspirin and ibuprofen work as well as prescription painkillers and muscle relaxants, and cause fewer side effects.
- Among treatments not recommended, due to lack of evidence that they work, are traction, acupuncture, massage, ultrasound, and transcutaneous electrical nerve stimulation.
- Spinal manipulation by a chiropractor or other therapist can be helpful when symptoms begin, but patients should be re-evaluated if they haven't improved after four weeks of treatment.

Tests for Muscular Fitness

How can you measure your muscular fitness? Many tests have been developed to measure muscular strength, muscular endurance, and flexbility. Some of these use very sophisticated equipment, but good results can be obtained by using common tests such as sit-ups or curl-ups, pull-ups, push-ups, grip strength, bench press, vertical jump, and the sit-and-reach flexibility test. Table 6.2 summarizes norms for muscular endurance, muscular strength, and flexibility tests for college students.

One Minute Bent-Knee Sit-Ups

Strong abdominal muscles improve posture and appearance, enhance sports performance, and aid in the prevention and treatment of low-back pain. Sit-ups are an excellent test for abdominal muscle fitness.

To perform the one minute bent-knee sit-up with your arms crossed over the chest, follow these instructions (figure 6.2):

- Start on your back, with knees flexed, feet on the floor, and the heels 12 to 18 inches from the buttocks.
- Your arms should be folded and crossed on your chest, with your hands on the opposite shoulders.
- Your feet should be held firmly on the ground by a partner.
- During the sit-up, arm contact with your chest must be maintained. Your buttocks must remain on the mat at all times.

FIGURE 6.2
The one-minute timed bent-knee sit-up test.

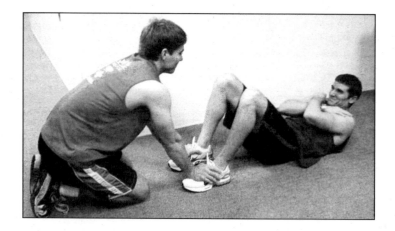

- In the up position, your elbows and forearms must touch the thighs (without your arms pulling away from your chest).
- In the down position, your midback makes contact with the floor.
- Your score equals the number of correctly executed sit-ups performed in one minute.

See Table 6.2 for your classification according to norms. Notice that an "excellent" rating is given for males performing more than 47 sit-ups in one minute, and 41 for females.

Partial Curl-ups

Partial curl-ups (also called "abdominal crunches" or "half-sit-ups") place less strain on your lower back than traditional sit-ups, and focus more directly on the abdominal muscle group. In other words, when testing or exercising the abdominal muscles, partial curl-ups are safer and more effective.

The partial curl-up test is conducted as follows (figure 6.3):

- Apply masking tape and string across a gym mat in two parallel lines 10 cm apart.
- Start by lying down on your back, with your head resting on the mat, arms straight and fully extended at your sides and parallel to your trunk, palms of your hands in contact with the mat, and the middle finger tip of both hands at the 0 mark line. Your knees should be bent at a 90 percent angle. Your heels must stay in contact with the mat, and the test is performed with your shoes on.

TABLE 6.2   Norms for Muscular Endurance, Muscular Strength, and Flexibility Tests: College Students*

Fitness Test	Gender	Poor	Below Average	Average	Above Average	Excellent
I-min sit-ups	Male	less than 33	33–37	38–41	42–47	Above 47
	Female	less than 27	27–31	32–35	36–41	Above 41
Partial curl-ups	Male	less than 16	16–20	21–22	23–24	25
	Female	less than 16	16–20	21–22	23–24	25
Pull-ups	Male	less than 5	5–7	8–11	12–14	Above 14
	Female	less than 0	less than 0	less than 0	1	Above 1
Parallel bar dips	Male	less than 4	4–8	9–13	14–20	Above 20
Push-ups	Male	less than 18	18–22	23–28	29–38	Above 38
	Female	less than 17	12–17	18–24	24–32	Above 32
Grip (R&L) strength (kg)	Male	less than 84	84–94	95–102	103–112	Above 112
	Female	less than 54	54–58	59–63	64–70	Above 70
I-RM bench press (weight ratio)	Male	less than 0.77	0.77–0.89	0.90–1.06	1.07–1.19	Above 1.19
	Female	less than 0.42	0.42–0.53	0.54–0.58	0.59–0.65	Above 0.65
Vertical jump (kgm/second)	Male	less than 61	61–72	73–87	88–103	Above 103
	Female	less than 51	51–57	58–66	67–73	Above 73
Sit & Reach Test (inches, footline at 0)	Male & Female	less than 3	-3 to -0.25	0 to 3.75	4 to 6.75	7 and greater
Shoulder Flexibility Test (inches, average of left and right sides)	Male & Female	Under -1	-1 to -0.25	0 to 1.75	2 to 4.75	5 and greater
Trunk Rotation Test (inches, average of left and right sides)	Male & Female	less than 13	13 to 15.75	16 to 18.75	19 to 21.75	22 and greater

* See text for an explanation of test procedures.

FIGURE 6.3
The one-minute partial curl-up test.

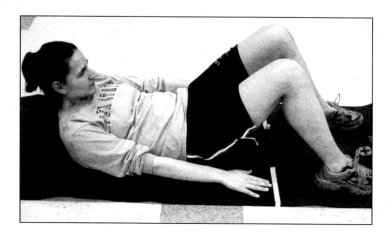

- Set a metronome to a cadence of 50 beats per minute. Perform as many consecutive curl-ups as possible, without pausing, at a rate of 25 per minute. The test is terminated after one minute.
- During each curl-up, the upper spine should be curled up so that the middle finger tips of both hands reach the 10 cm mark. During the curl-up your palms and heels must remain in contact with the mat. Anchoring of your feet is not permitted. On the return, your shoulder blades and head must contact the mat, and the finger tips of both hands must touch the 0 mark. The movement is performed in a slow, controlled manner at a rate of 25 per minute.
- The test is terminated before one minute if you experience undue discomfort, are unable to maintain the required cadence, or are unable to maintain the proper curl-up technique (e.g., heels come off the floor) over two consecutive repetitions.

Norms for the partial curl-up test are in Table 6.2.

Pull-ups

Pull-ups are an excellent test for measuring the muscular strength and endurance of your arms and shoulders. The traditional pull-up test uses the following procedures:

- Start in a hanging position, with your arms straight, and hands in an *overhand* position (palms away) as depicted in Figure 6.4.
- Pull your body upward until your chin is over the bar.
- After each pull-up, return to a fully extended hanging position. Your knees should stay straight during the entire test.
- Swinging and snap-up movements are not allowed during the test.
- A partner can hold an extended arm to help prevent swinging during the test.

The score is the total number of pull-ups until you are exhausted. Norms are listed in Table 6.2. Notice that a classification of "excellent" is given when college males perform more than 14 pull-ups, and females more than 1.

Parallel Bar Dips

The parallel bar dip test measures the muscular strength and endurance of the arms and shoulders of college males. Norms have not been developed for college females. To perform the test, follow these steps (figure 6.5):

- Assume a straight arm support position between parallel bars, with your legs straight.
- Lower your body until your elbows form a right angle, with your upper arm parallel to the floor. A partner can indicate when the proper position is reached.

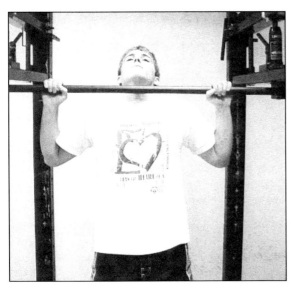

FIGURE 6.4
The pull-up test.

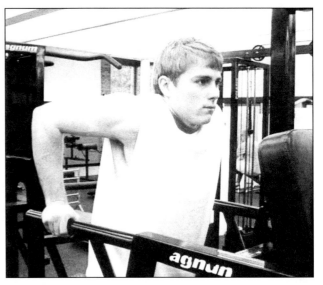

FIGURE 6.5
The parallel bar dip test.

- Push back up to a straight-arm support and continue for as many repetitions as possible.
- Rest is permitted in the up position. No swinging or kicking is allowed during the test.
- The score is the total number of bar dips until you are exhausted. An "excellent" classification is 21 or more bar dips.

Push-ups

Push-ups are a common test used to assess upper-body muscle strength and endurance. To perform the push-up test, follow these steps (figure 6.6):

- Assume the standard position for a push-up, with your body rigid and straight, toes tucked under, and your hands approximately shoulder-width apart and straight under your shoulders. Females can perform the test from the bent-knee position as depicted in Figure 6.6. Table 6.2 provides norms for the regular push-up for males, and the bent-knee push-up for females. In the Air Force, females are expected to perform the regular push-up with legs straight.
- A partner should place a fist on the floor beneath your upper chest. Lower down until your chest touches the fist, and then push up to the starting position.
- Your back must stay rigid and straight throughout the entire push-up test. Rest is allowed only in the up position.
- The score is the total number of push-ups until you are exhausted. There is no time limit. (See norms in Table 6.2). An "excellent" classification is more than 38 and 32 push-ups for males and females, respectively.

Grip Strength

The purpose of the grip strength test is to measure the strength of the grip squeezing muscles in your forearm and hand. Both the right and left hands should be measured separately, with the scores added prior to comparison with the norms listed in Table 6.2. A hand-grip dynamometer (as shown in figure 6.8) is required, and should be supplied by your instructor (most Physical Education departments have them).

To perform the grip strength test, follow these steps:

- First dry and chalk both of your hands (to ensure a good grip).
- Adjust the hand dynamometer to fit your hand.

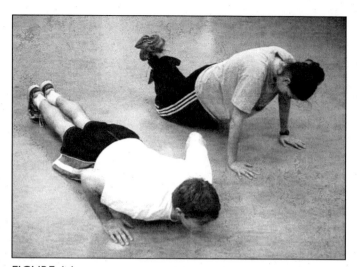

FIGURE 6.6
The push-up test for males and females.

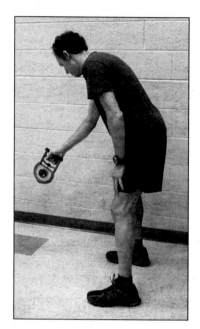

FIGURE 6.7
The hand-grip strength test.

- Assume a slightly bent forward position, with the hand to be tested out in front of your body, arm slightly bent (as depicted in Figure 6.7). Your arm and hand should not touch your body.
- The test involves an all-out gripping effort for 2–3 seconds, first with your right hand and then your left. Allow 2–4 trials for each hand. No swinging or pumping of your arm is allowed.
- The score is the sum of the separate tests of both hands, based on the best of 2–4 trials. The scale is read in kilograms. (See the norms in Table 6.2). An "excellent classification is above 112 kg for males, and above 70 kg for females.

One-Repetition Maximum Bench Press Test

The muscular strength of the chest and arms can be measured with the one-repetition maximum (1-RM) bench press test (the greatest weight that can be bench pressed once). The use of machine weights allows for safer and easier testing sessions. The norms for this test were developed using the Universal Gym machine (see figure 6.8), and results will be less accurate if other types of machines or free weights are used.

To perform the 1-RM bench press test, follow these steps:

- First, become familiar with the bench-press manuever by practicing several lifts using light weights.
- Begin the test by lying on your back on the bench, with arms extended and hands gripping the bar about shoulder-width apart.
- Lower the bar until it is approximately chest level, and then push it straight up with maximum effort until your arms are locked once again. Breathe in as the bar is lowered, and breathe out when the bar is raised. (This helps avoid undue buildup of pressure in the chest).
- Try the 1-RM bench press test several times until a true maximum effort is achieved. Allow 2 to 3 minutes between trials.
- The best lifting score is divided by your body weight to derive the weight ratio. For example, if a 160-pound male can bench press 145 pounds, the weight ratio equals 145/160 or 0.91. (Norms are listed in Table 6.2). An "excellent" rating is a weight ratio above 1.19 for males, and above 0.65 for females.

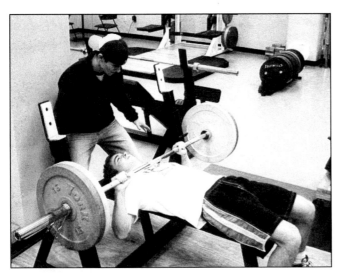

FIGURE 6.8
The 1-RM bench press test.

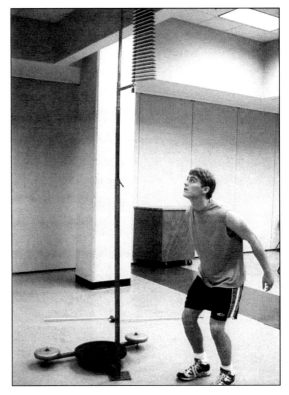

FIGURE 6.9
The vertical jump test.

Vertical Jump

The vertical jump is a simple yet effective test for measuring your muscular power, and has been used as an index of sports ability. Typically, athletes from sports such as basketball, volleyball, and football are able to jump higher than athletes from endurance sports such as running, cycling, and swimming.

To perform the vertical jump test, follow these steps:

- Stand facing sideways to a wall on which a measuring tape has been attached. Special equipment can be used for measuring vertical jump as shown in Figure 6.9.
- Standing erect with your feet flat on the floor, reach as high as possible on the tape with your arm and fingers fully extended and your palm toward the wall. This is recorded as the beginning height.
- Standing about a foot away from the wall, bring your arms downward and backward while bending your knees to a balanced semi-squat position, and then jump as high as possible with your arms moving forward and upward.
- The tape should be touched at the peak height of the jump with the fingers of the arm facing the wall. Record the highest jump from three trials, with a rest period of 10 to 15 seconds between trials. Subtract the beginning height from the peak height to determine the height jumped in centimeters, and then convert to meters.
- Calculate leg power using this equation:
  Leg power (kg-m/second) = 2.21 × weight kg × $\sqrt{\text{vertical jump meters}}$
  For example, if a 22-year-old female weighing 60 kg vertical jumps 0.35 meters, then her leg power would be calculated as follows:
  Leg power = 2.21 × 60 × $\sqrt{0.35}$ = 78.4 kg-m/second.

Leg power can be classified using the age and gender group standards presented in Table 6.2. For example, this 22-year-old female with a leg power of 78.4 kg-m/second would be given an "excellent rating."

Go to Health and Fitness Activity 6.3, and with the help of your instructor take all of the tests described in this chapter, and record your results and classifications.

How to Measure Flexibility

As emphasized earlier, good flexibility in one joint does not necessarily carry over to other joints. At least three different flexibility tests are recommended, because there is no general flexibility test for the whole body.

Sit-and-Reach Flexibility Test

Hip joint and hamstring flexibility is important for sports performance and may decrease risk of low back pain (although this is by no means well documented). One of the standard tests for hamstring and lower back flexibility is the sit-and-reach test.

To perform this test, a flexibility box is needed. It is 12 inches high, and has an overlap in front, so that minus readings can be obtained when the person being tested is unable to reach the footline. A ruler can be set on the box, with the footline set at zero, and plus or minus readings marked in centimeters or inches (see Figure 6.10).

To perform the sit-and-reach flexibility test, follow these procedures:

- First, warm up with aerobic exercise (for example, five minutes on a stationary cycle) and 3 to 4 minutes of static stretching. Warm muscles can stretch more safely and effectively.
- Remove your shoes, and sit facing the flexibility box with your knees fully extended, feet four inches apart. Your feet should be flat, heels touching, against the end board.
- To perform the test, extend your arms straight forward, with your hands on top of each other, fingertips perfectly even. Reach forward as far as possible (without bouncing), and hold the position of maximum reach for 1 to 2 seconds. A partner should determine the distance in front of or beyond the footline. Record the best score following four separate trials. Norms for classification are listed in Table 6.2. It is considered "good" to reach four or more inches beyond the footline, with seven or more inches rated as "excellent."

Shoulder Flexibility Test

The shoulder joints are used in many different sports movements, work activities, and activities of daily living. To perform the shoulder flexibility test, follow these procedures after warming up (figure 6.11):

- Raise one arm, bend the elbow, and reach down across your back as far as possible, as shown in figure 6.11.

FIGURE 6.10
The sit-and-reach flexibility test.

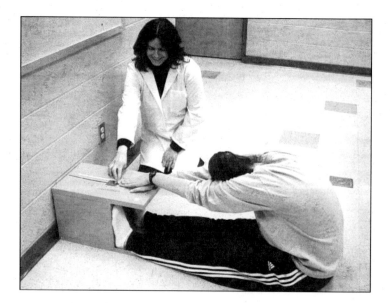

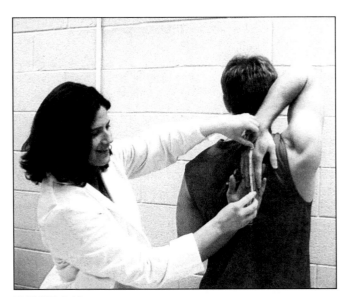

FIGURE 6.11
The shoulder flexibility test.

FIGURE 6.12
The trunk rotation flexibility test.

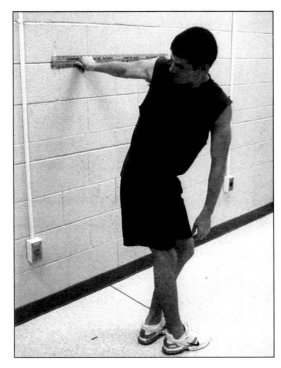

- At the same time, extend the other arm down and then up behind your back, trying to cross the fingers over those of the other hand.
- Measure the distance of finger overlap to the nearest one-quarter inch. If the fingers overlap, score as a plus; if they fail to meet, score as a minus.
- Repeat with your arms crossed in the opposite direction. Average the two scores, and use Table 6.2 for classification.

Trunk Rotation Flexibility Test

The trunk rotation flexibility test measures flexibility across several joints of the body. To perform this flexibility test, follow these procedures after warming up (figure 6.12):

- Tape two yardsticks to the wall at shoulder height, one right side up, and the other upside down. Draw a line on the floor perpendicular to the wall at the 15-inch marks on the rulers.
- Stand with your feet shoulder-width apart, toes on the line, left shoulder to the wall at arm's length (fist closed).
- With the left arm at your side, raise your right arm to shoulder height and rotate the trunk to the right as far as possible, reaching along the yardstick with fist closed and palm down. Reach as far as possible, and then hold the final position for two seconds. During the test, your knees should be slightly bent, with your feet always pointing straight ahead and on the toe line.
- A partner should record the distance reached by the knuckle of the little finger to the nearest one-quarter inch. Perform the test twice, and average the two scores.
- Next, perform the test facing the opposite direction, using the upside down yardstick (the greater the rotation, the higher the score). Perform two trials, and average. Then average the scores from both directions and use Table 6.2 to classify the results.

Summary

1. Muscular strength is the maximum one-effort force that one can generate against a resistance, while muscular endurance is the ability of the muscles to repeat a submaximal effort over and over. Flexibility is defined as the capacity of the joints to move through a full range of movement.

2. A basic strength program is performing two sets of 8 to 12 repetitions of 8 to 10 exercises two to three times per week for persons under 50 years of age and the same regimen using 10 to 15 repetitions for persons over 50 years of age. To develop flexibility, static stretching exercises should be repeated 2 to 4 times for each major muscle group and joint of the body, with a minimum of 2 to 3 sessions per week.

3. Development of muscular fitness has several important health-related benefits, including increased bone density (lowering risk of osteoporosis or brittle bones in old age), muscle size, and connective tissue strength, improved self-esteem, lowered risk of low back pain, and decreased frailty in old age.

4. Flexibility has several benefits, including enhanced performance; relaxation of mental stress and tension; improved body fitness, posture, symmetry, and self-image; and prevention and treatment of injury.

5. There is little evidence to suggest that weight lifting reduces the risk for heart disease, cancer, diabetes, high blood pressure, or high blood cholesterol.

6. Many tests have been developed to measure muscular strength and endurance. Some of these use very sophisticated equipment, but good results can be obtained by using common tests such as sit-ups, curl-ups, pull-ups, push-ups, grip strength, bench press, and vertical jump. Procedures for these tests were reviewed in this chapter.

7. Flexibility can be measured in three simple ways: the sit-and-reach, shoulder, and trunk rotation flexibility tests.

8. At some point in their lives, 60 to 80 percent of all Americans and Europeans will experience a bout of low back pain, ranging from a dull, annoying ache to intense and prolonged pain.

9. There are many risk factors for low back pain. Most low back pain is due to unusual stresses on the muscles and ligaments that support the spine of people with weak muscles. When the body is in poor shape, weak spinal and abdominal muscles may be unable to support the spine properly during certain types of lifting or physical activities.

10. Prevention of low back pain is based on recommendations for improving muscular fitness, weight loss, avoidance of smoking, proper lifting techniques, maintenance of proper posture, stress management, and comfortable seats and beds.

11. Recommendations to treat low back pain are still being debated, but the most important goal is to return to normal activities as soon as it is safe. Bed rest usually isn't necessary, and shouldn't last longer than two to four days.

12. Osteoporosis is characterized by reduced bone mass and increased susceptibility to fractures. The mainstays of treatment include estrogen replacement, adequate life-long calcium intake, and appropriate exercise.

HEALTH AND FITNESS ACTIVITY 6.1
Rating Your Posture

Good posture depends on good muscle tone and balance throughout your body, and flexible but sturdy joints. There are a number of poor postural habits and practices in standing, sitting, walking, and working which, if indulged over the years, will cause strain and changes in your postural muscles. Some muscles will lose their tone, while others become shortened and tight resulting in malalignment of the body segments. Habits and practices causing poor posture include sitting and standing with the back curved or slumped, sleeping with a sagging mattress, insufficient sleep and chronic fatigue, general muscle weakness and tightness due to lack of strengthening and stretching exercise, excess body weight, wearing poorly designed shoes, and a poor mental attitude (e.g., lack of self-confidence). See Figure 6.13 for an example of good standing posture.

Use Figure 6.14 to grade your posture. Follow these steps:

- Dress in a swim suit, with long hair pinned up or away from the ears.
- Breathe deeply and exhale several times to feel relaxed before having your posture checked.
- Stand in front of a mirror. Do not stand too rigidly or too relaxed. With the help of a friend, score your posture using Figure 6.15. Use these norms for classification:

Posture Norms	
Perfect posture	80 points
Good posture	65–79
Fair posture	35–64*
Poor posture	less than 35*

* Strengthen back and abdominal muscles, and work on hip and neck flexibility

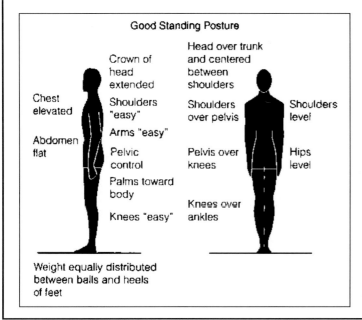

Good Standing Posture

Crown of head extended

Head over trunk and centered between shoulders

Chest elevated

Shoulders "easy"

Shoulders over pelvis

Shoulders level

Arms "easy"

Abdomen flat

Pelvic control

Pelvis over knees

Hips level

Palms toward body

Knees "easy"

Knees over ankles

Weight equally distributed between balls and heels of feet

FIGURE 6.13

Good posture is the correct alignment and balance of the various body segments: the head balanced over the shoulders and trunk, the trunk balanced over the thighs, the thighs balanced over the knees, which are balanced over the feet.

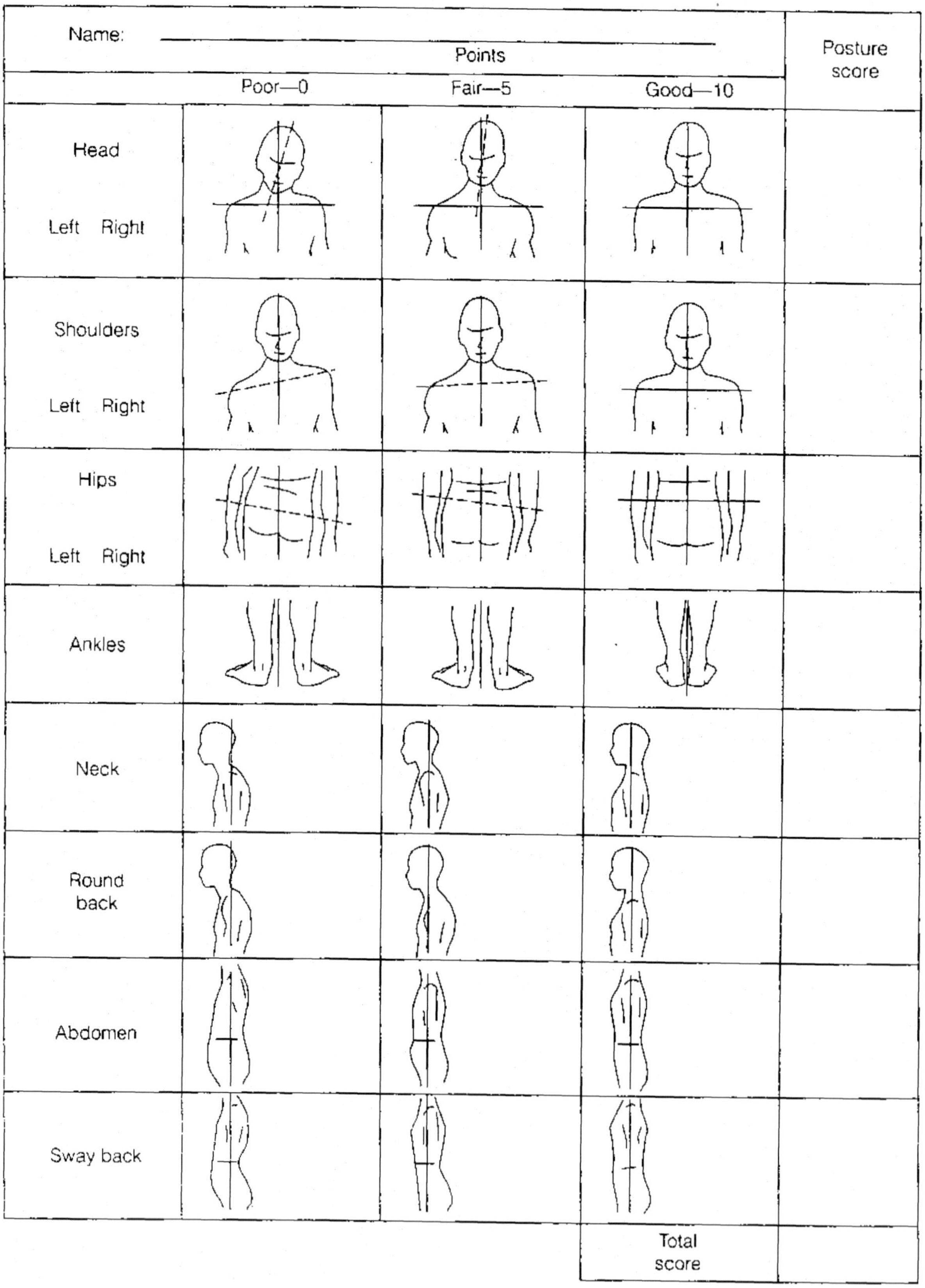

Name:		Points		Posture score
	Poor—0	Fair—5	Good—10	
Head Left Right				
Shoulders Left Right				
Hips Left Right				
Ankles				
Neck				
Round back				
Abdomen				
Sway back				
			Total score	

FIGURE 6.14
Rate your posture using this score sheet.

HEALTH AND FITNESS ACTIVITY 6.2
Risk of Low Back Pain

Score your risk of low back pain by answering the question listed below. Check "yes" if you engage in the behavior on a regular basis.

YES   NO

❑   ❑   1.   Your trunk muscles (back and abdomen) are weak from lack of weight training, heavy manual labor, or intense sports.

❑   ❑   2.   You are overweight (body mass index of 25 and higher), and your stomach sticks out.

❑   ❑   3.   You have poor joint flexibility, especially in the hip and back areas.

❑   ❑   4.   You engage in heavy lifting with bending and twisting motions.

❑   ❑   5.   When lifting, you bend over and lift with straight legs (versus squatting and lifting with your leg muscles).

❑   ❑   6.   You have long periods of sitting or driving, especially with vibrations, or you sit and stand in one position for long periods of time without breaks.

❑   ❑   7.   You smoke heavily (25 cigarettes a day or more).

❑   ❑   8.   Your sleeping mattress is too soft.

❑   ❑   9.   You have poor posture.

❑   ❑   10.   You have high levels of mental stress and anxiety.

Count up your "yes" answers and apply to these norms:

0   Excellent! (risk of low back pain is very low)
1–2   Average risk of low back pain
3–4   Above average risk of low back pain
5–10   High risk of low back pain

HEALTH AND FITNESS ACTIVITY 6.3
Assessment of Muscular Fitness

With the help of your class instructor, take each of the tests of muscular fitness listed below. After taking each test, record your score, and then use the norms in Table 6.2 to classify your results.

Fitness Test	Your Score	Classification
1-min sit-ups		
Partial curl-ups		
Pull-ups		
Parallel bar dips		
Push-ups		
Grip (right and left hands) strength (kg)		
1-RM bench press (weight ratio)		
Vertical jump (kgm/second)		
Sit-&-Reach Test (inches, footline at 0)		
Shoulder Flexibility Test (inches, average of left and right sides)		
Trunk Rotation Test (inches, average of left and right sides)		

Name _____ Date _____

Osteoporosis—Are You at Risk for Weak Bones?

Learn more about this bone-thinning disease that causes debilitating fractures of the hip, spine, and wrist. Complete the following questionnaire to determine your risk for developing osteoporosis.

Check any of these that apply to you.

- ❑ I'm older than 65.
- ❑ I've broken a bone after age 50.
- ❑ My close relative has osteoporosis or has broken a bone.
- ❑ My health is "fair" or "poor."
- ❑ I smoke.
- ❑ I am underweight for my height.
- ❑ I started menopause before age 45.
- ❑ I've never gotten enough calcium.
- ❑ I have more than two drinks of alcohol several times a week.
- ❑ I have poor vision, even with glasses.
- ❑ I sometimes fall.
- ❑ I'm not active.

- ❑ I have one of these medical conditions:

    Hyperthyroidism
    Chronic lung disease
    Cancer
    Inflammatory bowel disease
    Chronic hepatic or renal disease
    Hyperparathyroidism
    Vitamin D deficiency
    Cushing's disease
    Multiple sclerosis
    Rheumatoid arthritis

- ❑ I take one of these medicines:

    Oral glucocorticoids (steroids)
    Cancer treatments (radiation, chemotherapy)
    Thyroid medicine
    Antiepileptic medications
    Gonadal hormone suppression
    Immunosuppressive agents

If you have any of these "red flags," you could be at high risk tor weak bones. Talk to your doctor, nurse, pharmacist, or other health-care professional.

Source: U.S. Department of Health and Human Services. *Bone Health and Osteoporosis: A Report of the Surgeon General.* Rockville, MD: U.S. Department of Health and Human Services, Office of the Surgeon General, 2004.

CHAPTER 6 QUIZ
Assessment of Musculoskeletal Fitness

Note: Answers are given at the end of the quiz.

1. Clinical evience points towards lack of flexibility in the lower back hamstring area, combined with relatively weak _____ muscles, as the causes of a majority of low back pain cases.
   A. neck
   B. chest
   C. thigh
   D. abdominal
   E. upper back

2. _____ is the maximal one-effect force that can be exerted against a resistance.
   A. Muscular strength
   B. Muscular endurance
   C. Flexibility

3. For question #2, what test would be the best measure?
   A. one-minute timed, bent-knee sit-ups
   B. pull-ups
   C. 1-RM bench press
   D. sit-and-reach

4. Which one of the following tests is the best test for flexibility?
   A. one-minute timed, bent-knee sit-ups
   B. pull-ups
   C. 1-RM bench press
   D. sit-and- reach

5. T   F   The majority of Americans will experience at least one episode of acute back pain within their lifetime.

6. Which one of the following is *not* considered to be a risk factor associated with increased risk of osteoporosis?

   A. Age

   B. Bedrest

   C. Obesity

   D. Use of steroids

   E. Removal of ovaries

   F. Low dietary calcium intake

   G. Cigarette smoking

PART THREE

Conditioning for Physical Fitness

chapter seven

An Exercise Program for Total Fitness

For substantial health benefits, adults should do at least 150 minutes (2 hours and 30 minutes) a week of moderate-intensity, or 75 minutes (1 hour and 15 minutes) a week of vigorous-intensity aerobic physical activity, or an equivalent combination of moderate- and vigorous-intensity aerobic activity.

—U.S. Department of Health and Human Services,
2008 Physical Activity Guidelines for Americans

Exercise Program Basics

What is the best type of exercise program to build your physical fitness? During the first half of the 20th century, exercise programs to build muscular strength and size were extremely popular, led by stalwart promoters such as Charles Atlas and Jack LaLanne. During the 1970s and 1980s, the pendulum swung the other way to something totally new—aerobic fitness. During this era, muscular fitness took a back seat.

The modern-day aerobic fitness movement is more than 40 years old. It started in 1968, when Kenneth Cooper, at that time a physician for the Air Force, published his book *Aerobics*. In this book, Cooper challenged Americans to take personal charge of their lifestyles and counter the epidemics of heart disease, obesity, and rising healthcare costs through regular exercise. Millions took up the "aerobic challenge" and began running, cycling, walking, and swimming their way to better health. Muscular fitness became a forgotten concept.

The more recent focus has been a comprehensive approach to physical fitness in which three major components—aerobic fitness, muscular fitness, and body composition—are given balanced attention. In other words, to have total fitness, pay attention to all of the muscles of your body, both inside (heart) and out (skeletal), and keep lean by balancing calories burned with those eaten.

Developing Physical Fitness

How can your physical fitness be developed? Early on, emphasis was placed on a rigid and formal exercise program that demanded equipment, know-how, time, and lots of motivation. Few Americans were willing to stick to such a program over the long term, and fitness experts were left scratching their heads wondering what to do next. (Review Chapter 1). In surveys, adults cited several reasons why they did not exercise:

- not enough time
- too inconvenient
- lacked motivation
- did not find the exercise enjoyable
- found the exercise to be boring
- feared being injured
- lacked confidence in their ability to stick with an exercise program

Well, fortunately, recent research has shown that an informal, lifestyle approach to physical activity has many health benefits, and is much more attractive to most adults.

Today, you can pick one of two systems for building your fitness, or better yet, participate in both: (1) the lifestyle approach; (2) the formal exercise program. The lifestyle approach seeks to increase opportunities for physical activity throughout the daily routine, while the formal exercise program builds aerobic and muscular fitness to high levels through an exercise system based on specific frequency, intensity, and time guidelines. The *Activity Pyramid* will help you better understand how the lifestyle and formal exercise approaches to physical fitness can complement each other (see figure 7.1 and Health and Fitness Activity 7.1). The Activity Pyramid is similar to the Food Guide Pyramid (see Chapter 8), and puts all of the recommendations into a simple and easy-to-understand package.

FIGURE 7.1

The Activity Pyramid.

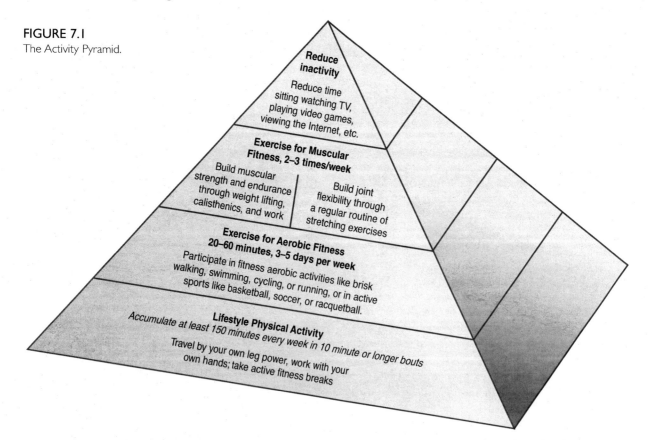

Reduce inactivity
Reduce time sitting watching TV, playing video games, viewing the Internet, etc.

Exercise for Muscular Fitness, 2–3 times/week
Build muscular strength and endurance through weight lifting, calisthenics, and work

Build joint flexibility through a regular routine of stretching exercises

Exercise for Aerobic Fitness 20–60 minutes, 3–5 days per week
Participate in fitness aerobic activities like brisk walking, swimming, cycling, or running, or in active sports like basketball, soccer, or racquetball.

Lifestyle Physical Activity
Accumulate at least 150 minutes every week in 10 minute or longer bouts
Travel by your own leg power, work with your own hands; take active fitness breaks

Notice several key features about the Activity Pyramid:

- The lifestyle approach to fitness is at the base of the Activity Pyramid, meaning that everyone should try to accumulate at least 150 minutes of physical activity every week. This is a good start, and brings basic health and fitness benefits. But higher levels of aerobic and muscular fitness can be achieved by working up the Activity Pyramid.
- The formal exercise program is summarized on levels 2 and 3 of the Activity Pyramid. Aerobic fitness is increased by brisk walking, swimming, cycling, running, or engaging in active sports for 20 to 60 minutes, 3 to 5 days per week.
- Muscular fitness means having strong and enduring muscles, and flexible joints. Muscular fitness is gained by lifting weights, doing calisthenics, engaging in hard physical labor (e.g., chopping wood), and stretching 2 to 3 times per week.
- We should all seek to reduce sitting time. We spend far too much time sitting watching TV, playing video games, viewing the Internet, driving our cars, and watching other people play sports.

The Lifestyle Approach

If you do not like setting aside 20 to 60 minutes in the midst of your busy schedule for exercise, or dressing in trendy exercise clothes and shoes, or counting your heart rate to keep within the training zone, or running in circles on a track, then the lifestyle approach is for you. Since 1993, most fitness and health organizations, including the Surgeon General's office, have urged that everyone should attempt to accumulate 30 minutes or more of moderate-intensity physical activity over the course of most if not all days of the week. Recently the *2008 Physical Activity Guidelines* adapted this to accumulating at least 150 minutes per week of moderate-intensity activity in 10 minute or longer bouts. This is the minimum amount of physical activity that improves the quality of life while decreasing the risk of most chronic diseases. Additional health and fitness benefits can be achieved by adding more time in moderate-intensity activity, or by substituting more vigorous activity.

An active lifestyle does not require a regimented, vigorous exercise program. Instead, you can make small changes to increase daily physical activity throughout the entire day. Many people have the perception that they must engage in vigorous exercise for 20 to 60 continuous minutes to reap health benefits. This is not true. What is important is moving your legs and arms at every opportunity, and accumulating activity minutes in 10 minute or longer bouts so that they total at least 30 nearly every day. Mix aerobic activities like climbing stairs or brisk walking with calisthenics or vigorous gardening to build both aerobic and muscular fitness. Develop an exercise mentality to counter the technology that can keep you sitting for hours.

The lifestyle approach to fitness has several advantages:

- Lack of time is the greatest barrier people give for not exercising regularly. By spreading physical activity throughout the day (e.g., three 10-minute walking breaks), you will find it easier to put in your 30 minutes a day rather than finding a full 30-minute segment to exercise in the midst of a busy schedule.
- To stick with your physical activity program for a lifetime, it must be convenient. The lifestyle approach to fitness is very convenient because it is easy to be physically active during the work day or leisure time. Examples include taking the stairs at every opportunity, walking during work breaks, cycling back and forth from work, working with your hands in the garden or around the home, walking the dog, or playing sports with the kids.
- Studies show that the lifestyle approach builds basic fitness, improves quality of life, and decreases the risk of chronic disease. These are improved even more by adding a formal exercise program to your routine.

The Formal Exercise Program

Although most people prefer a less technical, lifestyle approach to exercise, others enjoy the challenge of pushing themselves to build aerobic and muscular fitness to high levels. The formal exercise program is based on specific guidelines, each of which will be reviewed in detail later:

- *Aerobic fitness:* To build heart and lung fitness, and to keep lean, exercise aerobically 3 to 5 days per week (frequency), at 50 to 85 percent $\dot{V}O_{2max}$ (intensity), for 20 to 60 minutes each session (time).
- *Muscular fitness:* Perform a minimum of 8 to 10 separate exercises that train the major muscle groups. Perform 2–4 sets of 8 to 12 repetitions of each of these exercises to the point of fatigue, and do this at least 2 to 3 days per week. For flexibility, stretch at least 2 to 3 days a week and involve 2–4 repetitions of several stretches that are held 10 to 30 seconds at a position of mild discomfort.

Building Aerobic Fitness

The cornerstone of a comprehensive physical fitness program is aerobic exercise. As defined in Chapters 2 and 4, aerobic fitness is the ability to continue or persist in strenuous tasks involving large muscle groups for extended periods of time. In other words, aerobic fitness is the ability of the heart, blood vessels, blood, and lungs to supply oxygen to the working muscles during such activities as brisk walking, running, swimming, cycling, and other moderate-to-vigorous activities. Many health benefits have been related to regular, aerobic activity, and these will be reviewed in Part 4 of this book.

The aerobic or cardiorespiratory stage of a comprehensive physical fitness program consists of three segments: the warm-up, aerobic exercise (that conforms to frequency, intensity, and time guidelines), and the cool-down (Figure 7.2). See Health and Fitness Activity 7.2 to set up your own aerobic exercise program.

Warm-Up

A warm-up is the 5-to-20-minute transition period that precedes your aerobic exercise session. The primary purpose of the warm-up is to prepare your body for vigorous exercise. In general, your warm-up should entail mild-to-moderate aerobic exercise that causes an increase in your body's core temperature, heart rate, and sweat rate.

For example, if you are a runner, you should first walk briskly for about 1 to 2 minutes, then jog easily for 3 to 18 minutes (with the duration depending on air temperature and clothing). Your running speed can be slowly increased to the training level. If you are a cyclist, you should first cycle easily for 5 to 20 minutes, with the speed gradually increasing to the final training level. A swimmer could first warm-up for 5 to 10 minutes on an indoor stationary bicycle or cross-country ski simulator prior to entering the pool to swim laps. The first 5 to 10 minutes of swimming should be at an easy pace prior to reaching the training level.

As a general rule of thumb, a good warm-up consists of the same specific exercise that you will engage in during the aerobic session, but at a moderate intensity, allowing for a gradual increase in your body's temperature and heart rate. This warm-up not only warms your body, but it also directs your blood and nervous flow to the muscles that will be exercised vigorously.

Is it a good idea to stretch first before warming up? The answer is "no." Stretching exercises should always be preceded by a moderate aerobic warm-up (figure 7.3). The increase in body temperature makes stretching both safer and more productive. A good plan, especially if you like to exercise at a high intensity, is to exercise aerobically at an easy pace for 5 to 20 minutes (while dressed in cotton sweat pants and pullover). Next stretch for 5 to 10 minutes, then dress down, and finally start training at a high intensity.

An Exercise Program to Build Aerobic Fitness

Step 1 Warm-Up

Slowly elevate the pulse and body temperature to an aerobic training level by first engaging in 5 to 20 minutes of easy-to-moderate aerobic activity.

Step 2 Aerobic Exercise

A. F.I.T. Guidelines: *Based on your desire to exercise moderately or vigorously, follow the F.I.T. guidelines below.*

F.I.T. Guidelines	Moderate	Vigorous	Combination
Frequency (sessions/week)	≥5	≥3	≥3 to 5
Intensity (% HR reserve)	40–59%	≥60%	40–85%
Time (minutes/day) or (minutes/week)	30–60 ≥150	20–60 ≥75	20–60 ≥75–150

B. Intensity: *Calculate personal training heart rate using this formula:*

Training heart rate   = [(Maximum HR − resting HR) × intensity %] + resting HR

= [(_____ − _____) × _____] + _____

C. Aerobic Exercise Mode: Select 2–3 exercise modes based on personal goals.

Primary mode _____

Secondary mode _____

Backup mode _____

D. Build Exercise into Daily Schedule: *Note exercise time on specific days.*

Sun _____   Mon _____   Tues _____   Wed _____

Thurs _____   Fri _____   Sat _____

Step 3 Cool-Down

Slowly decrease the heart rate and body temperature by engaging in mild-to-moderate aerobic activity for 5–15 minutes.

FIGURE 7.2

The exercise program to build aerobic fitness consists of three steps: the warm-up, aerobic exercise, and the cool-down.

FIGURE 7.3
Flexibility exercises are best conducted when the body is warm from aerobic activity.

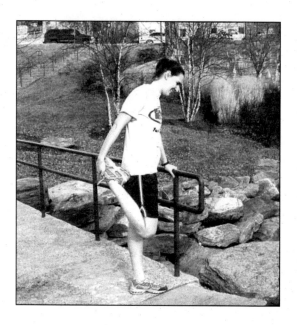

Aerobic F.I.T. Guidelines

To build your heart and lung fitness to a high level, engage in aerobic exercise 3 to 5 days per week (frequency), at 50 to 85 percent of your maximum heart rate reserve or $\dot{V}O_{2max}$ (intensity), for 20 to 60 minutes each session (time). In terms of minutes per week, aim for at least 150 minutes each week if engaging in moderate-intensity exercise, at least 75 minutes each week if engaging in vigorous-intensity exercise, or 75–150 minutes when moderate and vigorous exercise are combined. In other words, follow these F.I.T. guidelines, and you are certain to build aerobic endurance.

Frequency

Frequency of exercise refers to the number of exercise sessions per week in your exercise program. To build both aerobic fitness and keep body fat at healthy levels, you need to exercise at least 3 to 5 days each week. Aim for exercise nearly every day for optimal results.

When starting an aerobic exercise program, it is a good idea to work out every other day (in other words, allow two days between exercise sessions). This is especially important if you have largely avoided aerobic exercise most of your life. If you suddenly start exercising aerobically every day after years of inactivity, muscle soreness, fatigue, and injury are sure to follow. If you desire to build aerobic fitness to high levels, gradually increase your frequency of exercise to five or more days a week. Elite athletes take this a step further and work out twice a day on most days of the week, mixing easy and hard intensity days to avoid overtraining.

Intensity

To develop and maintain your aerobic fitness, your intensity of exercise should be between 50 percent and 85 percent of the maximum heart rate reserve. If your fitness level is low, intensity of effort can start at 40 percent, with a gradual progression toward a higher intensity (figure 7.2).

Intensity of exercise can be summarized as follows:

- **Light intensity** is 40 to 59 percent of the maximum heart rate reserve. This intensity range is reserved for those starting an exercise program after years of inactivity.
- **Moderate intensity** is 60 to 74 percent of the maximum heart rate reserve. This is the normal training range for most people.
- **High or vigorous intensity** is 75 percent and higher of the maximum heart rate reserve. This level of effort is for athletes desiring a high level of fitness.

FIGURE 7.4

The Karvonen formula calculates the training heart rate using a percentage of the "heart rate reserve," which is the difference between the maximum and resting heart rates.

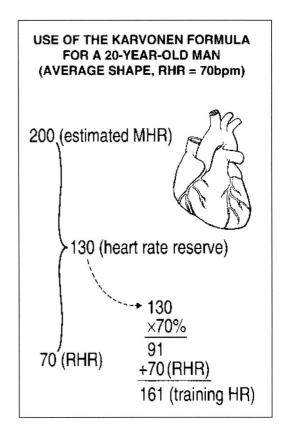

USE OF THE KARVONEN FORMULA
FOR A 20-YEAR-OLD MAN
(AVERAGE SHAPE, RHR = 70bpm)

200 (estimated MHR)

130 (heart rate reserve)

130
×70%
91
+70 (RHR)
161 (training HR)

70 (RHR)

What is the maximum heart rate reserve? As summarized in the Karvonen formula in Figure 7.4, the maximum heart rate reserve is the difference between the maximum heart rate and the resting heart rate.

To determine your maximum heart rate reserve, you must first estimate or measure your maximum and resting heart rates. As defined in Chapter 4, the maximum heart rate is the maximum attainable heart rate at the point of exhaustion from all-out exertion. For example, if you increase the speed and grade of a treadmill every 2 to 3 minutes and keep running, the maximum heart rate would be measured at the point of exhaustion and near-collapse. Another method is to run up a steep hill as fast as possible for 5 to 8 minutes (after a good warm-up), and then take your pulse rate when feeling completely exhausted.

The maximum heart rate can be estimated by using the formula 220 minus the age. For example, the maximum heart rate for a 20-year-old college student would be 220 – 20 = 200 beats/minute. This formula is not precise, however, with a variation of plus or minus 12 beats/minute for two thirds of the population of a given age. For example, two thirds of 20-year-olds have maximum heart rates that vary between 188 and 212 beats/minute; thus, it is best to directly measure your own maximum heart rate.

The resting heart rate is best measured in the morning just after waking up. Sit on the edge of the bed, and count your pulse for one minute. Try this three mornings in a row. (See Chapter 4 for a review).

Once you have your maximum and resting heart rates, you can calculate your maximum heart rate range. For example, if your maximum heart rate is 200 beats per minute and your resting heart rate is 70 beats per minute, the maximum heart rate reserve is 130 beats per minute. To determine the proper exercise training heart rate, multiple your chosen intensity level times the maximum heart rate reserve, and then add back the resting heart rate. (See Health and Fitness Activity 7.2).

In summary, the formula to estimate your exercise training heart rate is:

Training heart rate = [(maximum HR – resting HR) × 0.50 to 0.85] + resting HR.

Maximal heart rates and the training heart rate zone for people of varying ages using the Karvonen formula. The resting heart rate is assumed to be 70 bpm.

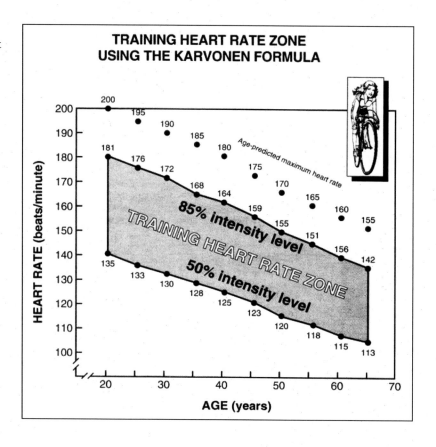

For example, if your maximum heart rate is 200 beats/minute and resting heart rate 70 beats/minute, and you wish to exercise at an intensity of 70 percent, the training heart rate would be calculated this way:

161 beats/minute = [(200 beats/minute – 70 beats/minute) × 0.70] + 70 beats/minute.

The training heart rate zone is the heart rate range between 50 percent and 85 percent of maximum heart rate range for all age groups. Figure 7.5 gives the training heart rate zone for ages 20 to 65 years using age-predicted maximum heart rates (220 – age) and an assumed resting heart rate of 70 beats per minute.

How to Measure Your Exercise Heart Rate   Your exercise heart rate can be measured by directly counting your pulse at the neck (figure 7.6) or by using a heart rate monitor (figure 7.7). Measuring the heart rate by counting the carotid pulse in the neck is safe and accurate. Place two fingers of one hand lightly on one side of the neck next to the voice box area, count for exactly 10 seconds, and then multiply by six to get the total beats per minute. Many different types of heart rate monitors are available, but the best ones (starting at $50) use chest-strap transmitters the wirelessly signal the heart rate to a monitor on the wrist.

You may not like to count the heart rate during exercise. Another system of monitoring exercise intensity is the rating (R) of perceived (P) exertion (E) scale (RPE). The RPE scale is very easy to use, relates well to your exercise heart rate, and teaches you to "listen" to your body (Table 7.1). Just simply pick out a number and descriptor that best indicates how you feel at a given moment during the exercise bout. To build good aerobic fitness, your exercise exertion should be perceived at 12 to 14 or "somewhat hard." When exercising at an RPE of 12 to 14, you are definitely working, but you can think, talk with a partner, and look around and enjoy the scenery.

When exercising at an RPE of 15 or higher, the pulse is very high, and it is difficult to talk or exercise for prolonged periods of time. Athletes often exercise at this level to prepare for competition. When exercising below an RPE of 12, the exercise stimulus is

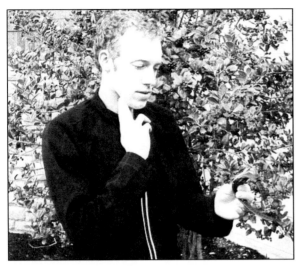

FIGURE 7.6
To measure the training heart rate during exercise, the participant should stop periodically and count his pulse, using the carotid pulse.

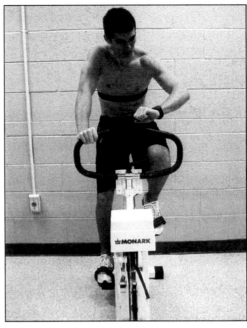

FIGURE 7.7
Heart rates can be accurately monitored using chest-strap transmitters that wirelessly signal the heart rate to a monitor on the wrist.

TABLE 7.1   Rating of Perceived Exertion Scale

	Light Intensity	
6	No exertion at all	
7	Extremely light	
8		
9	Very light	
10		
11	Light	

	Moderate Intensity	
12		
13	Somewhat hard	
14		

	Vigorous Intensity	
15	Hard (heavy)	
16		
17	Very hard	
18		
19	Extremely hard	
20	Maximal exertion	

too low to develop good aerobic fitness for most people (except those with very low fitness), but does enhance health and help prevent disease (see figure 7.8).

Time

Time refers to the duration in minutes of the exercise session or minutes exercised each week. As summarized in Figure 7.2, a formal aerobic exercise program entails at least 20 to 60 minutes per day of moderate- to vigorous-intensity exercise, on at least 3 to

FIGURE 7.8
The RPE scale is a good indicator of exercise intensity.

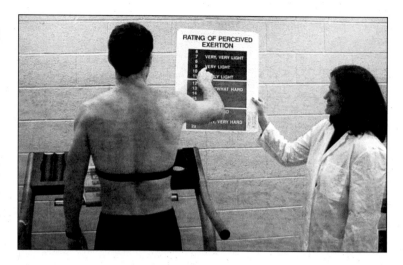

5 days a week. A key recommendation of the *2008 Physical Activity Guidelines* is that the health benefits of physical activity depend mainly on total weekly energy expenditure due to purposeful physical activity of at least 150 minutes a week of moderate-intensity, or 75 minutes a week of vigorous-intensity aerobic physical activity. These minutes can be accumulated throughout the week in episodes of at least 10 minutes.

Low activity is defined as fewer than 150 minutes of moderate-intensity physical activity a week or the equivalent amount (75 minutes) of vigorous-intensity activity. Medium activity is 150 minutes to 300 minutes of moderate-intensity activity a week (or 75 to 150 minutes of vigorous-intensity physical activity a week). High activity is more than the equivalent of 300 minutes of moderate-intensity physical activity a week.

There is insufficient scientific evidence to determine whether the health benefits of 30 minutes on 5 days a week are any different from the health benefits of 50 minutes on 3 days a week. As a result, the *2008 Physical Activity Guidelines* allow a person to accumulate 150 minutes a week in various ways. When adults do the equivalent of 150 minutes of moderate-intensity aerobic activity each week, the health and disease prevention benefits are substantial, but additional benefits are experienced as a person moves from 150 toward 300 minutes a week. The benefits continue to increase when a person does more than the equivalent of 300 minutes a week of moderate-intensity aerobic activity. Many adults will need to do more than 150 to 300 minutes a week of moderate-intensity aerobic physical activity to lose weight or keep it off.

Intensity and time work together to build aerobic fitness. As shown in Figure 7.9, as intensity increases, time of exercise can decrease, and vice versa. An important goal is to burn at least 150 calories each exercise session at an intensity of 50 percent and higher, or about 1,000 calories each week. Notice from figure 7.9 that you can burn about 150 calories by climbing stairs vigorously for 15 minutes, bicycling five miles in 30 minutes, or washing and waxing your car for 45 to 60 minutes.

Some athletes push themselves at a high intensity for prolonged periods of time each day. There is a delicate balance, however, between positive exercise training and overtraining. Overtraining, defined as pushing exercise training beyond your ability to recover, can accumulate over time, leading to incapacitating fatigue, injury, and a loss of desire to exercise.

Aerobic Exercise Mode

There are many different types of aerobic activities or modes that can build heart and lung fitness. The best aerobic activities use large muscle groups throughout the body, and can be maintained in a rhythmical fashion for 20 minutes or more. As emphasized earlier, a "total fitness" program attempts to build both aerobic and muscular fitness, while burning enough calories to keep body fat at optimal levels. Some modes of aerobic exercise are excellent in this regard, including rowing, cross-country skiing, swimming, and aerobic dance. See Table 7.2 for a rating of how well different physical activities build aerobic and muscular fitness.

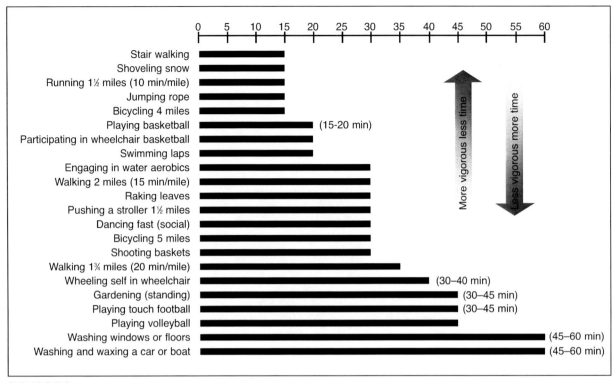

FIGURE 7.9

Number of minutes of physical activity to burn 150 calories.

Achieving the recommended amount of physical activity can be accomplished by engaging in a variety of moderate- or vigorous-intensity activities. The less vigorous the activity, the more time needed to burn the recommended number of Calories. The more vigorous the activity, the less time needed to burn the same number of Calories. *Source:* U.S. Department of Health and Human Services. *Physical Activity and Health: A Report of the Surgeon General.* Atlanta, GA: U.S. Department of Health and Human Services, Centers for Disease Control and Prevention, National Center for Chronic Disease Prevention and Health Promotion, 1996.

TABLE 7.2   The Aerobic and Muscular Fitness Value of Different Physical Activities

Physical Activity The table shows how well each activity builds aerobic fitness, burns energy, and builds muscle fitness (1 = not at all, 2 = a little, 3 = moderately, 4 = strongly, and 5 = very strongly).	**Calories per Hour** (150 lb person)	**Aerobic Fitness**	**Muscular Fitness** Activity is rated high if both upper and lower body muscles are improved.
Aerobic dance (vigorous)	474	4	4
Basketball (competitive)	545	4	2
Cycling (fast pace)	680	5	3
Rope jumping (moderate to hard)	680	5	3
Rowing (fast pace)	815	5	4
Running (brisk pace, 8 mph)	920	5	2
Shoveling dirt, digging	580	4	4
Skiing (cross-country, brisk)	610	5	4
Splitting wood	410	4	4
Stair climbing	610	5	3
Swimming laps (vigorous)	680	5	3
Tennis (competitive)	475	4	3
Walking (brisk, 4 mph)	270	3	2
Weight training	205	2	5

Cross-training is a system of training that grew in popularity during the late 1980s. In cross-training, you participate in several different types of aerobic activities to build fitness. For example, on three days of the week you may play intramural basketball, run on two other days, and mountain bike on another day. Several benefits of cross-training include:

- Decreased risk of injury
- Reduced boredom
- Increased long-term adherence to your exercise program
- Increased overall fitness.

To stay active over a lifetime, it is critical that you choose modes of physical activity that fit well into your schedule, meet your personal fitness goals, and are enjoyable and convenient. Brisk walking is the most popular form of physical activity in America because it is easily incorporated into the daily schedule, does not require any special skills or equipment, can be enjoyed with friends, and is much less apt to cause injuries than running. Sports such as basketball, racquetball, tennis, or soccer are also popular choices for many adults because they are fun, competitive, and social. Box 7.1 summarizes tips for exercising success.

The home aerobic fitness equipment market has exploded in recent years. Treadmills, cross-country ski machines, steppers/climbers, rowing machines, and stationary bicycles each provide an excellent aerobic workout. Exercisers tend to burn more calories on treadmills compared to other equipment. Rowing and cross-country ski machines are especially valuable because they build aerobic fitness while also giving the entire body musculature a good workout (figure 7.10).

Buying fitness equipment for home workouts can represent a sizeable financial commitment (typically $500 to $2000) as well as a lifestyle change. Unfortunately, some companies sell equipment that is largely worthless for improving aerobic fitness. The Federal Trade Commission suggests you ask yourself the following questions before purchasing fitness equipment:

- What are your fitness goals? Will this equipment help you meet them? Whether you want to build strength, improve aerobic endurance, or enhance your health, look for equipment that meets your personal goals.
- Will you really use the indoor exercise equipment? In theory, exercising at home sounds great, but if you don't use the equipment on a regular basis, it can burn a hole in your pocket without burning off any calories. Before you buy, prove to yourself that you're ready to stick to an ongoing fitness program.
- Can you see through outrageous claims? Any ads that promise "easy" or "effortless" results are false. Some companies claim you can get results by using their equipment for three or four minutes a day, three times a week—again, this is false. Exercise good judgment and common sense when evaluating advertising claims for fitness products. If it sounds too good to be true, it usually is.
- Can you try the equipment before you buy? Before you buy any exercise equipment, try it out. Test different types of equipment at a local gym or recreation center. Before you buy, shop around.

Cool-Down

The purpose of the cool-down is to slowly decrease your heart rate that was elevated during the aerobic phase. This is safely and effectively accomplished by keeping your feet and legs moving for 5 to 15 minutes by walking, jogging lightly, or cycling slowly. In other words, the cool-down is the warm-up in reverse. Mild activity following intensive aerobic exercise keeps the leg muscle "pumps" going, preventing the blood from pooling in the legs, and preventing feelings of lightheadedness.

BOX 7.1

Obstacles to Exercise and Tips for Exercise Success

Maintaining a regular exercise routine is all about getting around or removing the obstacles. Here are the 10 most common obstacles adults cite for not staying physically active:

1. *Do not have enough time to exercise.* Lack of time is consistently the number one reason people give for not exercising. But really, is it lack of time or lack of desire? A case in point is that the average American adult now averages 4 to 5 hours a day viewing television.
2. *Find it inconvenient to exercise.* For example, changing clothes, driving to the fitness center, parking, working out, showering, dressing, and driving back to the office or home becomes so onerous that many stop exercising (to the benefit of the fitness center that takes your money and signs up more people than they can handle, knowing many will fail to stick with it).
3. *Lack self-motivation.* In other words, I know I should exercise but the benefits don't outweigh the costs in terms of time, pain, and money.
4. *Do not find exercise enjoyable.* I never noticed the so-called "runner's high," and exercise feels too much like work.
5. *Find exercise boring.* For example, looking at a black line while swimming laps drives me nuts.
6. *Lack confidence in their ability to be physically active.* I'm too fat, people will stare, the pain hurts too much, and I like sitting on the couch.
7. *Fear being injured or have been injured recently.* I would play sports but too many people I know injured their knees.
8. *Lack self-management skills.* In other words, inability to set personal goals, monitor progress, or set up rewards for reaching goals.
9. *No support from significant others.* Lack encouragement, support, or companionship from family and friends.
10. *No place to exercise.* I do not have parks, sidewalks, bicycle trails, or safe and pleasant walking paths near my home or office, and the fitness center is too far away.

It's easy to stop exercising when these obstacles get in the way. But if you are wise and determined, you can make exercise a part of your daily routine, just like eating and sleeping. Here are six strategies to improve long-term compliance to an exercise regimen:

- Maximize convenience in terms of time, travel, and disruptions in family relationships. For example, establish an exercise room in your house, complete with aerobic and muscular fitness building equipment.
- Exercise with a partner or group. The social interaction often becomes a major stimulus for sticking with the routine.
- Emphasize variety and enjoyment in the exercise program.
- Involve your family in some way.
- Establish reasonable exercise goals, highlight these in a contract (with a witness signature from your spouse), and set up a reward system when the goals are achieved. For example, you may decide to brisk walk for 30 to 45 minutes every evening after dinner with your significant other. If you average five days a week for 10 weeks (verified with a progress chart), reward yourselves with a dinner out at the most expensive restaurant in town. If you fail, you get a frozen TV dinner (every day for a week).
- Support every initiative to establish walking and biking trails in your town, recreational parks, and sidewalks. Another plan is to band together with fellow workers to obtain work release time for exercise. For example, if you use the worksite fitness center or a local YMCA, ask your boss to reduce your work day from 8 to 7.5 hours.

The bottom line is that you will find the time to exercise if you really want to. Regular exercise makes you feel better mentally, and has multiple health benefits. You are not being selfish when you take time to exercise—you are being smart.

Building Muscular Fitness

As described earlier, muscular fitness includes an emphasis on flexibility and muscular strength and endurance. You can include both aerobic and muscular fitness activities in your daily workout routine, or emphasize aerobics on one day and then muscular fitness on the next day. A good "total fitness" workout routine that would take about 1 to 1.5 hours to complete could be organized as follows:

- Warm-up: 5 to 10 minutes of easy-to-moderate aerobic activity.
- Aerobic exercise: 20 to 30 minutes of moderate-to-vigorous aerobic activity.
- Cool-down: 5 to 10 minutes of mild-to-moderate aerobic activity.
- Stretching: 5 to 15 minutes of static stretching, emphasizing all major muscle groups and joints.
- Weight lifting: 20 to 30 minutes of weight lifting, two sets of 8 to 12 repetitions of 8 to 10 different exercises covering all the major muscle groups.

This routine could also be split into two days, with the first four stages completed during the first day, and the weight training completed the next (with an appropriate warm-up).

Flexibility Exercises

A program of flexibility exercises improves the range of motion around your body's joints and allows your muscles to move more efficiently. Without flexibility, gymnasts and ballet dancers could not perform their feats of strength and skill. As reviewed in Chapter 6, there are several other benefits in becoming flexible, including alleviation of stress and tension, improved body posture and symmetry, and prevention of injury.

There are several ways to stretch, but static stretching is preferred. Static stretching involves slowly applying stretch to a muscle group and then holding it in a lengthened position for 10 to 30 seconds and repeating 2–4 times. During this stretch, try to relax and focus attention on the muscles being stretched. As the seconds pass, the feeling of tension will slowly subside. Relax and then repeat this cycle four times, always stopping short of your pain threshold during the stretch. Always try to warm your body up through aerobic activity before stretching. You will be able to get through your flexibility routine more safely and effectively this way.

Flexibility is unique to each joint and muscle group. Try to hold at least 8 to 10 different stretches that affect all of the major muscle groups, as depicted in Box 7.2 and Appendix A. You should go through this routine about 2 to 3 times a week, or better yet, after each aerobic session. See Health and Fitness Activity 7.3 to experiment with this flexibility exercise program.

How to Build Muscular Strength and Endurance

As reviewed in Chapter 6, development of muscular fitness has several important health-related benefits, including increased bone density, muscle size, and connective tissue strength, and improved self-esteem. Strength training promotes a high quality of life for young and old alike.

The minimum strength training program is performing 2–4 sets of 8 to 12 repetitions of 8 to 10 exercises 2 to 3 times per week. The same regimen using 10 to15 repetitions is recommended for persons more than 50 years of age. This is a basic program, however, and you can experience greater gains in muscular strength and power using higher intensity (fewer repetitions with greater weight) with multiple sets (e.g., 3 sets of 6 reps to fatigue).

Principles of Weight Training

When you follow basic weight training guidelines and principles, you should experience a 25 to 30 percent increase in strength within the first six months. There are three major principles of weight training:

BOX 7.2

An Exercise Program to Build Flexibility

Step 1 Warm-up aerobically:
Never stretch unless the muscles and joints are warm from 5–15 minutes of moderate aerobic activity.

Step 2 Follow these minimum flexibility program guidelines:
A. *Frequency:* 2–3 days per week, or after each aerobic workout.
B. *Time:* Hold each position short of the pain threshold for 10–30 seconds, and repeat 2–4 times (total time, about 10–15 minutes). Relax totally, letting your muscles slowly go limp as the tension of the stretched muscle slowly subsides. Be sure that you do not stretch to the point of pain to avoid injury and a tightening recoil of the muscle.
C. *Stretching positions:* Improve flexibility in several body areas with 8 specific stretching exercises. Follow the order listed below, using the figures in Appendix A. To conduct each stretching exercise, follow the explanations in Appendix A. Do not be worried if you seem "tighter" than other people when practicing these stretches. Flexibility is an individual matter.

Back/hips/hamstrings/legs/calves
1. Lower back-hamstring rope stretch
2. Calf rope stretch
3. Groin stretch
4. Quad stretch
5. Spinal twist
6. Downward dog

Shoulders/arms/upper body
7. Upper-body rope stretch
8. Standing side stretch

- *Overload principle:* To develop muscular strength and endurance, you need to push your muscles to fatigue, lifting weights that are heavier than you are accustomed to. This is called the "overload principle." In other words, your muscles will not get bigger or stronger unless you challenge and fatigue them.
- *Progressive resistance principle:* The resistance or pounds of weight against which your muscles work should be increased periodically as gains in strength and endurance are made until you reach your desired level. This is called the "progressive resistance principle." In other words, if you can bench press 120 pounds eight times, increase the weight after a week or two of training to 130 pounds. Your repetitions may drop as you switch to the higher weight, but slowly increase them as you adjust to the higher weight. Over time, your muscles will enlarge and adapt to the new workload, and then increase the weight by another 10 pounds. Keep this up until you are bench pressing the weight that matches your personal goals.
- *Principle of specificity:* The development of muscular fitness is specific to the muscle groups that you exercise and the intensity of training. This is called the "principle of specificity." If you train your biceps (front on the upper arm) with heavy weights using arm curls, they will grow strong, but not your triceps (back of the upper arm). Decide what areas of your body need to be built up and then plan your workout accordingly. If you need stronger legs, emphasize leg lifts in your weight lifting routine.

Systems of Weight Training

As described earlier, strength exercise such as weight training and calisthenics is based on sets and repetitions. A repetition is defined as one weight-training or calisthenic movement, with a set defined as a certain number of these repetitions. Typically, the strength movement is continued until complete fatigue. In fact, your muscles cannot increase in size, strength, or endurance unless you lift to the point where you cannot perform even one more repetition. For example, six repetitions maximum (abbreviated 6-RM) is the greatest amount of weight that you can lift six times. A program based on 10-RM means that you choose a weight that you can lift only 10 times. At first this takes some experimentation until you find just the right weight for each specific strength exercise.

Muscular strength is developed when the weight is heavy and the repetitions to maximum are low, about 4 to 6. This is called high-intensity weight lifting. Muscular endurance is developed when the weight is somewhat light and the repetitions to fatigue are high, about 15 to 20. This is called low-intensity weight lifting. When the weight is moderate and the repetitions are 8 to 15, both muscular strength and endurance are developed to some degree, and this is called moderate-intensity weight lifting. This is summarized in figure 7.10.

As emphasized earlier, a basic muscular strength and endurance program should involve 2–4 sets of 8 to 12 repetitions to fatigue of 8 to 10 different exercises performed two or three days a week. This is a moderate intensity weight lifting program that should give you basic muscular strength and endurance. Box 7.3 outlines a weight lifting routine, giving specific instructions on how to perform 11 different strength exercises. See Health and Fitness Activity 7.4 to experiment with this muscular strength and endurance exercise program. If you want more strength, lower the repetitions to six so that you can use heavier weights. If you want more endurance, increase the repetitions to 15 so that you can use lighter weights. Two sets provide a good stimulus for muscular fitness gains, but 3–4 sets can add a bit more. Body builders often perform five to eight sets to repeatedly bring a muscle group to the point of complete fatigue. Calisthenics, if performed correctly, can build muscular strength and endurance without the need for equipment.

There are several other guidelines that you should follow when lifting weights to maximize increases in muscular fitness and ensure your safety:

- Perform every weight lifting exercise through a full range of motion.
- Adhere as closely as possible to the specific techniques listed for each exercise.
- Perform both the lifting and the lowering portion of the resistance exercises in a controlled manner.
- Maintain a normal breathing pattern, because breath holding can induce excessive

FIGURE 7.10

The intensity of lifting and the number of repetitions lifted to fatigue determine whether muscular strength and/or endurance will be developed.

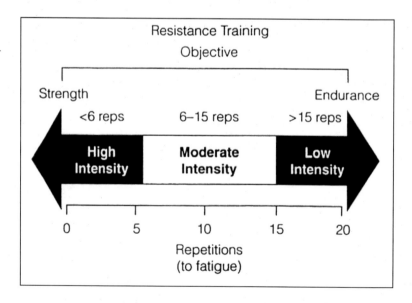

BOX 7.3

An Exercise Program to Build Muscular Strength and Endurance

Step 1 Warm up aerobically: Never strength train unless the muscles and joints are warm from 5 to 15 minutes of moderate aerobic activity.

Step 2 Follow these minimum strength training program guidelines:
A. *Frequency:* Strength train at least 2–3 days per week.
B. *Set and Reps:* Perform a minimum of 2–4 sets, 8 to 12 repetitions to the point of volitional fatigue for each exercise.
C. *Strength Exercises:* Perform a minimum of 8 to 10 different exercises that condition all of the major muscle groups. Try the routine described below. Perform each exercise through a full range of motion. Perform both the lifting and lowering portion of each exercise in a controlled manner. Maintain a normal breathing pattern because breath holding can induce excessive increases in blood pressure. If possible, exercise with a training partner who can provide feedback, assistance, and motivation.

Strength exercise	Part of body benefited	Equipment
#1. Lat pull-down	Side of back (lats) and shoulders	Pulley machine

Description: Kneel below the handle with your hands grasping it, arms straight. Forcefully pull down behind the head. Let the bar rise slowly and under control to the starting position, and repeat.

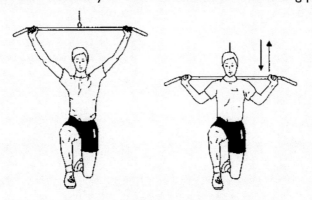

Strength exercise	Part of body benefited	Equipment
#2. Leg press	Front of the thigh and buttocks	Leg press machine

Description: While sitting with the feet on the pedals and hands grasping the handles on the seat, push the foot pedals forward. Keep your buttocks on the seat, and then move the foot pedals backward slowly and under control to the starting position, and repeat.

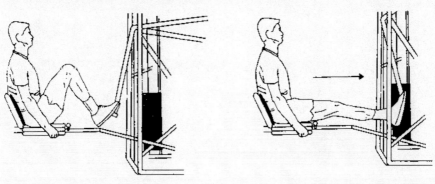

Strength exercise	**Part of body benefited**	**Equipment**
#3. Bench press	Front of the chest and back of upper arms (triceps)	Barbell, bench with rack

Description: Lie down on the bench with your knees bent and feet flat on the floor. Grasp the bar, signal the spotter, and move the bar off the bar shelf. Position the bar over your chest, elbows fully extended. Lower the bar slowly and under control until the bar touches your chest, and then push the bar up to full elbow extension, and repeat.

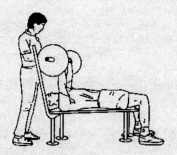 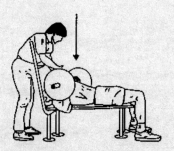 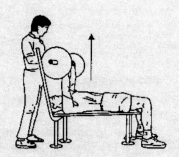

Strength exercise	**Part of body benefited**	**Equipment**
#4. Abdominal crunch	Abdomen.	Padded bench and floor mat

Description: Lie on the mat with your knees hooked over the bench and arms crossed over the chest. Tuck your chin to your chest and curl your upper body toward the thighs until your upper back is off the mat. Lower your shoulders slowly and under control, and repeat.

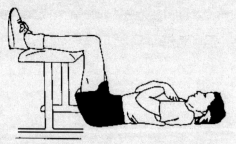 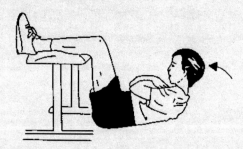

Strength exercise	**Part of body benefited**	**Equipment**
#5. Shoulder press	Shoulders and back of upper arms (triceps)	Shoulder press machine

Description: Face the machine while seated and push the handles up until the arms are fully extended. Lower the handles slowly and under control to shoulder level, and repeat.

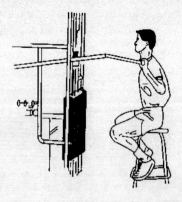 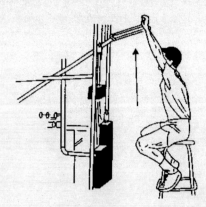

Strength exercise	**Part of body benefited**	**Equipment**
#6. Seated row	Upper back, shoulders, front of upper arms (biceps)	Pulley machine

Description: Sit facing the pulley machine with your feet on the foot supports. With your knees slightly flexed and body erect, pull the handles to your ribs, and then return them slowly and under control, and repeat.

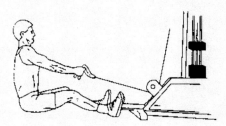 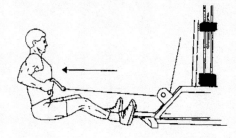

Strength exercise	**Part of body benefited**	**Equipment**
#7. Leg extension	Front of thigh (quadriceps)	Leg extension machine

Description: Sit on the machine with your ankles locked under the roller pad. With hands grasping the seat handles, extend your legs at the knees until they are straight, and then lower them slowly and under control to the starting position and repeat.

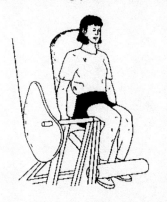 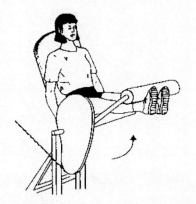

Strength exercise	**Part of body benefited**	**Equipment**
#8. Leg curl	Buttocks and back of legs (hamstrings)	Leg curl machine

Description: Lie down on the bench with your heels locked under the padded roller, hands grasping the handles. Keep your hips on the bench as you flex your legs at the knees and pull your heels as close to the buttocks as possible. Lower the roller pad slowly and under control to the starting position and repeat.

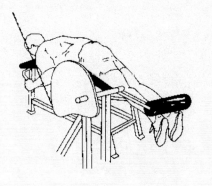 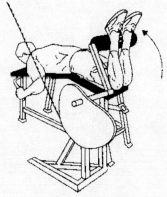

Strength exercise   **Part of body benefited**   **Equipment**
#9. Biceps curl   Front of upper arm (biceps)   Barbell

Description: With your hands grasping the bar, palms forward, raise the bar in an arc by flexing the arms at the elbows. Keep your upper arms and elbows stationary while maintaining your upright body position. After raising the bar to your shoulders, slowly lower the bar to the starting position and repeat.

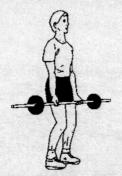 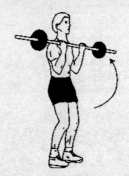

Strength exercise   **Part of body benefited**   **Equipment**
#10. Triceps pushdown   Back of upper arm (triceps)   Pulley machine

Description: Grasp the bar with your elbows flexed, palms facing downward. Push the bar down to full elbow extension while keeping your elbows next to your body. Allow the bar to slowly rise up to the starting position, and repeat.

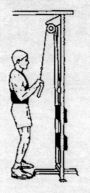 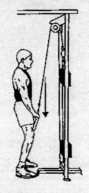

Strength exercise   **Part of body benefited**   **Equipment**
#11. Standing Heel Raise   Back of lower legs (calves)   Barbell, safety rack, and
    two inch platform

Description: Perform this exercise inside of a squat rack with two spotters. Position the bar on your shoulders at the base of your neck. Position the balls of your feet on the raised platform, with your heels down. Push up on your toes as high as possible in a slow, controlled manner while keeping the legs straight. Return under control to the starting position, and repeat.

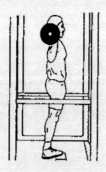 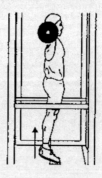

increases in blood pressure.

- Exercise with a training partner who can provide feedback, assistance, and motivation. For safety during some types of lifts with free weights, use a spotter. Err on the side of safety.

Don't forget that muscular fitness should complement your aerobic fitness program. Total fitness means that you give appropriate and balanced attention to both muscular and aerobic fitness as depicted in the Activity Pyramid (figure 7.1). You don't want to be a muscular person who gets out of breath climbing a long flight of stairs, nor do you want to be able to run five miles swiftly but be too weak to use your strength during emergencies.

HEALTH AND FITNESS INSIGHT
Taking Action: Increasing Physical Activity Levels of Americans: Recommendations from the *2008 Physical Activity Guidelines for Americans*

Most American adults are not exercising to the levels recommended in the *2008 Physical Activity Guidelines for Americans*. Experts claim that to turn this around, regular physical activity needs to be made the easy choice for Americans. To accomplish this goal, the "socio-ecologic" approach is needed, involving action at all levels of society: individual, interpersonal, organizational, community, and public policy. Example actions include:

- Personal goal setting (individual level);
- Support and encouragement from family and friends to be active (interpersonal level);
- Promotion of physical activity as part of worksite health promotion programs (organizational);
- Good access to parks and recreational facilities in neighborhoods (community); and
- Promotion of policies that support families who want their children to walk or bike to school (public policy).

Adults need to identify benefits of personal value to them. For many people, the health benefits, which are the focus of the *Physical Activity Guidelines for Americans,* are compelling enough. For others, different reasons are key motivators to be active. For example, physical activity:

- Provides opportunities to enjoy recreational activities, often in a social setting;
- Improves personal appearance;
- Provides a chance to help a spouse lose weight;
- Improves the quality of sleep;
- Reduces feelings of low energy; and
- Gives older adults a greater opportunity to live independently in the community.

Organizations and communities can provide many opportunities for physical activity, such as walking trails, bicycle lanes on roads, sidewalks, and sports fields. Schools, places of worship, worksites, and community centers can provide opportunities and encouragement for physical activity. Strategies at the community level include:

- Community-wide campaigns that combine physical activity messaging (distributed through television, newspapers, radio, and other media) with activities such as physical activity counseling, community health fairs, and the development of walking trails.
- Physical education classes to increase activity. Physical education classes should use a curriculum that increases the amount of time students are active during class.

- Interventions that increase social support for physical activity. These interventions start or enhance social-support networks, and include efforts such as organizing a buddy system (two or more people who set regular times to do physical activity together), walking groups, and community dances.
- Programs to create or enhance access to places to be physically active. This can include building walking trails and providing public access to school gymnasiums, playgrounds, or community centers. This also includes worksite activity programs that provide access to onsite or offsite fitness rooms, walking breaks, or other opportunities to engage in physical activity. Interventions to improve access should also include outreach that increases awareness of the opportunity to be active.

Summary

1. A comprehensive approach to physical fitness gives balanced attention to each of the major components—aerobic fitness, muscular fitness, and body composition.
2. There are two systems for building your fitness: (1) the lifestyle approach, and (2) the formal exercise program. The lifestyle approach seeks to increase opportunities for physical activity throughout the daily routine, while the formal exercise program builds aerobic and muscular fitness to high levels through an exercise system based on specific frequency, intensity, and time guidelines. The Activity Pyramid depicts how the lifestyle and formal exercise approaches to physical fitness can complement each other.
3. The lifestyle approach to fitness places an emphasis on accumulating at least 150 minutes of moderate-intensity physical activity over the course of each week.
4. The formal exercise program is based on specific guidelines for aerobic and muscular fitness. To build aerobic fitness, and to keep lean, exercise aerobically 3 to 5 days per week (frequency), at 50–85 percent $\dot{V}O_{2max}$ (intensity), for 20 to 60 minutes each session (time). To build muscular fitness, perform a minimum of 8 to 10 separate exercises that train the major muscle groups. Perform 2–4 sets of 8 to 12 repetitions of each of these exercises to the point of fatigue, and do this at least 2 to 3 days per week. For flexibility, stretch at least 2 to 3 days a week and involve at 2–4 repetitions of several stretches that are held 10 to 30 seconds at a position of mild discomfort.
5. The aerobic or cardiorespiratory stage of a comprehensive physical fitness program consists of three segments: the warm-up, aerobic exercise (that conforms to frequency, intensity, and time guidelines), and the cool-down. The formula to estimate your exercise training heart rate is: Training heart rate = [(maximum HR − resting HR) × 0.50 to 0.85] + resting HR.
6. The best aerobic activities use large muscle groups throughout the body, and can be maintained in a rhythmical fashion for 20 minutes or more.
7. There are several ways to stretch, but static stretching is preferred. Static stretching involves slowly applying stretch to a muscle group and then holding it in a lengthened position for 10 to 30 seconds.
8. There are three major principles of weight training: (1) overload principle, (2) progressive resistance principle, (3) principle of specificity.
9. Muscular strength is developed when the weight is heavy and the repetitions to maximum are low, about 4 to 6. Muscular endurance is developed when the weight is somewhat light and the repetitions to fatigue are high, about 15 to 20.

HEALTH AND FITNESS ACTIVITY 7.1
The Activity Pyramid: How Do You Rate?

This chapter emphasized a comprehensive approach to physical fitness in which three major components—aerobic fitness, muscular fitness, and body composition—are given balanced attention. In other words, to have total fitness, pay attention to all of the muscles of your body, both inside (heart) and out (skeletal), and keep lean by balancing calories burned with those eaten. This comprehensive approach to physical fitness is summarized in the Activity Pyramid (figure 7.1).

How comprehensive is your approach to physical fitness? Fill in the blanks below, total your points, and then compare them to the norms to determine how well you adhere to the recommendations of the Activity Pyramid. Give yourself 5 points for each "yes" answer, and 0 points for each "no" answer.

Yes 5 points	No 0 points	
❑	❑	**Level 1: Lifestyle Physical Activity.** Do you accumulate at least 150 minutes of physical activity every week?
❑	❑	**Level 2: Exercise for Aerobic Fitness.** Do you engage in brisk walking, swimming, cycling, running, active sports, or other aerobic activities for 20 to 60 minutes, 3 to 5 days per week?
		Level 3: Exercise for Muscular Fitness.
❑	❑	A. **Muscular strength and endurance exercise.** Do you lift weights, engage in strength calisthenics (push-ups, sit-ups, pull-ups, etc.), or work hard physically (e.g., chopping wood, lifting heavy objects, shoveling dirt) for about 20 to 30 minutes, 2 to 3 times per week?
❑	❑	B. **Flexibility exercise.** Do you engage in a regular stretching routine that affects major muscle groups and joints for about 10 to 20 minutes, 2 to 3 times per week?
❑	❑	**Level 4: Reduce Inactivity.** Do you make a conscious effort to reduce sitting time on most days by limiting watching TV, playing video games, viewing the Internet, etc.?

Your total points: _____

Norms Points	Classification
25	**Excellent**
15 or 20	**Good**
10	**Fair**
0 or 5	**Poor**

HEALTH AND FITNESS ACTIVITY 7.2
Your Aerobic Exercise Program

This chapter emphasized that aerobic exercise is the cornerstone of a comprehensive physical fitness program. The aerobic stage of a comprehensive physical fitness program consists of three segments: the warm-up, aerobic exercise (that conforms to frequency, intensity, and time guidelines), and the cool-down. This is summarized in Figures 7.1 and 7.2.

Go to Figure 7.2 and perform these tasks:

1. **Intensity Level:** Circle under "step 2" your desire to exercise moderately, vigorously, or both.

2. **Training Heart Rate:** Using the intensity range listed for your fitness level, go to step 2, B (intensity), and calculate your personal training heart rate. Use the maximum heart rate and resting heart rate that you measured from Chapter 4.

3. **Aerobic Exercise Mode:** Under step 2, C (aerobic exercise mode), write down your primary aerobic exercise mode (the one you use most often), a secondary mode, and a backup mode. Consult Table 7.1 if you are starting an exercise program and want guidelines on making good choices.

4. **Daily Schedule:** As emphasized in this chapter, half the challenge in exercising regularly is finding the time. Lack of time is the exercise barrier most frequently listed by people in surveys. Based on your current schedule, go to step 2, D (build exercise into daily schedule), and write down the specific times on the specific days you can exercise.

HEALTH AND FITNESS ACTIVITY 7.3
Your Flexibility Exercise Program

In this chapter, several specific guidelines were given for developing flexibility:

Frequency: 2 to 3 days per week, or after each aerobic workout.

Time: Hold each position short of the pain threshold for 10 to 30 seconds, and repeat 2–4 times (total time, about 10–15 minutes).

Stretching positions: Improve flexibility in several body areas with specific stretching exercises.

   In Appendix A, instructions for flexibility exercises are summarized. With the help of your class instructor, try the stretches listed below, and provide your personal comments on how they felt and areas of needed improvement.

Flexibility Exercise	How This Exercise Felt to You	Improvement in This Area Is Needed (Check "yes" or "no").
1. Lower back-hamstring rope stretch		❏ Yes ❏ No
2. Calf rope stretch		❏ Yes ❏ No
3. Groin stretch		❏ Yes ❏ No
4. Quad stretch		❏ Yes ❏ No
5. Spinal twist		❏ Yes ❏ No
6. Downward dog		❏ Yes ❏ No
7. Upper-body rope stretch		❏ Yes ❏ No
8. Standing side stretch		❏ Yes ❏ No

HEALTH AND FITNESS ACTIVITY 7.4
Your Muscular Strength and Endurance Exercise Program

In this chapter, guidelines for building muscular strength and endurance were described, including these:

Step 1 Warm-up aerobically: Never strength train unless the muscles and joints are warm from 5–15 minutes of moderate aerobic activity.

Step 2 Follow these minimum strength training program guidelines:

A. Frequency: Strength train at least 2 to 3 days per week.

B. Set and Reps: Perform 2–4 sets of 8 to 12 repetitions to the point of volitional fatigue for each exercise.

C. Strength Exercises: Perform a minimum of 8 to 10 different exercises that condition all of the major muscle groups.

With the help of your class instructor, try the routine described in Box 7.1. Perform each exercise through a full range of motion. Perform both the lifting and lowering portion of each exercise in a controlled manner. Maintain a normal breathing pattern because breath holding can induce excessive increases in blood pressure. Use a class-mate as a spotter. Try each of the strength exercises listed in Box 7.3, and provide your personal comments on how they felt and areas of needed improvement.

Flexibility Exercise	How This Strength Exercise Felt to You	Improvement in This Area Is Needed (Check "yes" or "no").
1. Lat pull-down		❏ Yes ❏ No
2. Leg press		❏ Yes ❏ No
3. Bench press		❏ Yes ❏ No
4. Abdominal crunch		❏ Yes ❏ No
5. Shoulder press		❏ Yes ❏ No
6. Seated row		❏ Yes ❏ No
7. Leg extension		❏ Yes ❏ No
8. Leg curl		❏ Yes ❏ No
9. Biceps curl		❏ Yes ❏ No
10. Triceps pushdown		❏ Yes ❏ No
11. Standing heel raise		❏ Yes ❏ No

CHAPTER 7 QUIZ

An Exercise Program for Total Fitness

Note: Answers are given at the end of the quiz.

1. The first step of a good warm-up is:
   A. stretching.
   B. low-intensity aerobic activity.
   C. resistance training.
   D. isometrics.

2. If a 30-year old individual has a maximal heart rate of 185 and a resting heart rate of 65, what is the heart rate reserve?
   A. 135
   B. 120
   C. 250
   D. 220

3. The exercise pulse is best counted using the _____ artery:
   A. radial
   B. carotid
   C. aorta
   D. femoral

4. Which mode listed below does not improve aerobic fitness to a significant level?
   A. weight lifting
   B. running
   C. cross-country skiing
   D. bicycling
   E. swimming

5. There are three major principles of weight training. Which one listed below is NOT included?
   A. specificity
   B. overload principle
   C. Valsalva's maneuver
   D. progressive resistance principle

6. What is the recommended rating of perceived exertion (RPE) during exercise training for the average person?
   A. very hard
   B. very, very hard
   C. somewhat hard
   D. very light
   E. light

7. To develop and maintain cardiorespiratory fitness, people should exercise at an intensity of 40/50–85% heart rate reserve for _____ minutes a session, 3–5 days a week.
    A. 10–15
    B. 30–75
    C. 5–30
    D. 20–60*
    E. 40–80

8. What is the estimated maximal heart rate of a 39-year-old man?
    A. 145
    B. 165
    C. 181
    D. 143

9. A minimum muscular strength and endurance program involves 2–4 sets, 8–12 repetitions of 8–10 different weight lifting exercises conducted at least days a week.
    A. 4–5
    B. 3–6
    C. 2–3
    D. 5–7
    E. 1–2

10. Three women, each 35 years of age, train at a heart rate of 150 bpm, 30 minutes/session, 5 days a week. One cycles, one runs, and the other uses a rowing machine. Which one will develop the best aerobic fitness?
    A. woman who cycles
    B. woman who runs
    C. woman who rows
    D. All will develop the same level of heart and lung fitness.
    E. None will improve their fitness because their training program is too easy.

11. A basic stretching program be followed at least 2–3 days a week, and involve 2–4 repetitions of several static stretches that are held _____ seconds.
    A. 1–5
    B. 10–30
    C. 45–60
    D. 60–120

chapter eight

Nutrition, Health, and Physical Performance

"Get a copy of the Food Guide Pyramid, and paste it on your refrigerator. By following this handy, simple guide, you'll reduce your risk of heart disease, stroke, cancer, and diabetes."
—Dr. Richard Deckelbaum of the American Heart Association

Introduction

Perhaps you are familiar with the adage proclaiming that "what you eat today will be walking and talking tomorrow." Day-to-day food choices indeed have much to do with how we live . . . and die. In the short term, the foods we eat provide the nutrients that build and maintain our bodies and fuel our daily activities. In the long term, daily food choices have a significant impact on our risk of developing major chronic diseases.

Your diet—the amount and type of food you typically eat—is influenced by many factors, including your cultural background and personal food preferences. On average, however, Americans tend to eat too much energy in the form of fat, especially the hard saturated fat commonly found in animal products. We also have diets too low in starch and fiber, found in plant foods like whole grains, fruits, and vegetables. Such dietary patterns help explain why Americans have high rates of obesity, heart disease, high blood pressure, stroke, diabetes, and certain forms of cancer.

Nutrition is the science that looks at how the foods we eat affect the functioning and health of our bodies. Although research into the relationship between diet and health is ongoing, scientists have identified the nutrients necessary for good health, and the foods that provide them. In this chapter, we'll focus on the key dietary guidelines for eating smart to maintain lifelong health and fitness. Before turning to these guidelines, however, let's look at a few basic nutrition concepts.

Nutrition Basics

The foods you eat contain a variety of compounds that provide energy, build and maintain organs and tissues, and regulate life-sustaining body functions. The energy in food is measured in kilocalories—one kilocalorie represents the amount of heat needed to raise one kilogram of water from 14.5°C to 15.5°C. In common usage, the term Calorie is used in place of kilocalorie to represent the amount of energy in food, even though a

Calorie is actually a much smaller unit of energy. In this text, we'll use the common term Calorie to refer to the energy content of foods. Most American adults consume between 1600 and 2500 Calories per day.

Essential Nutrients

For good health, your body needs adequate amounts of all the essential nutrients—the nutrients that your body cannot make on its own and thus must obtain from foods. There are more than 40 essential nutrients, classified into six groups: carbohydrates, fats, proteins, vitamins, minerals, and water. Three groups of essential nutrients supply energy:

- **Carbohydrates** are compounds made up of carbon, hydrogen, and oxygen; they are a main source of energy for the body, providing 4 Calories per gram. Carbohydrates are typically classified into two groups: simple sugars, which are made up of one or two basic sugar units, and complex carbohydrates, or starches, which are made up of long chains of sugar units. Carbohydrates are found in grains, fruits, vegetables, and milk.
- **Fats** are the most energy-rich of the nutrients, providing 9 Calories per gram. Fats have other functions in addition to providing energy: They enhance the aroma and flavor of foods, contribute to feelings of fullness, and transport certain vitamins; in the body, fats cushion the body's vital organs and help make up cell membranes. Fats are found in animal tissues and in some plants, including grains, nuts, and seeds.
- **Proteins** are made up of long strands of amino acids, compounds that contain carbon, hydrogen, oxygen, and nitrogen. Proteins form important parts of all the cells and tissues in your body, including skin, muscles, bones, and organs; as enzymes, hormones, and immune cells, proteins help regulate body processes, and protect you from infection. Proteins can also supply energy; like carbohydrates, they provide 4 Calories per gram. Proteins are found in animal foods, legumes, nuts, and grains.

Alcohol, although not an essential nutrient, also supplies energy at 7 Calories per gram.

The recommended breakdown of daily energy intake is 45 to 65 percent of total Calories from carbohydrate, 20 to 35 percent of total Calories from fat, and 10 to 35 percent of total Calories from protein (Figure 8.1). This breakdown is advocated for Americans of all activity levels, including sedentary people, fitness enthusiasts, and nearly all types of competitive athletes. (Sports nutrition principles, including carbohydrates and protein needs of athletes, will be reviewed later in the chapter).

The other classes of essential nutrients do not supply energy, but they perform many other critical functions in the body:

- **Vitamins** are organic (carbon-containing) substances that are present in minute amounts in foods. Vitamins are essential to the body because they promote specific chemical reactions in cells, reactions involved in such key processes as digestion, muscular movement, tissue growth, wound healing, and the production of energy. Vitamins

FIGURE 8.1
The healthy diet is primarily carbohydrate, with a moderate amount of fat and protein.

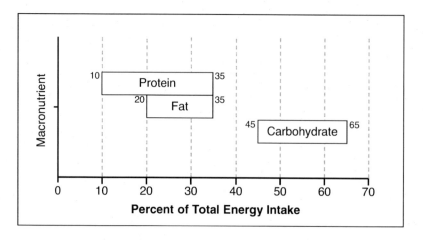

are classified as either water soluble or fat soluble, depending on whether they dissolve in water or fat; solubility affects how vitamins are transported and stored in your body. The fat-soluble vitamins are vitamins A, D, E, and K; the water-soluble vitamins are vitamin C and the B-complex vitamins. Refer to Table 8.1 for more information about the recommended intake levels and good food sources of specific vitamins.

TABLE 8.1   Recommended intakes and food sources vitamins and minerals.

Nutrient (other names)	Recommended Dietary Allowance (RDA)	Daily Value (DV)	Good Sources	Upper Level (UL)	Selected Adverse Effects
Vitamins					
Vitamin A (retinol)	Women: 700µ g Men: 900µ g	5,000 IU* (1,500 µ g)	Liver, fatty fish, fortified foods (milk, breakfast cereals, etc.)	10,000 IU (3,000 µ g)	*Liver toxicity, birth defects.* Inconclusive; bone loss
Carotenoids (alph-carotene, beta-carotene, beta-cryptoxanthin, lutein, lycopene, zeaxanthin)	None. (NAS advises eating more cartotenoid-rich fruits and vegetables)	None	Orange fruits & vegetable (alpha- and beta-carotene), green leafy vegetables (beta-carotene and lutein), tomatoes (lycopene)	None. Panel said don't take beta-carotene, except to get RDA for vitamin A	Smokers who took high doses of beta-carotene supplements (33,000–50,000 IU a day) had higher risk of lung cancer
Thiamin (vitamin B₁)	Women: 1.1 mg Men: 1.2 mg	1.5 mg	Breads, cereals, pasta, & foods made with "enriched" or whole-grain flour; pork	None	None reported
Riboflavin (vitamin B₂)	Women: 1.1 mg Men: 1.3 mg	1.7 mg	Milk, yogurt, foods made with "enriched" or whole-grain flour	None	None reported
Niacin (vitamin B₃)	Women: 14 mg Men: 16 mg	20 mg	Meat, poultry, seafood, foods made with "enriched" or whole-grain flour	35 mg†	*Flushing (burning, tingling, itching redness), liver damage*
Vitamin B₆ (pyridoxine)	Ages 19–50: 1.3 mg Women 50+: 1.5 mg Men 50+: 1.7 mg	2 mg	Meat, poultry, seafood, fortified foods (cereals, etc.), liver	100 mg	*Reversible nerve damage (burning, shooting, tingling pains, numbness, etc.)*
Vitamin B₁₂ (cobalamin)	2.4 µ g	6 µ g	Meat, poultry, seafood, dairy foods, fortified foods (cereals, etc.)	None	None reported
Folate (folacin, folic acid)	400 µ g	400 µ g (0.4 mg)	Orange juice, beans, other fruits & vegetables, fortified cereals, foods made with "enriched" or whole-grain flour	1,000 mg† (1mg)	*Can mask or precipitate a B₁₂ deficiency, which can cause irreversible nerve damage*
Vitamin C (ascorbic acid)	Women: 75 mg Men: 90 mg (Smokers: add 35 mg)	60 mg	Citrus & other fruits, vegetables, fortified foods (cereals, etc.)	2,000 mg	*Diarrhea*
Vitamin D	Ages 19–50: 200 IU‡ Ages 51–70: 400 IU‡ Over 70: 600 IU‡	400 IU	Sunlight, fatty fish, fortified foods (milk, breakfast cereals, etc).	2,000 IU	*High blood calcium, which may cause kidney and heart damage*

Nutrient (other names)	Recommended Dietary Allowance (RDA)	Daily Value (DV)	Good Sources	Upper Level (UL)	Selected Adverse Effects
Vitamin E (alpha-tocopherol)	15 mg (33 IU—synthetic) (22 IU—natural)	30 IU (synthetic)	Oils, whole grains, nut	1,000 mg[†] (1,100 IU—synthetic) (1,500 IU—natural)	*Hemorrage* May lower risk of
Vitamin K (phylloquinone)	Women: 90 μ g[‡] Men: 120 μ g[‡]	80 μ g	Green leafy vegetables, oils	None	Interferes with coumadin & other anti-clotting drugs
Calcium	Ages; 19–50: 1,000 mg[3] Over 50: 1,200 mg[3]	1,000 mg	Dairy foods, fortified foods, leafy green vegetables, canned fish (eaten with bones)	2,500 mg	*High blood calcium,* which may cause kidney damage, kidney stones
Chromium	Women: 25 μ g Men: 35μ g	120 μ g	Whole grains, bran cereals, meat, poultry, seafood	None	Inconclusive: kidney or muscle damage
Copper	900 μ g	2 mg (2,000 μ g)	Liver, seafood, nuts, seeds, wheat-bran, whole grains, chocolate	10 mg (10,000 μ g)	*Liver damage*
Iron	Women 19–50: 18 mg Women 50+: 8 mg Men: 8 mg	18 mg	Red meat, poultry, seafood, foods made with "enriched" or whole-grain flour	45 mg	*Gastrointestinal effects (constipation, nausea, diarrhea)*
Magnesium	Women: 320 mg Men: 420 mg	400 mg	Green leafy vegetables; whole-grain breads, cereals, etc.; nuts	350 mg[†]	*Diarrhea*
Phosphorus	700 mg	1,000 mg	Dairy foods, meat, poultry, seafood, foods (processed cheese, colas, etc.) made with phosphate additives	Ages 19–70: 4,000 mg Over 70: 3,000 mg	*High blood phosphorus,* which may damage kidneys and bones
Selenium	55 μ g	70 μ g	Seafood, meat, poultry, grains (depends on levels in soil)	400 μ g	Nail or hair loss or brittleness
Zinc	Women: 8 mg Men: 11 mg	15 mg	Red meat, seafood, whole grains, fortified foods (cereals, etc.)	40 mg	*Lower copper levels,* HDL ("good") cholesterol, and immune response

Note: Recommended dietary allowance (RDA). RDAs for adults only.

Daily value (DV). These levels appear on food and supplement labels. Unlike the RDAs, there's only one daily value for everyone over age 4.

Tolerable upper intake level (UL). These levels are upper safe daily limits. ULs for adults only.

Selected adverse effects. What happens if you take too much. *The UL is based on fire adverse effect listed in italics.* "Inconclusive" adverse effects are based inconsistent or sketchy evidence.

Other tolerable upper intake levels.

Boron: 20 mg	Manganese: 11 mg
Choline: 3.5 g	Molybdenum: 2,000 μ g (2 mg)
Flouride: 10 mg	Nickel: 1 mg
Iodine: 1,100 μ g (1.1 mg)	Vanadium: 1.8 mg

[*]We get vitamin A both from retinol and carotenoids, but this number assumes that all of the vitamin A comes from retinol.
[†]From supplements and fortified foods only.
[‡]Adequate intake (AI). The National Academy of Sciences (NAS) had too little data to set an RDA.

Source: Food and Nutrition Information Center, www.nal.usda.gov/fnic

- **Minerals** are inorganic (non-carbon-containing) substances that represent a small but important fraction of the weight of your body (about five pounds). Minerals are a part of many cells and tissues, including your bones, teeth, and nails. Like vitamins, minerals can also promote chemical reactions and regulate body processes. Major minerals, those present in the body in amounts greater that 5 grams, include calcium, phosphorus, magnesium, sodium, chloride, and potassium. The dozen or so trace minerals, present in the body in amounts less than 5 grams, include iron and zinc. Table 8.1 gives recommended intake levels and good food sources of key minerals.
- Water makes up about 60 percent of your body's weight and has many important functions. Water serves as a solvent and a lubricant, provides a medium for transporting key chemicals, participates in chemical reactions, and aids in the control of body temperature. Water balance is critical for health and exercise performance. You need about 8 cups of water or other liquids each day; fluid needs of physically active individuals will be described later in the chapter. Water is found in fruits, vegetables, and other liquids.

Guidelines for Nutrient Intake: Recommended Dietary Allowances (RDAs) and Dietary References Intakes (DRIs)

As stated earlier, an adequate intake of all essential nutrients is necessary for the proper functioning of the body. What exactly is an adequate intake? For more than 50 years, the Food and Nutrition Board of the National Academy of Sciences has been reviewing nutrition research and defining nutrient requirements for healthy people. Until recently, one set of nutrient intake levels reigned supreme: the **Recommended Dietary Allowances (RDAs).** When the RDAs were first created in 1941, their primary goal was to prevent diseases caused by vitamin and mineral deficiencies. If a vitamin or mineral is lacking in the diet, characteristic symptoms of deficiency develop based on the particular role that vitamin or mineral plays in the body. For example, an inadequate supply of vitamin C can result in scurvy, a collection of symptoms that includes excessive bleeding, loose teeth, and swollen gums. Fortunately, diseases caused by vitamin and mineral deficiencies are now rare in the United States and other developed nations.

Since the development of the RDAs, scientists have discovered that certain vitamins and minerals are important not just for preventing deficiency diseases but also for preventing chronic diseases such as heart disease, cancer, high blood pressure, diabetes, and osteoporosis. Because the RDAs were not designed to consider these common chronic diseases, the Food and Nutrition Board developed an ambitious plan for revamping the old RDAs. The new standards, known as the **Dietary Reference Intakes (DRIs),** include intakes for optimal health based on the prevention of both deficiencies *and* chronic diseases. The new focus on chronic diseases has led to increased intake recommendations for some nutrients. For example, the recommended intake for calcium has been raised for both men and women to reflect new research on the link between calcium intake and reduced risk of osteoporosis. The **RDA/DRI** is defined as "the average daily dietary nutrient intake level sufficient to meet the nutrient requirement of nearly all health individuals." The new DRIs also include the **Tolerable Upper Intake Level (UL),** defined as the highest average daily nutrient intake level that is likely to pose no risk of adverse health effects to most individuals. The RDA/DRI and UL levels for key nutrients are summarized in Table 8.1.

As a general rule, most Americans don't need vitamin and mineral supplements for good health, and pills and capsules are no substitute for healthy dietary habits. Supplements of some nutrients, if taken regularly in large amounts, can be harmful; some nutrients are directly toxic if taken in excess; large doses of nutrients can also cause problems by interfering with the absorption of other vitamins and minerals. In part because of concerns about people taking high doses of supplements, the DRIs also include standards for upper intake limits, the highest level of daily nutrient intake that is likely to pose no risks of adverse health effects to most individuals. (The use of supplements and performance aids by fitness enthusiasts and athletes will be discussed later in the chapter).

BOX 8.1

Web Links for Nutrition

- Government Health Web Site *http://www.health.gov*
  www.health.gov is a portal to the Web sites of a number of multi-agency health initiatives and activities of the U.S. Department of Health and Human Services (HHS) and other Federal departments and agencies.
- Tufts University Nutrition Navigator *http://navigator.tufts.edu*
  Provides a rating of the accuracy of nutrition content and usability of nutrition Web sites.
- Mayo Health Oasis *http://www.mayohealth.org*
  Provides consumers with good nutrition information in a fun, user-friendly format.
- Consumer Information Center *http://www.pueblo.gsa.gov*
  Provides access to hundreds of educational materials.
- U.S. Food and Drug Administration (FDA) *www.fda.gov*
  Provides government updates on food and nutrition issues, and basic nutrition guidelines.
- Meals for You (My Menus) *http://www.MealsForYou.com*
  Provides thousands of recipes with menu plans, shopping lists, and nutritional analysis.
- USDA Food and Nutrition Information Center *http://www.fnic.nal.usda.gov*
  Connects readers to the vast nutrition-related resources of the National Agricultural Library.
- Healthfinder *http://www.healthfinder.gov*
  Organizes the health and nutrition information from federal and state agencies.
- Vegetarian Resource Group *http://www.vrg.org*
  Provides nutrition information and recipes for those interested in the vegetarian diet.
- American Dietetic Association *http://www.eatright.org*
  A link for nutrition information for both consumers and dietitians.
- Cyberdiet *http://www.cyberdiet.com*
  Gives information on foods, recipes, vitamins and minerals, and food planning.

The first group of DRIs was released in 1997; additional reports were released through the year 2003. For more information on the DRIs, visit the Web site of the Food and Nutrition Board (see Box 8.1 Web Links for Nutrition" for this and other helpful nutrition-related sites). See Table 8.1 to review the current RDA/DRI levels. Daily Values represent the standards for nutrient intake currently used in food labels.

Dietary Guidelines for Health and Disease Prevention

All individuals, whether sedentary or very active, should consume a prudent diet to enhance quality of life and prevent disease. For our purposes in this text, a prudent diet is one that conforms to the *Dietary Guidelines for Americans,* developed by the U.S. Department of Agriculture (USDA), as well as the nutrition recommendations from the National Research Council, the American Heart Association, and the American Cancer Society. Let's take a closer look at the major guidelines in the *Dietary Guidelines for Americans.*

The *2005 Dietary Guidelines* seek to lower risk of chronic disease and promote health through 9 focus areas. Taken together, these focus areas encourage Americans to eat fewer calories, be more active, and make wiser food choices. Here are the 9 focus areas (key recommendations will be listed in the focus area sections that follow):

1. Weight Managment
2. Physical Activity
3. Food Groups to Encourage
4. Carbohydrates
5. Food Safety
6. Fats
7. Adequate Nutrients within Calorie Needs
8. Sodium and Potassium
9. Alcoholic Beverage

Weight Management and Physical Activity

Key Recommendations

- To maintain body weight in a healthy range, balance calories from foods and beverages with calories expended.
- To prevent gradual weight gain over time, make small decreases in food and beverage calories and increase physical activity.
- Engage in regular physical activity and reduce sedentary activities to promote health, psychological well-being, and a healthy body weight.
  - To reduce the risk of chronic disease in adulthood: Engage in at least 30 minutes of moderate-intensity physical activity, above usual activity, at work or home on most days of the week.
  - For most people, greater health benefits can be obtained by engaging in physical activity of more vigorous intensity or longer duration.
  - To help manage body weight and prevent gradual, unhealthy body weight gain in adulthood: Engage in approximately 60 minutes of moderate- to vigorous-intensity activity on most days of the week while not exceeding caloric intake requirements.
  - To sustain weight loss in adulthood: Participate in at least 60 to 90 minutes of daily moderate-intensity physical activity while not exceeding caloric intake requirements. Some people may need to consult with a healthcare provider before participating in this level of activity.
  - Achieve physical fitness by including cardiovascular conditioning, stretching exercises for flexibility, and resistance exercises or calisthenics for muscle strength and endurance.

Obesity rates in the United States doubled during the past quarter century. Eating fewer calories while increasing physical activity are the keys to controlling body weight. Caloric intake is about 250 calories/day higher than it was in 1970. Table 8.2 summarizes current intakes with recommended levels for energy and important nutrients.

Americans tend to be relatively inactive. One in four adult Americans do not participate in any leisure time physical activities, and 4 in 10 students in grades 9 to 12 view television 3 or more hours per day. To reduce the risk of chronic disease, it is recommended that adults engage in at least 30 minutes of moderate-intensity physical activity on most, preferably all, days of the week. For most people, greater health benefits can be obtained by engaging in physical activity of more vigorous intensity or of longer duration.

Regular physical activity is also a key factor in achieving and maintaining a healthy body weight for adults and children. To prevent the gradual accumulation of excess weight in adulthood, approximately 60 minutes of moderate- to vigorous-intensity physical activity on most days of the week may be needed. While moderate-intensity physical activity can achieve the desired goal, vigorous-intensity physical activity generally provides more

TABLE 8.2 Current American Adult (ages 20–39 years) Dietary Intake Compared to Recommended Levels

	Males	Females	Recommended
Energy (Calories)	2,825	2,028	Varies*
Carbohydrate (% total energy)	50.0	52.6	45–65
Fat (% total energy)	32.1	32.3	20–35
Saturated fat (% total energy)	10.8	10.9	<10
Protein (% total energy)	14.9	14.6	10–35
Alcohol (% total energy)	2.6	1.4	Not established
Dietary fiber (g/day)	18.6	13.9	M: 38; F: 25
Cholesterol (mg/day)	350	241	<300
Sodium (mg/day)	4,329	3,161	<2,300
Antioxidants			
Vitamin A (μ g/day RAE)	878	961	M: 900; F: 700
Vitamin C (mg/day)	102	85	M: 90; F: 75
Vitamin E (mg/day α-T)	10.4	8.2	15
Vitamin B_6 (mg/day)	2.2	1.6	1.3; 50+ yr, M 1.7, F 1.5
Folate (μ g /day DFE)	435	327	400
Calcium (mg/day)	1025	797	1,000; 50+ yr, 1,200
Iron (mg/day)	17.9	13.7	M: 8; F: 18, 50+ yr, 8
Zinc (mg/day)	14.8	10.1	M: 11; F: 8

*Energy needs vary according to body size and physical activity, with the RDA average set at 2,900 Calories for males, and 2,200 for females. There is evidence that energy intake is underestimated in national surveys. Nonetheless, obesity prevalence is increasing which means that Americans tend to take in more energy than they expend.

RAE = retinol activity equivalent, DFE = dietary folate equivalents

Source: USDA's Continuing Survey of Food Intakes by Individuals. (Can be downloaded via the Internet at: www.barc.usda. gov/bhnrc/foodsurvey/home htm.)

benefits than moderate-intensity physical activity. Control of caloric intake is also advisable. However, to sustain weight loss for previously overweight/obese people, about 60 to 90 minutes of moderate-intensity physical activity per day is recommended.

The barrier often given for a failure to be physically active is lack of time. Setting aside 30 to 60 consecutive minutes each day for planned exercise is one way to obtain physical activity, but it is not the only way. Physical activity may include short bouts (e.g., 10-minute bouts) of moderate-intensity activity. The accumulated total is what is important—both for health and for burning calories. Physical activity can be accumulated through three to six 10-minute bouts over the course of a day. Elevating the level of daily physical activity may also provide indirect nutritional benefits. A sedentary lifestyle limits the number of calories that can be consumed without gaining weight. The higher a person's physical activity level, the higher his or her energy requirement and the easier it is to plan a daily food intake pattern that meets recommended nutrient requirements.

Food Groups to Encourage

Key Recommendations

- Consume a sufficient amount of fruits and vegetables while staying within energy needs. Two cups of fruit and 2½ cups of vegetables per day are recommended for a reference 2,000-calorie intake, with higher or lower amounts depending on the calorie level.
- Choose a variety of fruits and vegetables each day. In particular, select from all 5 vegetable subgroups (dark green, orange, legumes, starchy vegetables, and other vegetables) several times a week.
- Consume 3 or more ounce-equivalents of whole-grain products per day, with the rest of the recommended grains coming from enriched or whole-grain products. In general, at least half the grains should come from whole grains.
- Consume 3 cups per day of fat-free or low-fat milk or equivalent milk products.

The *MyPyramid Food Guidance System* provides food-based guidance to help implement the recommendations of the *Guidelines* (see Figure 8.2). *MyPyramid* provides specific recommendations for making food choices that will improve the quality of an average American diet. Taken together, they would result in the following changes from a typical diet:

- Increased intake of vitamins, minerals, dietary fiber, and other essential nutrients, especially of those that are often low in typical diets.
- Lowered intake of saturated fats, *trans* fats, and cholesterol and increased intake of fruits, vegetables, and whole grains to decrease risk for some chronic diseases.
- Calorie intake balanced with energy needs to prevent weight gain and/or promote a healthy weight.

Consuming an appropriate number of servings from each food group is important because foods from different groups tend to provide different essential nutrients. Grains and cereals should form the basis of each meal, supplemented with liberal servings of vegetables and fruit, and low-fat servings of meat and dairy products. Box 8.2 summarizes the suggested amounts of food to consume from the basic food groups, subgroups, and oils in *MyPyramid* to meet recommended nutrient intakes at 12 different calorie levels.

Within each group, foods vary in the amount of nutrients and calories they provide. Daily food choices should emphasize nutrient-dense foods, those that are high in nutrients relative to the amount of calories they contain. Within the breads and cereals food group, for example, a slice of whole-wheat bread has more nutrients and fiber, and fewer calories, than a croissant.

Fruits, vegetables, whole grains, and milk products are all important to a healthful diet and can be good sources of key nutrients. When increasing intake of fruits, vegetables, whole grains, and fat free or low fat milk and milk products, it is important to decrease one's intake of less nutrient dense foods to control calorie intake.

Carbohydrates

Key Recommendations

- Choose fiber-rich fruits, vegetables, and whole grains often.
- Choose and prepare foods and beverages with little added sugars or caloric sweeteners, such as amounts suggested by the USDA *MyPyramid.*
- Reduce the incidence of dental caries by practicing good oral hygiene and consuming sugar- and starch-containing foods and beverages less frequently.

Carbohydrates are part of a healthful diet. The recommended intake of carbohydrates is 45 to 65 percent of total calories. For an individual eating 2,000 calories a day, this would be 900 to 1,300 calories or 225 to 325 grams of carbohydrate (divide by 4, the number of calories per gram of carbohydrate). American male and female adults consume 50 and 53 percent of calories from carbohydrate, respectively (Table 8.2). Much of this carbohydrate is in the form of processed sugar instead of the preferable plant starch.

It is important to choose carbohydrates wisely. Carbohydrates come in 2 forms: simple and complex. Simple carbohydrates are sugars found within many foods like fruits, vegetables, and milk, and in concentrated form like processed sugars and honey. Complex carbohydrates are plant starches often found in wheat, rice, oats, and corn. Dietary fiber is a type of carbohydrate only found in plants that cannot be digested in the human intestinal tract. Grains and cereals are major sources of both starch and fiber. Whole grain products contain all of the original fiber while refined grain products have had it removed through processing procedures.

Foods in the basic food groups that provide carbohydrates—fruits, vegetables, grains, and milk—are important sources of many nutrients. Choosing plenty of these foods, within the context of a calorie-controlled diet, can promote health and reduce chronic disease risk. However, the greater the consumption of foods containing large amounts of

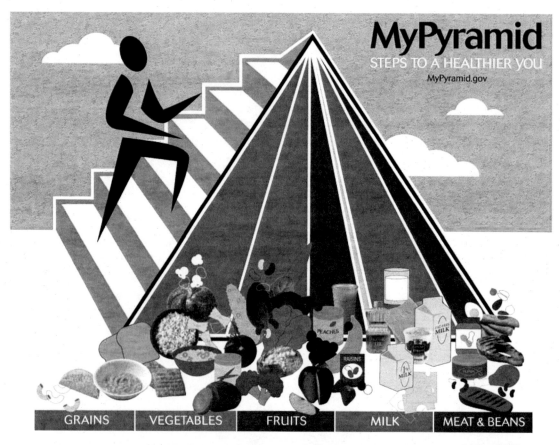

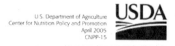

FIGURE 8.2

Food guide pyramid: A guide to healthy food choices. The food guide pyramid emphasizes that bread, cereals, rice, and pasta be included with each meal, and should form the foundation of a healthy diet. At least five servings of fruit and vegetables each day are recommended, supplemented with low-fat choices of dairy and meat products. *Source:* United States Department of Agriculture, The food guide pyramid. *Home and Garden Bulletin* 252, 1992.

BOX 8.2

Food Guide Pyramid: What Is a Serving?

MyPyramid

Food Intake Patterns

The suggested amounts of food to consume from the basic food groups, subgroups, and oils to meet recommended nutrient intakes at 12 different calorie levels. Nutrient and energy contributions from each group are calculated according to the nutrient-dense forms of foods in each group (e.g., lean meats and fat-free milk). The table also shows the discretionary calorie allowance that can be accommodated within each calorie level, in addition to the suggested amounts of nutrient-dense forms of foods in each group.

Daily Amount of Food From Each Group

Calorie Level[1]	1,000	1,200	1,400	1,600	1,800	2,000	2,200	2,400	2,600	2,800	3,000	3,200
Fruits[2]	1 cup	1 cup	1.5 cups	1.5 cups	1.5 cups	2 cups	2 cups	2 cups	2 cups	2.5 cups	2.5 cups	2.5 cups
Vegetables[3]	1 cup	1.5 cups	1.5 cups	2 cups	2.5 cups	2.5 cups	3 cups	3 cups	3.5 cups	3.5 cups	4 cups	4 cups
Grains[4]	3 oz-eq	4 oz-eq	5 oz-eq	5 oz-eq	6 oz-eq	6 oz-eq	7 oz-eq	8 oz-eq	9 oz-eq	10 oz-eq	10 oz-eq	10 oz-eq
Meat and Beans[5]	2 oz-eq	3 oz-eq	4 oz-eq	5 oz-eq	5 oz-eq	5.5 oz-eq	6 oz-eq	6.5 oz-eq	6.5 oz-eq	7 oz-eq	7 oz-eq	7 oz-eq
Milk[6]	2 cups	2 cups	2 cups	3 cups	3 cups	3 cups	3 cups	3 cups	3 cups	3 cups	3 cups	3 cups
Oils[7]	3 tsp	4 tsp	4 tsp	5 tsp	5 tsp	6 tsp	6 tsp	7 tsp	8 tsp	8 tsp	10 tsp	11 tsp
Discretionary calorie allowance[8]	165	171	171	132	195	267	290	362	410	426	512	648

1 **Calorie Levels** are set across a wide range to accommodate the needs of different individuals. The attached table "Estimated Daily Calorie Needs" can be used to help assign individuals to the food intake pattern at a particular calorie level.

2 **Fruit Group** includes all fresh, frozen, canned, and dried fruits and fruit juices. In general, 1 cup of fruit or 100% fruit juice, or 1/2 cup of dried fruit can be considered as 1 cup from the fruit group.

3 **Vegetable Group** includes all fresh, frozen, canned, and dried vegetables and vegetable juices. In general, 1 cup of raw or cooked vegetables or vegetable juice, or 2 cups of raw leafy greens can be considered as 1 cup from the vegetable group.

Vegetable Subgroup Amounts are Per Week

Calorie Level	1,000	1,200	1,400	1,600	1,800	2,000	2,200	2,400	2,600	2,800	3,000	3,200
Dark green veg.	1 c/wk	1.5 c/wk	1.5 c/wk	2 c/wk	3 c/wk	3 c/wk	3 c/wk	3 c/wk	3 c/wk	3 c/wk	3 c/wk	3 c/wk
Orange veg.	.5 c/wk	1 c/wk	1 c/wk	1.5 c/wk	2 c/wk	2 c/wk	2 c/wk	2 c/wk	2.5 c/wk	2.5 c/wk	2.5 c/wk	2.5 c/wk
Legumes	.5 c/wk	1 c/wk	1 c/wk	2.5 c/wk	3 c/wk	3 c/wk	3 c/wk	3 c/wk	3.5 c/wk	3.5 c/wk	3.5 c/wk	3.5 c/wk
Starchy veg.	1.5 c/wk	2.5 c/wk	2.5 c/wk	2.5 c/wk	3 c/wk	3 c/wk	6 c/wk	6 c/wk	7 c/wk	7 c/wk	9 c/wk	9 c/wk
Other veg.	3.5 c/wk	4.5 c/wk	4.5 c/wk	5.5 c/wk	6.5 c/wk	6.5 c/wk	7 c/wk	7 c/wk	8.5 c/wk	8.5 c/wk	10 c/wk	10 c/wk

4 **Grains Group** includes all foods made from wheat, rice, oats, cornmeal, barley, such as bread, pasta, oatmeal, breakfast cereals, tortillas, and grits. In general, 1 slice of bread, 1 cup of ready-to-eat cereal, or 1/2 cup of cooked rice, pasta, or cooked cereal can be considered as 1 ounce equivalent from the grains group. **At least half of all grains consumed should be whole grains.**

5 **Meat & Beans Group** in general, 1 ounce of lean meat, poultry, or fish, 1 egg, 1 Tbsp. peanut butter, 1/4 cup cooked dry beans, or 1/2 ounce of nuts or seeds can be considered as 1 ounce equivalent from the meat and beans group.

6 **Milk Group** includes all fluid milk products and foods made from milk that retain their calcium content, such as yogurt and cheese. Foods made from milk that have little to no calcium, such as cream cheese, cream, and butter, are not part of the group. Most milk group choices should be fat-free or low-fat. In general, 1 cup of milk or yogurt, 1 1/2 ounces of natural cheese, or 2 ounces of processed cheese can be considered as 1 cup from the milk group.

7 **Oils** include fats from many different plants and from fish that are liquid at room temperature, such as canola, corn, olive, soybean, and sunflower oil. Some foods are naturally high in oils, like nuts, olives, some fish, and avocados. Foods that are mainly oil include mayonnaise, certain salad dressings, and soft margarine.

8 **Discretionary Calorie Allowance** is the remaining amount of calories in a food intake pattern after accounting for the calories needed for all food groups—using forms of foods that are fat-free or low-fat and with no added sugars.

Estimated Daily Calorie Needs

To determine which food intake pattern to use for an individual, the following chart gives an estimate of individual calorie needs. The calorie range for each age/sex group is based on physical activity level, from sedentary to active.

	Calorie Range		
Children	**Sedentary**	→	**Active**
2–3 years	1,000	→	1,400
Females			
4–8 years	1,200	→	1,800
9–13	1,600	→	2,200
14–18	1,800	→	2,400
19–30	2,000	→	2,400
31–50	1,800	→	2,200
51+	1,600	→	2,200
Males			
4–8 years	1,400	→	2,000
9–13	1,800	→	2,600
14–18	2,200	→	3,200
19–30	2,400	→	3,000
31–50	2,200	→	3,000
51+	2,000	→	2,800

Sedentary means a lifestyle that includes only the light physical activity associated with typical day-to-day life.

Active means a lifestyle that includes physical activity equivalent to walking more than 3 miles per day at 3 to 4 miles per hour, in addition to the light physical activity associated with typical day-to-day life.

U.S. Department of Agriculture
Center for Nutrition Policy and Promotion
April 2005

added sugars, the more difficult it is to consume enough nutrients without gaining weight. Consumption of added sugars provides calories while providing little, if any, of the essential nutrients.

As mapped out by *MyPyramid,* more servings of grain products should be consumed at each meal than any other type of food, followed by fruits and vegetables. Grains (e.g., pasta, rice, wheat, cereals) should form the center of most meals. By choosing more whole grain products, fruits, and vegetables, intake of total carbohydrate and fiber will increase while intake of total fat, saturated fat, and cholesterol will decrease.

These strategies are recommended by the USDA to incorporate more foods from plant sources into the diet:

- Include grain products, fruits, or vegetables in every meal.
- Choose fruits and vegetables for snacks.
- Choose beans as an alternative to meat.
- Choose whole grains in preference to processed (refined) grains.

Dietary Fiber

Although dietary fiber provides no energy, it has many beneficial actions in the body and promotes a low risk of colon cancer, heart disease, and diabetes. There are 2 kinds of dietary fiber: soluble fiber which is soluble in water and forms a gel, and insoluble fiber which is insoluble in water. Soluble fiber is found in many fruits and vegetables, and in some grains like oats. The sticky residue in the bowl after eating oatmeal is the soluble fiber from the oat bran. Insoluble fiber is found in many vegetables and whole grains (e.g., wheat bran).

Soluble fiber controls the rate of blood glucose absorption in the intestine, promotes lower blood cholesterol levels, and improves the health of the colon. Insoluble fiber increases the rate at which food residue moves through the colon, reducing the risk of colon cancer.

The recommended dietary fiber intake is 14 grams per 1,000 calories consumed. Although male and female adults should consume an average of 38 and 25 grams of dietary fiber each day, respectively, to encourage good health and bowel movements, current intake is about 14 grams/day for females, and 19 grams/day for males (Table 8.2).

Most popular American foods are not high in dietary fiber. Dietary fiber is found solely in plant foods (none in animal-based foods including meats, eggs, and dairy products), and is abundant in legumes, nuts and seeds, whole grains, fresh and dried fruits, and vegetables (see Table 8.3).

The Food Label

In 1990, the Food and Drug Administration (FDA) approved a new procedure for nutrition labeling of processed foods and authorized appropriate health claims (see Figure 8.3). While the old food label emphasized vitamin and mineral content, the new food label focused on the real nutritional shortcomings of Americans, total fat, saturated fat, cholesterol, sodium, dietary fiber, and sugars. The Nutrition Facts food label uses the Daily Values to help consumers plan healthy diets. They serve as the nutrient reference values on the food label, combining information from the RDA/DRI and the *Dietary Guidelines for Americans.* The Daily Values are based on a 2,000 calorie diet, close to the average American intake. A Daily Value of 20 percent for total fat means that a serving of this particular food provides 20 percent of the total fat allowed for the average adult.

An important feature of the FDA's mandate to improve food labels is the regulation of nutrient content claims and health claims. Nutrient content claims describe the amount of nutrient in foods such as "cholesterol free," "low fat," "light," or "lean." These nutrient content claims are now based on precise definitions and specific portion sizes to avoid consumer confusion when comparing one food brand with another. For example, "low fat" means 3 grams of fat or less per serving, and "cholesterol free" indicates less than 2 mg of cholesterol per serving. Health claims that link foods with prevention of certain

TABLE 8.3   Selected Sources and Amounts of Dietary Fiber

Food	Amount	Soluble Fiber, g	Total Fiber, g
Legumes (cooked)			
Black beans	1/2 cup	2.1	7.5
Kidney beans	1/2 cup	2.3	5.7
Pinto beans	1/2 cup	2.7	7.4
Vegetables (cooked)			
Green peas	1/2 cup	1.2	4.4
Butternut winter squash	1/2 cup	0.4	3.4
Brussel sprouts	1/2 cup	1.3	2.9
Broccoli	1/2 cup	1.1	2.3
Zucchini	1/2 cup	0.3	2.3
Corn	1/2 cup	0.1	2.2
Spinach	1/2 cup	0.6	2.2
Green beans	1/2 cup	0.8	2.0
Potato	1/2 cup	0.2	0.9
Fruits (raw)			
Apple	1 medium	1.4	3.7
Orange	1 medium	2.1	3.1
Prunes	1/4 cup	1.3	3.0
Banana	1 medium	1.0	2.8
Blueberries	1/2 cup	0.6	2.0
Raisins	1/4 cup	0.5	1.7
Strawberries	1/2 cup	0.6	1.7
Mango slices	1/2 cup	0.9	1.5
Grapefruit	1/2 medium	0.8	1.3
Grapes	1 cup	0.1	0.8
Grains			
Oat bran (dry)	1/3 cup	2.0	4.4
Raisin bran (dry)	1/2 cup	0.5	3.6
Grape-Nuts (dry)	1/3 cup	2.0	3.6
Oatmeal (cooked)	1/2 cup	1.2	2.0
Whole-wheat bread	1 slice	0.4	1.9
Brown rice (cooked)	1/2 cup	0.2	1.8
Nuts and seeds			
Dry roasted almonds	1 oz	0.4	3.9
Dry roasted sunflower seeds	1 oz	1.0	3.1
Dry roasted peanuts	1 oz	0.6	2.3

Note: Within each category, the foods are listed from high to low in total fiber.

Source: USDA

diseases must be scientifically based. The FDA has approved about a dozen health claims, and these include the benefits of fiber on heart disease and cancer, the connection between diets low in saturated fat and cholesterol with heart disease, low-sodium foods and high blood pressure, fruits and vegetables with cancer, and sugar with dental caries.

Food Safety

Key Recommendations

- To avoid microbial food-borne illness:
  - Clean hands, food contact surfaces, and fruits and vegetables. Meat and poultry should not be washed or rinsed.
  - Separate raw, cooked, and ready-to-eat foods while shopping, preparing, or storing foods.
  - Cook foods to a safe temperature to kill microorganisms.

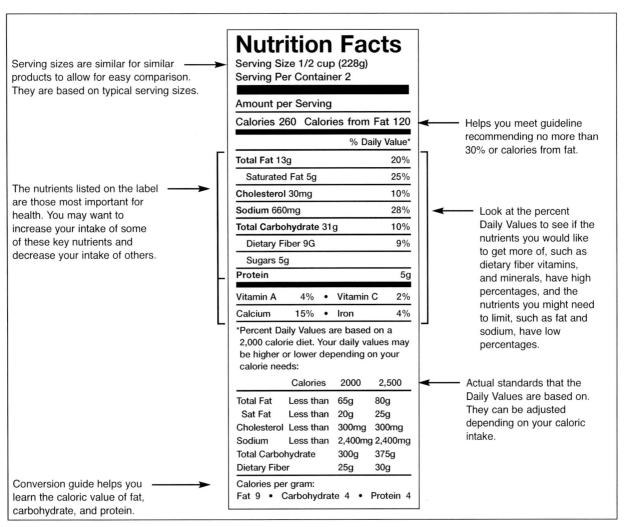

Serving sizes are similar for similar products to allow for easy comparison. They are based on typical serving sizes.

The nutrients listed on the label are those most important for health. You may want to increase your intake of some of these key nutrients and decrease your intake of others.

Conversion guide helps you learn the caloric value of fat, carbohydrate, and protein.

Nutrition Facts

Serving Size 1/2 cup (228g)
Serving Per Container 2

Amount per Serving

Calories 260   Calories from Fat 120

	% Daily Value*
Total Fat 13g	20%
Saturated Fat 5g	25%
Cholesterol 30mg	10%
Sodium 660mg	28%
Total Carbohydrate 31g	10%
Dietary Fiber 9G	9%
Sugars 5g	
Protein	5g

Vitamin A	4%	• Vitamin C	2%
Calcium	15%	• Iron	4%

*Percent Daily Values are based on a 2,000 calorie diet. Your daily values may be higher or lower depending on your calorie needs:

		Calories	2000	2,500
Total Fat	Less than		65g	80g
Sat Fat	Less than		20g	25g
Cholesterol	Less than		300mg	300mg
Sodium	Less than		2,400mg	2,400mg
Total Carbohydrate			300g	375g
Dietary Fiber			25g	30g

Calories per gram:
Fat 9 • Carbohydrate 4 • Protein 4

Helps you meet guideline recommending no more than 30% or calories from fat.

Look at the percent Daily Values to see if the nutrients you would like to get more of, such as dietary fiber vitamins, and minerals, have high percentages, and the nutrients you might need to limit, such as fat and sodium, have low percentages.

Actual standards that the Daily Values are based on. They can be adjusted depending on your caloric intake.

FIGURE 8.3
Guidelines for interpretation of the food label.

- Chill (refrigerate) perishable food promptly and defrost foods properly.
- Avoid raw (unpasteurized) milk or any products made from unpasteurized milk, raw or partially cooked eggs, or foods containing raw eggs, raw or undercooked meat and poultry, unpasteurized juices, and raw sprouts.

Avoiding foods that are contaminated with harmful bacteria, viruses, parasites, toxins, and chemical and physical contaminants are vital for healthful eating. The signs and symptoms of food-borne illness range from gastrointestinal symptoms, such as upset stomach, diarrhea, fever, vomiting, abdominal cramps, and dehydration, to more severe systemic illness, such as paralysis and meningitis. The USDA estimates that every year about 76 million people in the United States become ill from pathogens in food; of these, about 5,000 die. Consumers can take simple measures to reduce their risk of food-borne illness, especially in the home.

Food-borne illness is caused by eating food that contains harmful bacteria, toxins, parasites, viruses, or chemical contaminants. According to the USDA, bacteria and viruses, especially *Campylobacter, Salmonella* and Norwalk-like viruses, are among the most common causes of food-borne illness we know about today. Signs and symptoms after eating just a small portion of an unsafe food may appear within half an hour or may not develop for up to 3 weeks. Pregnant women, young children, older persons, and people with weakened immune systems or certain chronic diseases are at high risk of food-borne illness.

To keep food safe, people who prepare food should clean hands, food contact surfaces, and fruits and vegetables; separate raw, cooked, and ready-to-eat foods; cook foods to a safe internal temperature; chill perishable food promptly; and defrost food properly. For more important information on cooking, cleaning, separating, and chilling, see *www.fightbac.org.* Seven key steps should be followed to keep food safe:

1. Wash hands and surfaces often especially after handling raw meat, poultry, fish, shellfish, or eggs.
2. Separate raw, cooked, and ready-to-eat foods while shopping, preparing or storing.
3. Cook foods to a safe temperature. Reheat sauces, soups, marinades, and gravies to a boil, reheat leftovers thoroughly to at least 165°F, and cook whole poultry to 180°F. The danger zone for bacterial growth is 40°F to 140°F.
4. Refrigerate perishable foods promptly.
5. Serve safely by keeping hot foods hot (140°F or above) and cold foods cold (40°F or below).
6. Check and follow label safety instructions.
7. When in doubt, throw it out.

Fats

Key Recommendations

- Consume less than 10 percent of calories from saturated fatty acids and less than 300 mg/day of cholesterol, and keep *trans* fatty acid consumption as low as possible.
- Keep total fat intake between 20 to 35 percent of calories, with most fats coming from sources of polyunsaturated and monounsaturated fatty acids, such as fish, nuts, and vegetable oils.
- When selecting and preparing meat, poultry, dry beans, and milk or milk products, make choices that are lean, low-fat, or fat-free.
- Limit intake of fats and oils high in saturated and/or *trans* fatty acids, and choose products low in such fats and oils.

The amount and quality of dietary fat has a significant impact on risk of heart disease, cancer, obesity, and other health problems. Diets low in saturated fat and cholesterol decrease risk of heart disease, while high fat diets promote certain types of cancers and obesity.

Most of the fat in food is triglyceride, a molecule made up of 3 units known as fatty acids and 1 unit called glycerol. The fatty acids differ in length and the degree of saturation or the number of hydrogens in the chain.

The saturated fatty acid carries the maximum possible number of hydrogen atoms, with no points of unsaturation (see Figure 8.4). A saturated fat is a triglyceride that contains 3 saturated fatty acids. Saturated fats are found in all types of dietary fats, but are in greatest concentration in red meat, whole milk, butter, and tropical oils (e.g., palm kernel oil, coconut oil). Saturated fats raise blood cholesterol levels and increase the risk of heart disease.

In the monounsaturated fatty acid, there is one point of unsaturation where hydrogens are missing (Figure 8.4). If there are 2 or more points of unsaturation, then it is a polyunsaturated fatty acid. Olive and canola oils are particularly high in monounsaturated fats; most other vegetable oils, nuts, and high-fat fish are good sources of polyunsaturated fats. Both kinds of unsaturated fats reduce blood cholesterol when they replace saturated fats in the diet, and lower risk of heart disease.

American adults average about 32 percent total calories as fat (see Table 8.2). The most common sources of fat include beef, margarine, salad dressings and mayonnaise, oils, and dairy products. About 11 percent of total caloric intake is saturated fat, and more than one-third of the saturated fat Americans consume comes from cheese, beef, and milk.

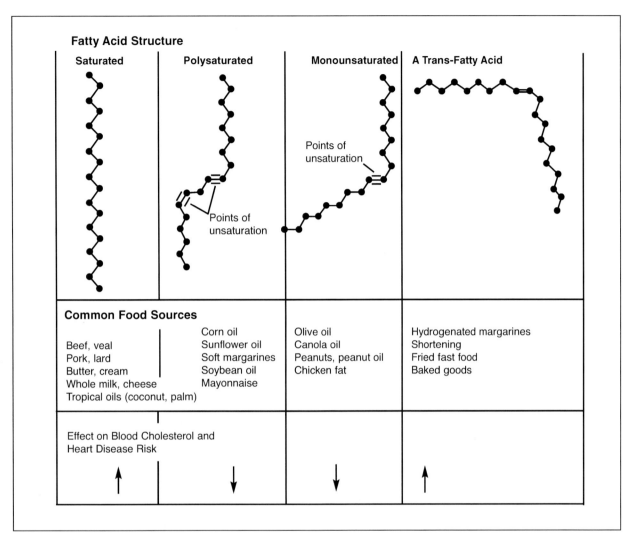

FIGURE 8.4
Fatty acid structure, common food sources, and influence on blood cholesterol levels and heart disease.

To meet the total fat recommendation of 20 to 35 percent of calories, most dietary fats should come from sources of polyunsaturated and monounsaturated fatty acids. The upper limit on the grams of fat in the diet depends on total caloric intake. For example, at 2,000 calories per day, the suggested upper limit for total fat is 700 calories (2,000 × 0.35). This is equal to 78 grams of fat (700 ÷ 9, the number of calories each gram of fat provides). For saturated fat, no more than 200 out of 2,000 calories should be ingested which is 22 grams (200 ÷ 9).

When manufacturers process foods, they often alter the fatty acids in the food through a process called hydrogenation. Hydrogenation is the process of adding hydrogen to unsaturated fatty acids to make fat stay fresher longer, more solid, and less greasy-tasting. Some of the unsaturated fatty acids, instead of becoming saturated during the hydrogenation process, end up changing their shapes into *trans*-fatty acids (Figure 8.4). *Trans*-fatty acids raise blood cholesterol levels, and are found in most margarines, shortening, fast foods like French fries, fried chicken, and fried fish, chips, and baked goods like muffins, cakes, doughnuts, crackers, and pies. *Trans*-fat levels must be listed on food labels, and this may prompt companies to provide products without these types of fats.

Cholesterol is a type of dietary fat found only in animal products. It is a soft waxy substance that is also made in the body for a variety of purposes, including the formation of cell membranes and certain types of hormones. Dietary cholesterol tends to raise blood cholesterol levels, but not as strongly as saturated fat. Cholesterol intake should be below 300 mg/day. Animal products are the source of all dietary cholesterol, egg yolks being one of the richest sources with each containing about 220 mg of cholesterol. Eggs and beef contribute to nearly one-half of all the dietary cholesterol Americans ingest.

Limiting Fat Intake

To limit intake of high-fat foods, especially those containing high amounts of saturated fat, follow these recommendations:

- Replace fat-rich foods with fruits, vegetables, grains, and beans.
- Eat smaller portions of meat and other high-fat foods.
- Choose baked and broiled foods instead of fried foods.
- Select nonfat and low-fat milk and dairy products.
- When eating meat, select lean cuts ("select" or "choice" USDA grade).
- Choose beans, seafood, and poultry as an alternative to beef, pork, and lamb.

Adequate Nutrients within Calorie Needs

Key Recommendations

- Consume a variety of nutrient-dense foods and beverages within and among the basic food groups while choosing foods that limit the intake of saturated and *trans* fats, cholesterol, added sugars, salt, and alcohol.
- Meet recommended intakes within energy needs by adopting a balanced eating pattern, such as the USDA Food Guide or the DASH Eating Plan.

An important goal is to choose meals and snacks that are high in nutrients but low to moderate in energy content. At the same time, limit saturated and *trans* fats, cholesterol, added sugars, and salt. An additional premise of the *Dietary Guidelines* is that the nutrients consumed should come primarily from foods. Foods contain not only the vitamins and minerals that are often found in supplements, but also hundreds of naturally occurring substances, including carotenoids, flavonoids, and isoflavones, and protease inhibitors that may protect against chronic health conditions.

Two examples of eating patterns that exemplify the *Dietary Guidelines* are the DASH Eating Plan and *MyPyramid*. These two similar eating patterns are designed to integrate dietary recommendations into a healthy way to eat and are used in the *Dietary Guidelines* to provide examples of how nutrient-focused recommendations can be expressed in terms of food choices. Both *MyPyramid* and the DASH Eating Plan differ in important ways from common food consumption patterns in the United States. In general, they include:

- *More* dark green vegetables, orange vegetables, legumes, fruits, whole grains, and low-fat milk and milk products.
- *Less* refined grains, total fats (especially cholesterol, and saturated and *trans* fats), added sugars, and calories.

As defined earlier, sugars are classified as simple carbohydrates while starch is defined as a complex carbohydrate. During digestion, the body breaks down all carbohydrates except fibers into sugars. Sugars and starches occur naturally in many foods, including milk, fruits, some vegetables, bread, cereals, and grains. These foods also supply many other important nutrients. On the other hand, so-called added sugars—those added during processing or at the table—supply calories but few nutrients. Foods rich in added sugars include things like soft drinks and desserts.

Carbonated drinks are the single biggest source of added sugars in the American diet (about 8 to 10 teaspoons per can), supplying one-third of all sugar ingested. Carbonated soft drink consumption has been soaring, and now accounts for more than one-fourth of Americans' beverage consumption.

Sugar is hidden in many other foods. One cup of yogurt, for example, has 7 teaspoons of sugar, 1 cup of canned corn has 3, and 1 tablespoon of ketchup has 1. Desserts often have more sugar than expected: a glazed donut has 6 teaspoons of sugar, 1 chocolate éclair or a piece of angel food cake each has 7, 2 ounces of chocolate candy has 8, a piece of iced chocolate cake or berry pie each has 10, and 4 ounces of hard candy has 20. To locate hidden sugars, check the list of ingredients on the food label: sugars are listed by many different names, including brown sugar, corn sweetener, corn syrup, fructose, fruit juice concentrate, glucose or dextrose, high-fructose corn syrup, honey, lactose, maltose, molasses, raw sugar, table sugar or sucrose, and syrup. If one of these appears near the top of the list, the food is probably high in added sugars. The total grams of sugar per serving listed on the Nutrition Facts panel includes both naturally occurring and added sugars.

The average American male and female ingest far too much sugar, about 22 and 16 teaspoons of added sugar on average each day, respectively. The USDA recommends that people learn to choose and prepare foods and beverages with little added sugars or caloric sweeteners. Total discretionary calories (see Box 8.2) should not exceed the allowance for any given calorie level. The discretionary calorie allowance covers all calories from added sugars, alcohol, and the additional fat found in even moderate fat choices from the milk and meat group. For example, the 2,000-calorie pattern includes only about 267 discretionary calories. At 29 percent of calories from total fat (including 18 g of solid fat), if no alcohol is consumed, then only 8 teaspoons (32 g) of added sugars can be afforded. This is less than the amount in a typical 12-ounce soft drink. If fat is decreased to 22 percent of calories, then 18 teaspoons (72 g) of added sugars is allowed. If fat is increased to 35 percent of calories, then no allowance remains for added sugars, even if alcohol is not consumed.

Sugar and Health

Sugars and starches can both promote tooth decay. The more often foods containing sugars and starches are eaten, and the longer these foods are in the mouth before the teeth are brushed, the greater the risk for tooth decay.

Despite widespread concerns, intake of sugar has not been associated with increased risk of heart disease, cancer, diabetes, or abnormal behavior. Some parents feel that sugar affects the behavior of their children, but there is no good scientific support for the belief that sugar causes hyperactivity, impairment in mental function, or abnormal behavior in children.

Sugar Substitutes

Sugar substitutes such as sorbitol, saccharin, and aspartame are ingredients in many foods, and have been shown to be safe by many different research teams and professional organizations. Most of the sugar substitutes do not provide significant calories and can be useful if one is trying to lose weight. Foods containing sugar substitutes, however, may not always be lower in calories than similar products that contain sugars. Thus, the food label should be reviewed carefully.

Sodium and Potassium

Key Recommendations

- Consume less than 2,300 mg (approximately 1 tsp of salt) of sodium per day.
- Choose and prepare foods with little salt. At the same time, consume potassium-rich foods, such as fruits and vegetables.
- *Individuals with hypertension, blacks, and middle-aged and older adults.* Aim to consume no more than 1,500 mg of sodium per day, and meet the potassium recommendation (4,700 mg/day) with food.

Sodium is an essential mineral that plays a role in the regulation of water balance, normal muscle tone, acid-base balance, and the conduction of nerve impulses. The human body needs about 500 mg of sodium per day, but Americans consume much more—about 4,000 to 6,000 per day. Sodium intake is a concern for health because for many people, high sodium intake is associated with high blood pressure, a form of cardiovascular disease and a key risk factor for heart attacks and strokes.

The *Dietary Guidelines* recommend that intake be limited to no more than 2,300 mg of sodium per day, the equivalent of a little more than a teaspoon of table salt. Salt or sodium chloride (NaCl) is 40 percent sodium. Thus 1 teaspoon of salt (about 5,000 mg) is approximately 2,000 mg of sodium.

Food labels list sodium rather than salt content. When reading a Nutrition Facts Panel on a food product, look for the sodium content. Foods that are low in sodium (less than 140 mg or 5 percent of the Daily Value [DV]) are low in salt. On average, the natural salt content of food accounts for only about 10 percent of total intake, while discretionary salt use (i.e., salt added at the table or while cooking) provides another 5 to 10 percent of total intake. Approximately 75 percent is derived from salt added by manufacturers. It is important to read the food label and determine the sodium content of food.

The richest sources of sodium are sauces, salad dressings, cheeses, processed meats, soups, and grain-cereal products. Table 8.4 gives sodium values for different types of foods. The USDA recommends several steps to keep sodium intake at healthy levels:

- Learn to read food labels, and limit foods high in sodium.
- Look for labels that say "low-sodium"—they contain 140 mg or less of sodium per serving.
- Choose more fresh fruits and vegetables (which are very low in sodium).
- Choose fresh or frozen fish, shellfish, poultry, and meat most often. They are lower in salt than most canned and processed forms.
- Reduce the use of salt during cooking, and use herbs, spices, and low-sodium seasonings.
- Avoid using the salt shaker on prepared foods at the table, and go easy on condiments such as soy sauce, ketchup, mustard, pickles, and olives.
- Limit the use of foods with visible salt on them (snack chips, salted nuts, crackers, etc.).

Alcoholic Beverages

Key Recommendations

- Those who choose to drink alcoholic beverages should do so sensibly and in moderation—defined as the consumption of up to 1 drink per day for women and up to 2 drinks per day for men.
- Alcoholic beverages should not be consumed by some individuals, including those who cannot restrict their alcohol intake, women of childbearing age who may become preg-

TABLE 8.4 Where's the Salt?

Food Groups	Sodium, mg
Bread, cereal, rice, and pasta	
Cooked cereal, rice pasta, unsalted, 1/2 cup	Trace
Ready-to-eat cereal, 1 oz	100–360
Bread, 1 slice	110–175
Vegetable	
Vegetables, fresh or frozen, cooked without salt, 1/2 cup	Less than 70
Vegetables, canned or frozen with sauce, 1/2 cup	140–460
Tomato juice, canned, 3/4 cup	660
Vegetable soup, canned, 1 cup	820
Fruit	
Fruit, fresh, frozen, canned, 1/2 cup	Trace
Milk, yogurt, and cheese	
Milk, 1 cup	120
Yogurt, 8 oz	160
Natural cheeses, 1 1/2 oz	110–450
Processed cheeses, 2 oz	800
Meat, poultry, fish, dry beans, eggs, and nuts	
Fresh meat, poultry, fish, 3 oz	Less than 90
Tuna, canned, water pack, 3 oz	300
Bologna, 2 oz	580
Ham, lean roasted, 3 oz	1,020
Other	
Salad dressing, 1 tbsp	75–220
Ketchup, mustard, steak sauce, 1 tbsp	130–230
Soy sauce, 1 tbsp	1,030
Salt, 1 tsp	2,000
Dill pickle, 1 medium	930
Potato chips, salted, 1 oz	130
Corn chips, salted, 1 oz	235
Peanuts, roasted in oil, salted, 1 oz	120

*Source: U.S. Department of Agriculture.

nant, pregnant and lactating women, children and adolescents, individuals taking medications that can interact with alcohol, and those with specific medical conditions.

• Alcoholic beverages should be avoided by individuals engaging in activities that require attention, skill, or coordination, such as driving or operating machinery.

About 55 percent of U.S. adults are current drinkers. The hazards of heavy alcohol consumption are well known and include increased risk of liver cirrhosis, hypertension, cancers of the upper gastrointestinal tract, injury, violence, and death. Alcoholic beverages supply calories but few or no nutrients. Alcohol may have beneficial effects when consumed in moderation. The lowest death rates for coronary heart disease occur at an intake of 1 to 2 drinks per day. While it is true that moderate amounts of alcohol lower risk of coronary heart disease, this must be balanced against all the health risks.

Individuals in some situations should avoid alcohol—those who plan to drive, operate machinery, or take part in other activities that require attention, skill, or coordination. Some people, including children and adolescents, women of childbearing age who may become pregnant, pregnant and lactating women, individuals who cannot restrict alcohol intake, individuals taking medications that can interact with alcohol, and individuals with specific medical conditions should not drink at all. Even moderate drinking during pregnancy may have behavioral or developmental consequences for the baby. Heavy drinking

TABLE 8.5   Blood Alcohol Content (BAC) and Symptoms

Blood Alcohol Content [g/100 ml of blood or g/(210 L) of breath]*	Symptoms
0.01–0.05	Normal behavior
0.03–0.12	Mild euphoria; increased confidence; slight decrease in attention, judgment, and control
0.09–0.25	Feelings of excitement; emotional instability; loss of critical judgment; impairment of perception, memory, and comprehension; slower reaction time; reduced peripheral vision; impaired balance; drowsiness
0.18–0.30	Confusion, disorientation, dizziness, vision disturbance, slurred speech, lack of coordination while walking, apathy, lethargy
0.25–0.40	Stupor, marked incoordination, inability to stand or walk, vomiting, sleep, inability to control urination
0.35–0.50	Coma, lack of reflexes, low body temperature, reduced heartbeat and breathing
0.45+	Death from inability to breathe

*Ranges overlap due to varying responses from one individual to another.

Source: Intoximeters Inc., at http://intox.com.

during pregnancy can produce a range of behavioral and psychosocial problems, malformation, and mental retardation in the baby.

If one chooses to drink alcoholic beverages, they should be consumed in moderate amounts, defined as no more than 2 drinks a day for men, and 1 drink a day for women. One serving of alcohol, commonly called a drink, delivers 0.5 ounces of pure alcohol and is found in:

- 12 ounces of regular beer (150 calories).
- 5 ounces of wine (100 calories).
- 1.5 ounces of 80-proof distilled spirits (100 calories).
- s10 ounces of a wine cooler (140 calories).

The amount of alcohol in actual mixed drinks varies widely. While a whiskey sour/highball has about 0.5 to 0.6 ounces of ethanol, a dry martini has about 1 ounce, and a Manhattan 1.15 ounces.

When ingested, alcohol passes from the stomach into the small intestine, where it is rapidly absorbed into the blood and distributed throughout the body. Peak blood alcohol levels are reached in fasting people within 30 minutes to 2 hours. As a rule of thumb, 1 standard alcoholic drink consumed within 1 hour will produce a blood alcohol level or content (called BAL or BAC) of 0.02 in a 150-pound male, but this varies depending on body size, gender, food taken along with the alcohol, and tolerance (i.e., less responsive to alcohol because of long-term use). Five beers consumed within 1 hour will cause the BAC to rise on average to 0.10, which violates the drinking and driving laws of most states. The liver enzyme system takes 3 hours on average to clear the body of alcohol from 2 to 3 drinks. Table 8.5 summarizes the relationship between BAC and clinical symptoms.

Sports Nutrition Recommendations for Fitness Enthusiasts and Athletes

Some college students are fitness enthusiasts, working out for 30 to 60 minutes, several times a week. Others are members of athletic teams, training at a high intensity for several days nearly every day. What adaptations beyond the prudent diet should be pursued by student fitness enthusiasts and athletes? Here are several common questions posed by fitness enthusiasts and athletes:

- Can diet changes improve exercise performance and athletic endeavor?
- What is the optimal diet for student athletes?
- Are the nutritional stresses imposed by heavy exertion greater than can be met by the traditional food supply? Are vitamin and mineral supplements needed?
- Do students who lift weights need protein supplements to maximize size and power?
- Are there performance-enhancing aids (called **ergogenic aids**) that are safe, beneficial, and ethical?

As time spent in intense exercise (running, swimming, bicycling, weight lifting, etc.) increases above one hour a day, several changes in the diet are recommended (above and beyond the dietary recommendations described earlier in this chapter). As will be emphasized in this section, however, the changes are actually quite few:

- Increase in energy intake (in other words, more food).
- Increase in the percent of calories coming from carbohydrate.
- Increase in fluid intake.

Vitamin and mineral supplements are not needed by athletes. Contrary to popular opinion, even protein supplements are not needed by strength athletes if they are eating a balanced diet that matches their energy needs.

Obtain More Energy Through Carbohydrate

For highly active individuals, energy intake must increase (unless weight loss is the desired goal). What type of fuel does the working muscle prefer during intense exercise like team sports, running, swimming, cycling, and weight lifting? The answer is carbohydrate, which functions as a high octane fuel for the working muscles. When dietary carbohydrate intake is low and sports drinks are avoided, body carbohydrate stores fall and the muscle reluctantly changes over to fat for fuel, decreasing the ability to exercise intensely. The result is premature fatigue, and a feeling of staleness.

Table 8.6 summarizes the recommended changes in energy, carbohydrate, and fat for people who exercise intensely more than one hour a day. Notice that endurance athletes (e.g., runners, cyclers, swimmers) should ingest enough carbohydrate to represent 60 to 70 percent of total energy intake. At the same time, the proportion of fat in the diet should decrease to 15 to 25 percent. This is more carbohydrate than most athletes normally ingest, so changes in diet are typically needed to reach this goal. Fitness enthusiasts, and team and power athletes (e.g., basketball, soccer, football, track and field athletes, weight lifters), should follow the basic dietary guidelines and get about 55 percent of calories from carbohydrate and 30 percent from fat while ensuring that caloric intake matches energy output.

TABLE 8.6 The Energy and Quality of Diet Recommended for People Who Exercise Compared to Average American Intake

	Calories*		% of Total Energy Intake		
	Males	Females	Carbohydrate	Fat	Protein
Actual intake of average American	2500	1600	51	33	16
Fitness enthusiasts	2900	2000	55	30	15
Endurance athletes	2,500–7,500	2,000–4,000	60–70	15–25	15
Team/power athletes	3,000–10,000	2,000–4,000	55	30	15

*Energy intake can vary widely depending on body size and amount of exercise.

To increase carbohydrate and lower fat intake—consume more of the following high-carbohydrate foods:

- grain products (pasta, bagels, breads, brown rice, cereals, etc.)
- tubers (potatoes, yams)
- legumes (kidney beans, pinto beans, etc.)
- dried fruits (raisins, dates, etc.)
- fresh fruits and vegetables, and juices

—and consume less of the following high-fat foods:

- free fats (margarine, oil, salad dressing, mayonnaise, etc.)
- high-fat dairy products (most cheeses, whole milk, butter, cream cheese, etc.)
- high-fat meats (fried meats, bacon, corned beef, ground beef, ham, sausages, etc.).

A high-carbohydrate diet is especially recommended prior to important endurance race events. The process of eating a very high carbohydrate diet while tapering down exercise prior to a race is called **carbohydrate loading,** and is practiced by most elite athletes.

Drink More Fluids

Water is vital for your life and optimal health. One can live for weeks without food, but only for several days without water. Every body function depends on an ample water supply. Everyone needs water, but this becomes an even more important practice if you exercise.

Water balance in your body means that your input of fluids equals output. About 2.7 and 3.7 liters of water is lost from the body of women and men, respectively, each day, most of it from urination, and the balance from sweat through the skin, moisture in the breath, and water in the fecal mass. To gain this back, you need to drink 80 percent of this back each day from drinking water and beverages (about 8 cups for women, and 12 cups for men), with water from food providing the rest.

The vast majority of healthy people adequately meet their daily hydration needs by letting thirst be their guide. Prolonged physical activity and heat exposure will increase water losses. During exercise, you lose water through the sweat glands. To stay in water balance, you must drink the same amount as lost in the sweat.

Exercise and Sweat

During exercise, heat builds up in the body. This heat must be released from the body, or heat exhaustion can occur within a half hour. During exercise, the evaporation of sweat on the skin is the major avenue of heat loss. Sweat rates depend on the intensity of exercise and environmental conditions, but usually range from 0.5 to 1.5 liters per hour of exercise. The efficiency of sweat evaporation, and thus heat loss, is greatly affected by humidity. If the humidity rises above 70 percent, the sweat rolls of the skin, and little heat is given off, increasing your risk of heat exhaustion.

How much fluid should you drink during exercise to avoid dehydration from sweat loss? A good habit is to measure your body weight before and after each exercise session and replace the loss in water. Each pound of weight lost during exercise should be replaced with two cups or one-half quart of fluid.

Your thirst desire lags behind actual body needs during exercise. So before, during, and after the exercise bout, you should drink fluid, even beyond what you feel like drinking. A good plan is to drink two cups of water or sports drink immediately before exercising, one cup every 15 minutes during exercise, and then two more cups afterwards.

Are sports drinks better than water? Water is the best fluid except when you exercise beyond one hour. Sports drinks have enough sugar in them (about 4–8 percent concentration) to delay fatigue and enhance endurance, and the small amount of sodium enhances taste and improves water absorption. When exercise is long-term, a sweetened, flavored, and cooled sports drink will stimulate you to take in more fluids, helping to keep you in water balance.

Nutrient Supplements Are Not Needed for Student Athletes

There is considerable misinformation and exaggeration regarding the relationship between nutrient supplements and exercise. Coaches' magazines, popular fitness journals, supplement companies, and training table practices of sports superstars send the message that high levels of vitamins, minerals, and other special nutrients are needed as an energy boost, to maximize performance, to compensate for less-than-optimal diets, to meet the unusual nutrient demands included by heavy exercise, and to help alleviate the stress of competition.

Exercise and Nutrient Needs

Many people who exercise feel that they need to use supplements because the exercise burns up their body's stores of vitamins and minerals faster than they can eat them. Does exercise create a need for certain nutrients that is greater than the amount you can get from your diet?

The answer for most people is "no." Heavy exercise does increase the need for some vitamins and minerals, but this can easily be met by eating a balanced diet that matches the extra calories expended. Student athletes eat a lot of food, especially if they are large and train several hours a day. As a result, vitamin and mineral intake generally exceeds RDA/DRI standards.

Some student athletes, however, are at risk of nutrient deficiency when they participate in sports that emphasize leanness (gymnasts, wrestlers, ballet dancers, body builders, female runners). In this case, the solution is eating more food in accordance with the recommendations of the Food Guide Pyramid.

Do Dietary Supplements Improve Performance?

There is no convincing support for the role of nutrient supplements in enhancing performance, hastening recovery, or decreasing the rate of injury in healthy, well-nourished athletes. If an athlete is eating poorly, however, nutrient deficiencies can develop, and then performance will suffer.

Guidelines for Evaluating Supplement Claims

How can the student athlete understand and interpret the claims often made by dietary supplement proponents and manufacturers? Unfortunately, misinformation abounds. The **Federal Trade Commission (FTC)** and the **Food and Drug Administration (FDA)** work together to review claims on product labeling and in advertising. Claims about any dietary supplement are supposed to be truthful, not misleading, and substantiated, but many fraudulent products are still available to the public, escaping FTC and FDA review.

The use of dietary supplements should be based on solid research. Often, college students are confused about the research claims pushed forward by companies selling the products. Here are some guidelines for judging the worth of any particular dietary supplement:

- Call a professor from a nutrition or exercise science department in a nearby university to get help in understanding the research claims behind the supplement.
- Visit the Internet sites listed in Box 8.1. Many of them have information on supplements. You can also visit the Internet site of the FTC *(http://www.ftc.gov)* or sites dedicated to quackery *(http://www.quackwatch.com)*.
- Be suspicious of claims that seem to good to be true (they generally are).
- If a new supplement comes out on the market, wait several months for public and scientific opinion on effectiveness and safety to be formulated.

Student Athletes Do Not Need Protein Supplements

Interest in the influence of dietary protein intake on athletic performance began in the days of the ancient Greeks and Romans. In those days, athletes and military recruits consumed meat-rich diets in the belief that they would achieve the strength of the consumed animal.

Modern research has shown that exercise has a strong influence on protein metabolism in the athlete's body. During long endurance exercise, the body can break down protein, which then acts as a fuel source, supplying 5 to 15 percent of all energy expended. During heavy strength training, extra protein is needed to build up muscles.

Despite the need for extra protein, the average American diet has more than enough protein to meet the demands of all types of exercise programs, even weight lifting. Many weight lifters feel that protein supplements are necessary to build muscle mass. While it is true that some weight trainers may need an extra 25 to 50 grams of protein a day during active muscle building phases, we now know this is easily obtained in the diet without the use of protein supplements.

The average individual who does not exercise needs about 0.8 grams of protein per kilogram of body weight each day (g/kg/d). For the average American adult man and woman, weighing 80 kg and 65 kg respectively, this translates into a recommended protein intake of 64 g/day for men and 52 g/day for women. The protein requirement increases to 1.0 g/kg/d for fitness enthusiasts, 1.2 g/kg/d for endurance athletes (who tend to burn protein for fuel), and 1.6 g/kg/d for power athletes (Table 8.7).

However, the average sedentary American is already ingesting enough protein to match the increased needs of endurance athletes (current average intake is 100 g/day for men and 66 g/day for women). In other words, we tend to eat a lot of protein, and this is more than enough for even the highly active runner or cyclist. Power athletes need substantial amounts of protein, but because they are already eating a lot of food to meet the energy needs of their large bodies and heavy exercise habits, they easily obtain the protein from their regular food. In fact, as long as the diet provides about 15 percent of calories as protein, the protein needs of all athletes, small or large, runner or weight lifter, will be met without supplements or an emphasis on high protein foods. The average American obtains 16 percent of calories in the form of protein (without even trying) (Table 8.2).

Use of Ergogenic Aids Is Unethical (and Usually of No Value)

For thousands of years, warriors and athletes have used a wide variety of substances in the attempt to enhance physical performance. The ancient Greek athletes used special herbs and mushrooms, ancient Muslim warriors used hashish, during World War II German soldiers experimented with steroids, and today athletes use a growing list of drugs, nutrients, and supplements.

TABLE 8.7   Estimated Protein Needs According to Exercise Habits

	Calories* (Body weight in kilograms)		Estimated Protein Needs*		
	Males	Females	g/kg body weight per day	Males, g/day	Females, g/day
Average adult	2,500 (80 kg)	1,600 (65 kg)	0.8	64	52
Fitness enthusiasts	2,900 (75 kg)	2,000 (60 kg)	1.0	75	60
Endurance athletes	3,500 (70 kg)	2,600 (58 kg)	1.2	84	70
Team/power athletes	4,500 (100 kg)	3,500 (80 kg)	1.6	160	128

*All protein requirements fall within 15% of total caloric intake.

Ergogenic aids are defined as substances or methods that tend to increase exercise performance capacity. Although there are many worthless ergogenic aids, others confer impressive benefits. Many of the best ergogenic aids are now banned, and their use is considered unethical. The **International Olympic Committee (IOC)** has prohibited the use of steroids, stimulants, growth hormone, testosterone, blood doping, and other types of drugs that influence performance. Athletes are constantly searching for a "performance edge" through the use of supplements and other ergogenic aids, and are often willing to use banned substances. Most athletes, however, do not use these aids because of their belief in ethical standards.

HEALTH AND FITNESS INSIGHT
Sugar Substitutes

We are born liking the sensation of sweetness. The claim that sugar causes an increase in heart disease, cancer, diabetes, or abnormal behavior is not true. Sugar provides energy without vitamins or minerals (i.e., "empty calories"), however, and can promote dental caries under the right conditions. Consumers want the taste of sugar without the added energy, and the food industry has responded to this demand by producing many energy-reduced or nonnutritive sweeteners (or more simply, sugar substitutes). The American Dietetic Association has reviewed the literature, and concluded that "consumers can safely enjoy a range of nutritive and nonnutritive sweeteners when consumed in moderation and within the context of a diet consistent with the *Dietary Guidelines for Americans.*"

Here is a summary of currently available and safe nonnutritive alternatives to sugar:

Sucralose *(Splenda).* Sucralose is actually made from sugar, but is chemically altered so that it slips undigested through the intestinal tract. The Food and Drug Association (FDA) has approved its use as a tabletop sweetener, and as an additive in beverages and desserts. Sucralose is used in very small quantities because it is 600 percent sweeter than normal table sugar.

Saccharin *(Sweet 'N Low).* In 1977, the FDA proposed banning saccharin because animal studies suggested a cancer risk. Pressured by the artificial-sweetener industry, Congress indefinitely suspended the proposed ban and mandated a warning label instead. In 1991, the FDA withdrew its proposed ban, but the warning label still remains. Saccharin is 200 percent to 700 percent sweeter than normal table sugar.

Aspartame *(Equal, NutraSweet).* Aspartame has been approved by the FDA as a general-purpose sweetener, and is 160 percent to 220 percent sweeter than table sugar. Heat tends to destroy the sweetness of aspartame, but newer forms can increase its sweetening power in cooking and baking.

Acesulfame potassium *(Sunette).* Acesulfame potassium (also known as ace-K) has been approved for use as a tabletop sweetener and as an additive in a variety of desserts and beverages. Ace-K is 200 percent sweeter than table sugar, and currently is used almost exclusively in soft drinks (notably *Pepsi One).*

Summary

1. The body requires more than 40 essential nutrients for good health, and foods are classified into six groups: carbohydrates, fats, proteins, vitamins, minerals, and water.
2. The new standards for nutrient intake are called Dietary Reference Intakes (DRIs). The DRIs include intakes for optimal health based on the prevention of both nutrient deficiencies and chronic diseases.
3. All Americans are urged to eat a diet with the proportion of total energy intake at 55 percent or more for carbohydrate, less than 30 percent for fat, and about 15 percent for protein.
4. Dietary guidelines have been advocated for disease prevention and enhanced quality of life.
5. The Nutrition Facts food label uses the Daily Values, a set of nutrient reference values, to help consumers plan healthy diets. The Daily Values are based on a 2,000-Calorie diet, close to the average American intake.
6. As time spent in intense exercise increases above one hour a day, several changes in the diet are recommended: Increase in energy intake (in other words, more food); increase in the percent of calories coming from carbohydrate; increase in fluid intake. Vitamin and mineral supplements are not needed by athletes. Protein supplements are not needed by strength athletes if they are eating a balanced diet that matches their energy needs.
7. A high-carbohydrate diet is probably the most important nutritional principle for people who exercise. When the body carbohydrate stores drop too low, ability to exercise intensely falls, and one can feel stale and tired.
8. Probably the second most important dietary principle for individuals who exercise is to drink large quantities of water.

HEALTH AND FITNESS ACTIVITY 8.1
Rating Your Diet by the Food Pyramid

The food pyramid shown early in this chapter is an excellent guide to help you eat healthfully while obtaining all known vitamins and minerals. How close is your diet to the recommendations of MyPyramid?

Step 1 Write down *everything* (all fluids and foods) that you ate yesterday. Be exact!

Food or Beverage	**How much (cups, tablespoons, slices, etc.)?**

Step 2 Refer to Chart 1 on the next page.* Go to www.mypyramid.gov for more information and to print out a calorie pattern based on your needs. Fill in the blanks.

*Note: This is for an individual needing 2,800 calories a day. See Box 8.2 and mypyramid.gov to find your calorie needs.

MyPyramid Worksheet

Check how you did today and set a goal to aim for tomorrow

MyPyramid.gov
STEPS TO A HEALTHIER YOU

Write in Your Choices for Today	Food Group	Tip	Goal Based on a 2800 calorie pattern.	List each food choice in its food group*	Estimate Your Total
	GRAINS	Make at least half your grains whole grains	**10 ounce equivalents** (1 ounce equivalent is about 1 slice bread, 1 cup dry cereal, or ½ cup cooked rice, pasta, or cereal)		_____ ounce equivalents
	VEGETABLES	Try to have vegetables from several subgroups each day	**3 ½ cups** Subgroups: Dark Green, Orange, Starchy, Dry Beans and Peas, Other Veggies		_____ cups
	FRUITS	Make most choices fruit, not juice	**2 ½ cups**		_____ cups
	MILK	Choose fat-free or low fat most often	**3 cups** (1 ½ ounces cheese = 1 cup milk)		_____ cups
	MEAT & BEANS	Choose lean meat and poultry. Vary your choices—more fish, beans, peas, nuts, and seeds	**7 ounce equivalents** (1 ounce equivalent is 1 ounce meat, poultry, or fish, 1 egg, 1 T. peanut butter, ½ ounce nuts, or ¼ cup dry beans)		_____ ounce equivalents
	PHYSICAL ACTIVITY	Build more physical activity into your daily routine at home and work.	At least **30 minutes** of moderate to vigorous activity a day, 10 minutes or more at a time.	*Some foods don't fit into any group. These "extras" may be mainly fat or sugar— limit your intake of these.	_____ minutes

How did you do today? ☐ Great ☐ So-So ☐ Not so Great

My food goal for tomorrow is: _____

My activity goal for tomorrow is: _____

CHART I
2,800 Calorie Food Plan

HEALTH AND FITNESS ACTIVITY 8.2
Analyzing Your Energy and Nutrient Intake Using the Internet

Directions: Take the food list from Physical Fitness Activity 8.1 (where you listed all foods and their amounts ingested during the previous day) and enter the foods into the USDA Internet diet analysis program, "MyPyramid Tracker": *http://www.mypyramidtracker.gov*
   Follow the simple instructions given at the Internet site. List your intake of Calories and nutrients below, and compare to recommended levels. What areas need special attention?

	Your Intake	**Recommended**
Energy (kilocalories)	_____	Varies*
Carbohydrate (percent total energy)	_____	45–65
Fat (percent total energy)	_____	20–35
Saturated fat (percent total energy)	_____	<10
Protein (percent total energy)	_____	10–35
Dietary fiber (gm)	_____	M: 38; F: 25
Cholesterol (mg)	_____	<300
Sodium (mg)	_____	<2,400
Vitamin C (mg)	_____	M: 90; F:75
Calcium (mg)	_____	1000; 50+ yr, 1200
Iron (mg)	_____	M: 8; F: 18

*Energy needs vary according to body size and physical activity, with RDA average set at 2,900 kilocalories for males, and 2,200 for females.

Comment on areas of needed improvement (consult the text for ideas):

_____

_____

_____

_____

_____

_____

_____

_____

_____

_____

HEALTH AND FITNESS ACTIVITY 8.3
Estimating Blood Alcohol Content

Go to the Internet site, *http://intox.com/,* and access the "drink wheel" page. Enter your gender, weight, and the amount of alcohol that you consumed during a given period of time at your last drinking occasion. If you do not drink, enter these data for a friend of yours who does. Enter your estimate blood/breath alcohol concentration and compare to Table 8.5. Notice the disclaimer that is attached to the "drink wheel" page (and listed in Table 8.5).

Your estimate blood/breath alcohol concentration is: ___ g/210 liters of breath
(Note: g/210 liters of breath is the same unit as g/100 ml blood).

HEALTH AND FITNESS ACTIVITY 8.4

Review of Internet Sites That Provide Information on Dietary Guidelines

Visit 2 to 3 of the Internet sites listed in Box 8.1, review information that is provided regarding Dietary Guidelines for Americans or similar material, and write a two-paragraph summary of what you learned.

_____

_____

_____

_____

_____

_____

_____

_____

_____

_____

_____

_____

_____

_____

_____

_____

_____

_____

_____

_____

_____

_____

_____

_____

_____

CHAPTER 8 QUIZ
Nutrition, Health, and Physical Performance

Note: Answers are given at the end of the quiz.

1. Three cans of beer contain about _____ ounces of pure alcohol.
   A. 0.5
   B. 1
   C. 1.5
   D. 2.0
   E. 0.8

2. If you lost 6 pounds during a long-endurance exercise bout, you should drink ____ cups to restore body water.
   A. 10
   B. 12
   C. 3
   D. 8
   E. 6

3. If you eat 2,800 calories, what is the maximum grams of fat you should include in this diet?
   A. 80
   B. 109
   C. 28
   D. 40
   E. 128

4. T   F   High sugar intake has been linked in well-designed studies to cancer.

5. Nutrient reference standards for _____ are called Daily Values.
   A. the United States
   B. food labels
   C. the United Kingdom
   D. Canada
   E. ADA

6. One teaspoon of table salt has ____ mg sodium.
   A. 1000
   B. 2500
   C. 2000
   D. 5000
   E. 900

7. Ten french fries have 158 calories, with 2.0 grams of protein, 19.8 grams of carbohydrate, and 8.3 grams of fat. What percent of calories are protein?
   A. 5
   B. 10
   C. 15
   D. 20
   E. 25

8. How many grams of protein are recommended for the average 70 kg American?
   A. 100
   B. 56
   C. 25
   D. 90
   E. 133

9. If an 80-kg man eats 3,400 Calories a day, at least _____ grams of carbohydrate is recommended.
   A. 244
   B. 340
   C. 383
   D. 425
   E. 150

10. T   F   According to the MyPyramid, fruits should be eaten in the greatest quantity each day.

11. Which one of the following concepts is not included in the USDA Dietary Guidelines for Americans:
    A. Eat five servings or more a day of foods high in protein.
    B. Choose a diet low in saturated fat and cholesterol and moderate in total fat.
    C. Choose and prepare foods with less salt.
    D. Aim for a healthy weight.
    E. Choose beverages and foods to moderate your intake of sugars.

12. Which food listed below does not have dietary fiber in it?
    A. watermelon
    B. lettuce
    C. filbert nuts
    D. whole grain bagels
    E. whole milk (4 percent)

PART FOUR

Physical Activity, Health and Disease Prevention

chapter nine

Prevention of Heart Disease

"The doctor of the future will give no medicine, but will interest his patients in the care of the human frame, in diet, and in the prevention of disease."

—Thomas Edison

Introduction

Your heart is a strong, muscular pump that, if given the chance, will beat nearly three billion times, pumping 42 million gallons of blood within your lifetime. Your heart, only the size of your closed fist, pumps over a gallon of blood per minute to your body. During intense exercise, your heart can pump out five gallons per minute. As you become fit, your heart grows larger. The sturdy hearts of some of the world's best athletes can pump out about 10 gallons each minute.

As shown in Figure 9.1, your heart has four chambers: the right and left atriums that pump blood to the lower heart, and the right and left ventricles that pump blood to the lungs and the body. Blood is received from the body into the right atrium, and is pumped through the right ventricle to the lungs where oxygen is added, and then to the left atrium and left ventricle where it is pumped strongly through a large blood vessel called the aorta to the body.

The heart muscle does not receive oxygen or nourishment from the blood passing through its chambers. Instead, it is fed through an intricate system called the coronary arteries, that branch off the aorta (figure 9.2). Your coronaries are not very large, only about the size of the lead inside a pencil at their largest width, and much smaller as they permeate the heart muscle. About one half a quart of blood, or one tenth of the blood leaving your heart, surges through your coronary blood vessels each minute as you rest. Five times this amount of blood passes through your coronaries during intense exercise. Unfortunately, the heart's small coronary blood vessels are easily clogged by poor lifestyle habits, cutting short the action of this mighty pump.

FIGURE 9.1
Your heart, only the size of your closed fist, is a strong pump that sends over a gallon of blood per minute to the rest of the body. During intense exercise, the heart of an endurance athlete can pump out about 10 gallons each minute.

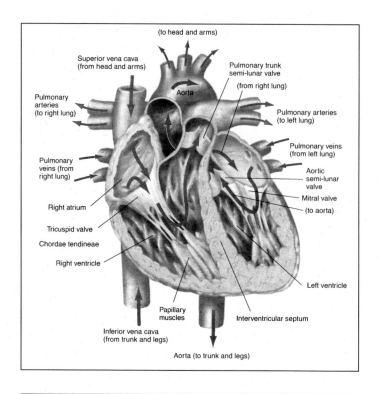

FIGURE 9.2
The first branches off your aorta are the coronary blood vessels, which feed the heart muscle. The carotid arteries supply blood and nourishment to the brain.

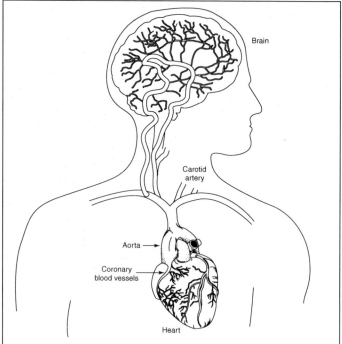

Diseases of the Heart and Blood Vessels: The Basics

The heart and its blood vessels can become diseased, a common health problem called **cardiovascular disease (CVD).** Most CVD is caused by deposits of material, often called **plaque,** that block the coronary arteries and the arteries that supply blood to the brain. These plaque deposits of cholesterol, fatty material, calcium, and other substances are called **atherosclerosis.** Over time, atherosclerosis narrows the coronary arteries and arteries in the brain, reducing the flow of oxygen-rich blood. Box 9.1 provides a glossary of terms that will be used in this chapter.

BOX 9.1

Glossary of Terms

angina pectoris Severe constricting pain in the chest, often radiating to a shoulder (usually left) and down the arm, due to coronary disease.

aorta A large artery which is the main trunk of the body's arterial system, arising from the base of the left ventricle of the heart.

atherosclerosis Lipid deposits in the inner lining of arteries. Atherosclerosis is a multistage process set in motion when the arteries are damaged as a result of high blood pressure, smoking, toxic substances in the environment, and other agents. Plaque develops when low-density lipoproteins accumulate at the site of arterial damage and platelets act to form a fibrous cap over this fatty core. Deposits block, or eventually entirely shut off, blood flow.

atria, left and right of heart The atrium of the right side of the heart receives the venous blood from the body; the atrium of the left side of the heart receives oxygenated blood from the lungs.

bile acids Bile is the yellowish brown or green fluid secreted by the liver and discharged into the small intestine, where it aids in fat digestion. Bile contains several types of bile acids and other substances.

cardiac rehabilitation A therapeutic program of exercise, lifestyle change, appropriate drug therapy, and group and family therapy for patients with heart disease.

cardiopulmonary resuscitation (CPR) Restoration of heart and lung function following a heart attack, using artificial respiration and chest compression.

cardiovascular disease (CVD) Includes a variety of diseases of the heart and blood vessels, coronary heart disease, stroke, high blood pressure, and other related diseases.

catheter A small, thin-walled tube suitable for injection of a special fluid used for visualizing deposits in the coronary arteries of the heart.

cerebrovascular disease or accident (CVA) CVA or stroke affects the blood vessels supplying blood to the brain. CVA occurs when a blood vessel bringing oxygen and nutrients to the brain bursts or is clogged by a blood clot. Because of this rupture or blockage, part of the brain does not get the flow of blood it needs and nerve cells in the affected area die.

cholesterol A waxy substance that circulates in the bloodstream. When the level of cholesterol in the blood is too high, some of the cholesterol is deposited in the walls of the blood vessels. Over time, these deposits can build up until they narrow the blood vessels, causing atherosclerosis, which reduces the blood flow. The higher the blood cholesterol level, the greater is the risk of getting heart disease.

coronary arteries The first arterial branches off the aorta are the coronary arteries, which feed the heart muscle. The right coronary passes around the right side of the heart, while the left coronary divides into two major branches that feed the front and back parts of the left heart.

coronary heart disease (CHD) A condition in which the flow of blood to the heart muscle is reduced. Like any muscle, the heart needs a constant supply of oxygen and nutrients that are carried to it by the blood in the coronary arteries. When the coronary arteries become narrowed or clogged, they cannot supply enough blood to the heart. If not enough oxygen-carrying blood reaches the heart, the heart may respond with pain called angina. The pain usually is felt in the chest or sometimes in the left arm or shoulder. When the blood supply is cut off completely, the result is a heart attack. The part of the heart muscle that does not receive oxygen begins to die, and some of the heart muscle is permanently damaged.

coronary artery bypass graft surgery Insertion of vein grafts that shunt blood from the aorta to branches of the coronary arteries, to increase the flow beyond the local obstruction.

embolus Clots that float in from other areas.

heart attack Also called myocardial infarction. Occurs when a coronary artery becomes completely blocked, usually by a blood clot, resulting in lack of blood flow to the heart muscle and therefore a loss of needed oxygen. As a result, part of the heart muscle dies. The blood clot usually forms over the site of a cholesterol-rich narrowing (called plaque).

heart disease The leading cause of death and a common cause of illness and disability in the United States. Coronary heart disease is the principal form of heart disease, which is the result of atherosclerosis, or the buildup of cholesterol deposits in the coronary arteries that feed the heart.

hemorrhagic stroke Strokes that occur when a blood vessel in the brain or on its surface ruptures and bleeds.

high density lipoproteins (HDL) Called the "good" cholesterol because the HDL carrier acts as a type of shuttle as it takes up cholesterol from the blood and body cells and transfers it to the liver, where it is used to form bile acids. A low level of HDL-cholesterol increases the risk for CHD, whereas a high HDL-cholesterol level helps protect against CHD.

lipoproteins Fat and protein compounds that carry cholesterol and fats in the blood.

low density lipoproteins (LDL) Cholesterol carried in the LDL (called LDL-cholesterol) is called "bad" cholesterol because it contributes to the buildup of atherosclerosis, increasing heart disease risk. The higher the level of LDL in the blood, the greater is the risk for CHD.

myocardial infarction (MI) See heart attack.

percutaneous transluminal coronary angioplasty (PTCA) A procedure designed to widen the narrowed coronary artery through use of small catheters and a balloon. The balloon is inflated at the arterial blockage to compress the plaque.

plaque See atherosclerosis.

risk factors Personal habits or characteristics that medical research has shown to be associated with an increased risk of disease.

stroke A form of cerebrovascular disease that affects the arteries of the central nervous system. A stroke occurs when blood vessels bringing oxygen and nutrients to the brain burst or become clogged by a blood clot or some other particle. Because of this rupture or blockage, part of the brain does not get the flow of blood it needs. Deprived of oxygen, nerve cells in the affected area of the brain cannot function, and die within minutes. When nerve cells cannot function, the part of the body controlled by these cells cannot function either.

thrombus Clots that form in the area of the narrowed brain blood vessels.

transient ischemic attack (TIA) A sudden loss of brain function with complete recovery usually within 24 hours; caused by a brief period of inadequate blood flow because of a clot in a brain artery.

ventricles, left and right of heart The two lower chambers of the heart. The right ventricle pumps venous blood to the lungs, and the left ventricle pumps oxygenated blood to the body.

Atherosclerosis begins with injury to the walls of the arteries. High blood cholesterol, high blood pressure, cigarette smoking, and other factors injure the inner lining of the arteries. In response, white blood cells collect in the inner lining of the arteries, engulf cholesterol and other debris, and release proteins that stimulate the formation of deposits. The net result is a progressive narrowing of the blood vessel.

Atherosclerosis often begins during childhood, and progresses from fatty streaks in the arteries to raised deposits within several decades. About three in four elderly Americans have plaque deposits in their coronary and brain arteries, a process that began early in life because of inactivity, high-fat diets, low fruit and vegetable intake, and excess weight gain.

CVD is the number one killer in the United States. In fact, the leading cause of death among Americans in every year since 1900 has been CVD. Every 37 seconds, an American dies of CVD, leading to nearly one million deaths each year. Four of every 10 coffins contain victims of CVD.

Coronary Heart Disease

There are several different types of diseases of the heart, which together are called **heart disease.** Heart disease is the leading cause of death in the United States, Canada, Europe, and other westernized nations (figure 9.3). Half of men and nearly one third of women will experience heart disease within their lifetimes. A woman's lifetime risk of heart disease is much greater than for breast cancer.

When atherosclerosis forms in the coronary arteries, this is called **coronary heart disease (CHD).** One of every five deaths in the United States is from CHD, the most common form of heart disease and CVD. Often, a blood clot forms in the narrowed coronary artery, blocking the blood flow to the part of the heart (figure 9.4). This causes a heart attack, or what doctors call a **myocardial infarction (MI).** Each year, more than one million Americans have a heart attack, and about one third of them will die.

As the deposits in the coronary arteries grow, parts of the heart muscle do not receive enough blood and oxygen. This causes chest pain called **angina** pectoris, and often is felt during stress, excitement, or exercise. The first indication of a heart attack may be any of several warning signals listed in Box 9.2.

FIGURE 9.3

The three leading causes of death in the United States for men and women. Heart disease is the leading cause of death, followed by cancer and stroke.

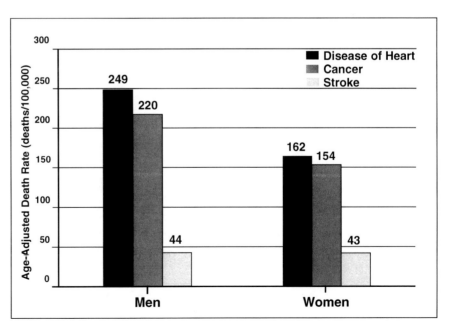

FIGURE 9.4

Coronary heart disease causes a progressive narrowing of the coronary artery. A clot can form in the narrowed coronary artery, causing a heart attack.

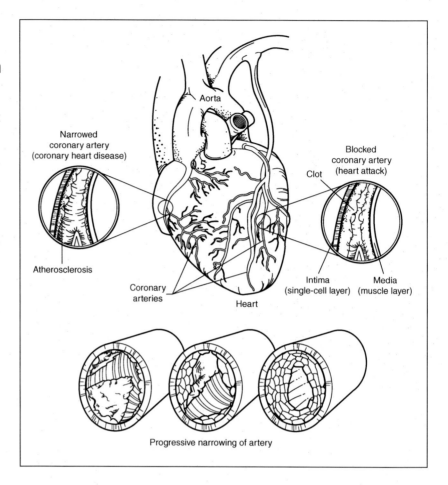

Treatment of a Heart Attack

When a heart attack occurs, it's critical to recognize the signals and respond immediately. Delaying may increase heart damage and reduce the chance of survival. Anyone experiencing the warning signals of a heart attack should be taken immediately to the nearest hospital with emergency cardiac care. People who become unconscious before reaching the emergency room may receive emergency cardiopulmonary resuscitation (CPR).

When a coronary artery gets blocked, the heart muscle doesn't die instantly. If a victim gets to an emergency room fast enough, clot-dissolving agents can be injected to dissolve a clot in a coronary artery and restore some blood flow. These drugs must be used within a few hours of a heart attack for best effect.

In the weeks following a heart attack, two invasive techniques may be used to improve blood supply to the heart muscle. One technique is percutaneous transluminal coronary angioplasty (PTCA), also known as angioplasty or balloon angioplasty. Another procedure is coronary artery bypass graft surgery.

Before performing either of these procedures, a doctor must find the blocked part of the coronary artery. A thin plastic tube called a catheter is guided through an artery in the arm or leg and into the coronary artery. Then the doctor injects a liquid dye visible in X-rays through the catheter, and identifies obstructions.

PTCA is a procedure designed to widen the narrowed coronary artery through use of small catheters and a balloon (see figure 9.5). The balloon is inflated at the arterial blockage to compress the plaque. In coronary artery bypass graft surgery, surgeons take a blood vessel from another part of the body and construct a detour around the blocked area of the coronary artery. One end of the vessel is attached above the blockage; the other, to the coronary artery just beyond the blocked area. This restores blood supply to the heart muscle (figure 9.5).

BOX 9.2

Warning Signs of a Heart Attack

Some heart attacks are sudden and intense—the "movie heart attack," where no one doubts what's happening. But most heart attacks start slowly, with mild pain or discomfort. Often people affected aren't sure what's wrong, and wait too long before getting help. Here are signs that can mean a heart attack is happening:

- Chest discomfort. Most heart attacks involve discomfort in the center of the chest that lasts more than a few minutes, or that goes away and comes back. It can feel like uncomfortable pressure, squeezing, fullness, or pain.
- Discomfort in other areas of the upper body. Symptoms can include pain or discomfort in one or both arms, the back, neck, jaw, or stomach.
- Shortness of breath. May occur with or without chest discomfort.
- Other signs: These may include breaking out in a cold sweat, nausea, or lightheadedness

If you or someone you're with has chest discomfort, especially with one or more of the other signs, don't wait longer than a few minutes (no more than 5) before calling for help. Call 9-1-1 . . . Get to a hospital right away.

Calling 9-1-1 is almost always the fastest way to get lifesaving treatment. Emergency medical services staff can begin treatment when they arrive—up to an hour sooner than if someone gets to the hospital by car. The staff are also trained to revive someone whose heart has stopped. Patients with chest pain who arrive by ambulance usually receive faster treatment at the hospital, too.

If you can't access the emergency medical services (EMS), have someone drive you to the hospital right away. If you're the one having symptoms, don't drive yourself, unless you have absolutely no other option.

Source: American Heart Association

Percutaneous Transluminal Coronary Angioplasty (PTCA)
A catheter is inserted into a groin artery and threaded up to the blocked coronary artery. The balloon is then inflated several times, compressing the plaque against the arterial wall.

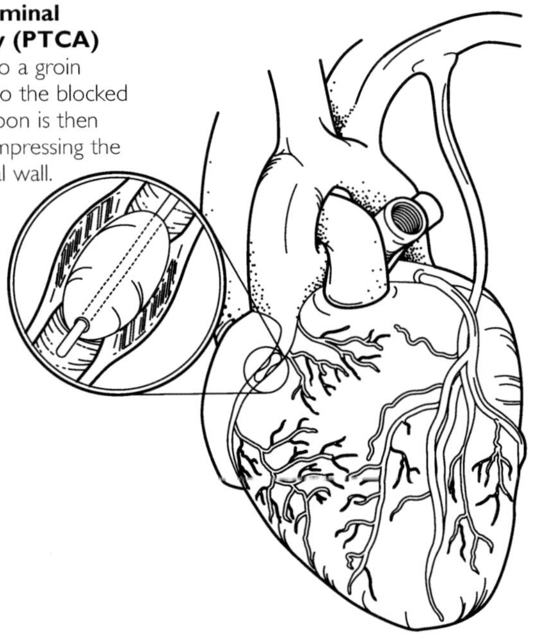

Coronary Artery Bypass Surgery
A segment of a blood vessel from another part of the body (the saphenous vein in the leg or the preferred choice, the internal mammary artery in the chest) is used as a graft. A venous graft is performed by sewing one end of the vein into the aorta and the other end into the blocked artery at a point beyond the obstructed coronary artery. Thus, blood is carried around the point of obstruction, effectively "Bypassing" the blockage. If necessary, multiple coronary artery blockages can be bypassed in a single operation.

FIGURE 9.5
Two Treatments for Coronary Heart Disease.

Stroke

The brain requires 20 to 25 percent of the heart's output of fresh blood. Unlike other organs, the brain cannot store energy, and if deprived of blood for more than a few minutes, brain cells die from energy loss and certain chemical interactions that are set in motion. The functions these brain cells control—speech, vision, muscle movement, comprehension—die with them.

Stroke is the common name for several disorders that occur within seconds or minutes after the blood supply to the brain is disturbed. The medical term is **cerebrovascular disease** or **accident (CVA).** The warning signals or symptoms of a stroke are very distinctive, and are summarized in Box 9.3.

About 10 percent of strokes are preceded by "little strokes" called **transient ischemic attacks** or **TIAs.** TIAs can occur days, weeks, or even months before a major stroke. About 36 percent of people who have experienced TIAs will later have a stroke. TIAs occur when a blood clot temporarily clogs an artery, with the symptoms occurring rapidly and lasting only a short time (most less than five minutes).

Most strokes occur because the arteries in the brain become narrow from a buildup of atherosclerosis. Clots that form in the area of the narrowed brain blood vessels (called a **thrombus**) or ones that float in from other areas (an **embolus**) can then totally block the blood flow, causing the stroke. Three fourths of strokes are caused by these clots that plug narrowed brain arteries.

Other strokes occur when a blood vessel in the brain or on its surface ruptures and bleeds (**hemorrhagic stroke**). Often the hemorrhage occurs when a spot in a brain artery has been weakened from atherosclerosis or high blood pressure. Hemorrhagic strokes are less common than those caused by clots, but are far more lethal.

About 780,000 Americans suffer a new or recurrent stroke each year. About three in 10 people who have a stroke die within a year, six in 10 within eight years. Each year, stroke kills over 150,000 people, accounting for one of every 16 U.S. deaths. It's the third largest cause of death, ranking behind diseases of the heart and cancer. Of those who survive, one-half suffer long-term disabilities, needing help caring for themselves or when walking. Here are the leading disabilities among stroke survivors:

- 50% have some one-sided paralysis.
- 35% have depressive symptoms.

BOX 9.3

Warning Signs of a Stroke

The American Stroke Association says these are the warning signs of stroke:

- Sudden numbness or weakness of the face, arm, or leg, especially on one side of the body
- Sudden confusion, trouble speaking or understanding
- Sudden trouble seeing in one or both eyes
- Sudden trouble walking, dizziness, loss of balance or coordination
- Sudden, severe headache with no known cause

If you or someone with you has one or more of these signs, don't delay! Immediately call 9-1-1 or the emergency medical services (EMS) number so an ambulance (ideally with advanced life support) can be sent for you. Also, check the time, so you'll know when the first symptoms appeared. It's very important to take immediate action. If given within three hours of the start of symptoms, a clot-busting drug can reduce long-term disability for the most common type of stroke.

- 26% are institutionalized in a nursing home.
- 26% are dependent in activities of daily living (grooming, eating, bathing, etc.).
- 19% have aphasia (trouble speaking or understanding the speech of others).

Risk Factors for Stroke

Risk factors are defined as personal habits or characteristics that medical research has shown to be associated with an increased risk of disease. Increasing age, male sex, ethnicity (African American), and family history of stroke are important risk factors for stroke that you cannot change. Other major risk factors for stroke can be changed, and these include:

- High blood pressure (by far, the most important risk factor for stroke).
- Cigarette smoking.
- Physical inactivity.
- Obesity.
- Excessive alcohol intake (increases the risk for hemorrhagic stroke).
- Elevated blood cholesterol.
- Diabetes mellitus.
- Illicit drug use (especially cocaine).

Heartening Facts About CVD

One of the greatest public health and medical success stories of the last several decades is the decrease in CVD death rates, now 64 percent lower than in 1950 (see figure 9.6). Death rates for stroke have fallen 74 percent since 1950. Men and women of all races have shared in this encouraging downturn.

What are the reasons for this success? There is no doubt that medical treatment of CVD has improved through use of new drugs and surgical procedures. The majority of the decline, however, is because of improvements in lifestyle by Americans, especially reductions in cigarette smoking, and improvements in dietary quality and exercise habits. Lifestyle habits have a strong effect on CVD. In fact, a healthy lifestyle can cut heart risk by as much as 70 percent.

FIGURE 9.6

Disease of the heart and stroke death rates have fallen strongly since 1950.

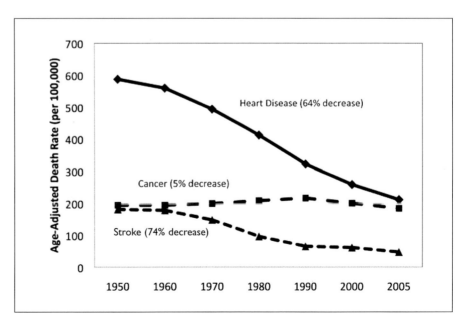

Risk Factors for Heart Disease

Why is heart disease so common in the United States, Canada, and Europe? Many factors, especially your lifestyle habits, are linked to heart disease. The American Heart Association has identified 13 heart disease risk factors (Table 9.1). Heredity, gender (being a male), race, and increasing age are major risk factors that you cannot change. You can change six risk factors: cigarette/tobacco smoke, high blood pressure, high blood cholesterol, physical inactivity, obesity, and diabetes. Notice that among the risk factors listed, overweight/obesity is the most prevalent, followed by physical inactivity. Your response to stress is listed as a "contributing factor" because research shows it has some effect on heart disease, but more study is needed to sort out conflicting information. Excessive alcohol and some illegal drugs also contribute to heart disease.

Your danger of heart attack increases with the number of risk factors. For example, smokers with high blood cholesterol and high blood pressure are 20 times more likely to die from CHD than nonsmokers with normal levels. Often those stricken with heart disease have several risk factors, each of which is only marginally abnormal. See Health and Fitness Activities 9.1 and 9.2 for more information on assessing heart disease risk.

The risk factors listed in Table 9.1 do not explain all heart disease. In fact, about half of heart disease deaths are not explained by these established risk factors. Many other factors are probably important, but not enough is known to include them at this time. These include short height, baldness, high blood levels of insulin, emotional distress, a hostile personality, inflammatory factors, clotting factors, and many others.

Major Risk Factors You Can't Change

Heredity, male sex, race, and increasing age are major heart disease risk factors that you cannot control or change. Increasing age is a powerful risk factor for heart disease, because many of the other risk factors take decades to promote enough plaque formation to cause a heart attack. Figure 9.7 shows that CHD death rates rise strongly with increase in age for both males and females.

- **Increasing Age** About four out of five people who die of CHD are age 65 or older. Heart disease does contribute to many deaths before the age of 65, ranking second only to cancer as an early cause of death. But most people who die of CHD are in their

TABLE 9.1   Risk Factors for Heart Disease According to the American Heart Association

Major Risk Factors That *Can't* Be Changed	% U.S. Adults with Risk Factor
1. Heredity	——
2. Male	——
3. Increasing age	13% (over age 65)
4. Race	

Major Risk Factors That *Can* Be Changed	
1. Cigarette/tobacco smoke	20%
2. High blood pressure	31% (≥140/90 mm Hg)
3. High blood cholesterol	17% (≥240 mg/dl)
4. Physical inactivity	39%
5. Obesity and overweight	66% (body mass index ≥25 kg/m²)
6. Diabetes	11%

Contributing Factor	
1. Individual response to stress	——
2. Excessive alcohol	
3. Some illegal drugs	

FIGURE 9.7
Coronary heart disease deaths rates rise strongly with increase in age for both males and females.

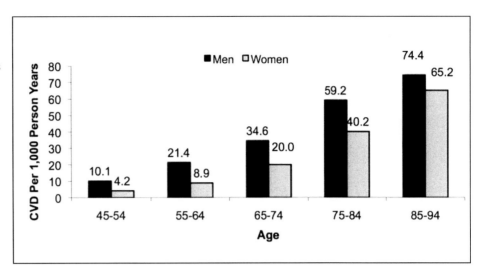

70s and 80s, reaping the harvest of poor health habits that were planted early in life. The odds of heart disease in old age are much lower for people who have practiced good health habits all their lives.

● **Male Sex** Men have a greater risk of heart attack than women, and they have attacks earlier in life. Even after menopause, when women's death rate from heart disease increases, it's not as great as men's. Female hormones are protective against heart disease, and many women live more healthfully than men, who tend to be risk takers.

● **Heredity and Race** Children of parents with heart disease are two to five times more likely to develop it themselves. The direct role of heredity is difficult to define precisely, however, because CHD risk factors tend to cluster within families. In other words, family members tend to have similar lifestyle habits. Thus, it is difficult to know whether genetics or health habits are more responsible when someone is stricken with heart disease. African Americans have a greater risk of heart disease than whites, and much of this is due to higher rates of severe high blood pressure.

Major Risk Factors You Can Change

Unlike heredity, male sex, and increasing age, the other risk factors for heart disease listed in Table 9.1 are based on your lifestyle habits, and can be changed. In other words, you can decide to avoid tobacco, be physically active, keep lean, and also eat in such a way that blood pressure and blood cholesterol are kept at optimal levels.

The Healthy People 2020 initiative described in Chapter 2 has targeted several heart disease risk factors. Government health officials hope to cut cigarette smoking and inactivity prevalence in half, and substantially reduce the proportion of adults who have high blood pressure, high blood cholesterol, and obesity. Reaching these targets for the year 2020 will require a concentrated effort by every American.

Cigarette and Tobacco Smoke

The Surgeon General regards cigarette smoking as the single most preventable cause of premature death in the United States. More than 443,000 people die from smoking each year, primarily from cancer and CVD (figure 9.8). Even secondhand smoke exposure increases your risk of heart disease. Your decision to avoid all exposure to tobacco smoke will add 15 years to your life when compared to those electing to smoke.

The proportion of U.S. adults who smoke has fallen strongly since the 1960s, such that today 20 percent still have the habit. However, the Healthy People 2020 target of 12 percent will require a tremendous effort at both the governmental and individual levels. Cigarette smoking is a major problem among certain minority groups, those with poor income and low education, and adolescents (see Table 9.2).

FIGURE 9.8

Cancer and CVD are the primary causes of death in smokers.

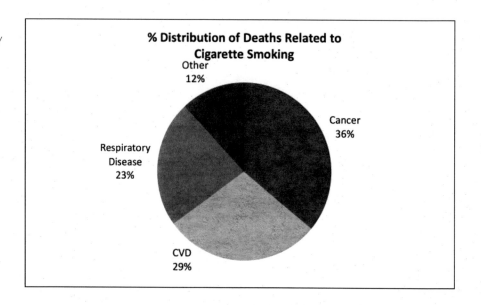

Table 9.2   Percent of Adults 18 years and Older Who Smoke Cigarettes

Group	Percent Cigarette Smoking	
	Males	**Females**
All adults	23	18
Race/Ethnicity		
American Indian or Alaska Native	37	36
Black or African American	25	16
White	23	20
Hispanic	18	8
Asian	16	4
Poverty level		
Below poverty level	32	26
At or above poverty level	23	18
Education		
Less than high school education	30	20
High school graduate	27	20
College degree	13	9
Graduate degree	6	6
Age group (yrs)		
18 to 24	25	19
25 to 44	26	20
45 to 64	23	20
65 and older	9	8

Source: Centers for Disease Control and Prevention, National Center for Health Statistics

Cigarette smoking almost always begins in the adolescent years. The nicotine found in tobacco is very addictive. More than one million young persons start to smoke each year, get hooked, and then keep on smoking. The prevalence of tobacco use among adolescents is 20 percent, similar to the adult prevalence.

High Blood Pressure

As described in Chapter 4, blood pressure is the force of the blood pushing against the walls of the arteries as the heart works. **High blood pressure** or **hypertension** is defined as a blood pressure of 140/90 mm Hg and above, and prehypertension 120–139/80–89 mm Hg. Fifty-eight percent of American adults have prehypertension

FIGURE 9.9

Prevalence of prehypertension
or hypertension among
American adults 18 years or
older.

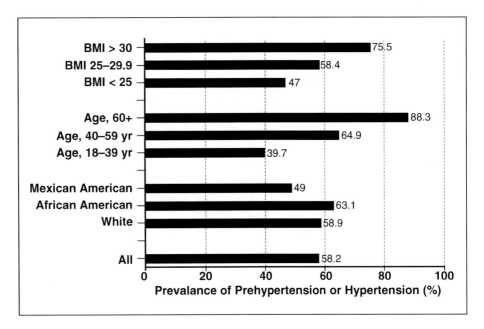

The National Heart, Lung, and Blood Institute of the National Institutes of Health

or hypertension. Of adults with hypertension, one third don't even know they have it. Only 31 percent of hypertensives have achieved control through lifestyle change or medication. Figure 9.9 shows that the elderly, obese, and African Americans have a high prevalence of prehypertension and hypertension.

High blood pressure usually doesn't give early warning signs, and for this reason is known as the "silent killer." High blood pressure increases the risk for CHD and other forms of heart disease, stroke, and kidney failure.

How You Can Prevent and Treat High Blood Pressure   High blood pressure is common in countries around the world where salt and alcohol intakes are high, potassium intake from fruits and vegetables is low, and physical inactivity and obesity are the norm. Prudent lifestyle habits lie at the foundation of both prevention and treatment of high blood pressure. You can do much for your blood pressure by following these recommendations:

- **Lose weight if overweight:** There is a strong relationship between your body weight and blood pressure. Being overweight more than triples your risk of developing high blood pressure. Weight loss is the most effective of all lifestyle strategies in normalizing blood pressure.
- **Reduce sodium intake to less than 2,300 mg per day:** When high salt intake is maintained all your life, your risk of high blood pressure climbs strongly (see Chapter 8).
- **Maintain adequate dietary potassium intake (fruits and vegetables):** Potassium, which is common in fresh fruits and vegetables, helps reduce blood pressure by increasing the amount of sodium that leaves the body in the urine. You should eat five to nine servings of fruits and vegetables each day to keep potassium intake at optimal levels.
- **Limit alcohol intake:** Heavy alcohol consumption (three drinks or more a day on average) increases the blood pressure. Keep your intake under two drinks a day if you are a male, and under one drink a day if you are female (see Chapter 8).
- **Exercise regularly:** Regular aerobic exercise is a powerful tool in both preventing and treating high blood pressure.

The National Heart, Lung, and Blood Institute of the National Institutes of Health advocates the DASH eating plan to lower blood pressure. Blood pressure reductions are seen within two weeks of starting the meal plan. This meal plan, called Dietary Approaches to Stop Hypertension, or DASH for short, is described in Box 9.4. The

BOX 9.4

Following the DASH Diet

The DASH eating plan given here is based on 2,000 calories a day. The number of daily servings in a food group may vary from those listed depending on your caloric needs.

Use this chart to help you plan your menus, or take it with you when you go to the store.

Food Group	Daily Servings (except as noted)	Serving Sizes	Examples and Notes	Significance of Each Food Group to the DASH Eating Plan
Grains and grain products	7–8	1 slice bread 1 cup dry cereal* 1/2 cup cooked rice, pasta, or cereal	Whole-wheat bread, English muffin, pita bread, bagel, cereals, grits, oatmeal, crackers, unsalted pretzels, and popcorn	Major sources of energy and fiber
Vegetables	4–5	1 cup raw leafy vegetable 1/2 cup cooked vegetable 6 oz vegetable juice	Tomatoes, potatoes, carrots, green peas, squash, broccoli, turnip greens, collards, kale, spinach, artichokes, green beans, lima beans, sweet potatoes	Rich sources of potassium, magnesium, and fiber
Fruits	4–5	6 oz fruit juice 1 medium fruit 1/4 cup dried fruit 1 1/2 cup fresh, frozen, or canned fruit	Apricots, bananas, dates, grapes, oranges, orange juice, grapefruit, grapefruit juice, mangoes, melons, peaches, pineapples, prunes, raisins, strawberries, tangerines	Important sources of potassium, magnesium, and fiber
Low-fat or fat-free dairy foods	2–3	8 oz milk 1 cup yogurt 1 1/2 oz cheese	Fat-free (skim) or low-fat (1%) milk, fat-free or low-fat buttermilk, fat-free or low-fat regular or frozen yogurt, low-fat and fat-free cheese	Major sources of calcium and protein
Meats, poultry, and fish	2 or less	3 oz cooked meats, poultry, or fish	Select only lean; trim away visible fats; broil, roast, or boil, instead of frying; remove skin from poultry	Rich sources of protein and magnesium
Nuts, seeds, and dry beans	4–5 per week	1/3 cup or 1 1/2 oz nuts 2 tbsp or 1/2 oz seeds 1/2 cup cooked dry beans	Almonds, fiberts, mixed nuts, peanuts, walnuts, sunflower seeds, kidney beans, lentils, and peas	Rich sources of energy, magnesium, potassium, protein, and fiber
Fats and oils†	2–3	1 tsp soft margarine 1 tbsp low-fat mayonnaise 2 tbsp light salad dressing 1 tsp vegetable oil	Soft margarine, low-fat mayonnaise, light salad dressing, vegetable oil (such as olive, corn, canola, or safflower)	Besides fats added to foods, remember to choose foods that contain less fats
Sweets	5 per week	1 tbsp sugar 1 tbsp jelly or jam 1/2 oz jelly beans 8 oz lemonade	Maple syrup, sugar, jelly, jam, fruit-flavored gelatin, jelly beans, hard candy, fruit punch, sorbet, ices	Sweets should be low in fat

*Serving sizes vary between 1/2–1 1/4 cups. Check the product's nutrition label.

†Fat content changes serving counts for fats and oils; for example, 1 tbsp of regular salad dressing equals 1 serving; 1 tbsp of a low-fat dressing equals 1/2 serving; 1 tbsp of a fat-free dressing equals 0 servings.

Source: www.nhlbi.nih.gov

DASH diet is low in sodium, saturated fat, total fat, and cholesterol, and rich in fruits, vegetables, and lowfat dairy foods. The key to the DASH diet is eating at least three servings of fruits and vegetables at each meal.

High Blood Cholesterol

High blood cholesterol is a major risk factor for heart disease. Cholesterol is a waxy substance that circulates in the bloodstream. Your body makes it own cholesterol, and also absorbs cholesterol from certain kinds of foods, specifically all animal products (i.e., meats, dairy products, and eggs) (see Chapter 8). Cholesterol is essential for the formation of bile acids (used in fat digestion) and some hormones, and is a component of cell membranes, and brain and nerve tissues.

Thus, some cholesterol is necessary to keep your body functioning normally. However, when blood cholesterol levels are too high, some of the excess is deposited in the artery walls, increasing your risk of heart disease.

Every adult should know their cholesterol level, and have it checked at least once every five years (or every year if heart disease risk is high). Blood cholesterol levels fall into one of three categories—desirable, borderline high risk, or high risk—as summarized in Table 9.3. Try to keep your blood cholesterol as low as possible. For all age groups, a blood cholesterol under 160 mg/dl is optimal because heart disease is rare below this level. At the very least, children and adolescents should keep their blood cholesterol under 170 mg/dl, and adults under 200 mg/dl.

Despite an impressive drop from the 1960s, 17 percent of American adults still have high-risk blood cholesterol levels (defined as 240 mg/dl and higher). The average American has a blood cholesterol level of 202 mg/dl (figure 9.10). Serum cholesterol levels peak in middle age among men, and in old age among women.

"Good" and "Bad" Cholesterol   Cholesterol is transported through the blood by carriers called lipoproteins. Two specific types of cholesterol carriers are called low-density lipoproteins (LDL) and high density lipoproteins (HDL). Cholesterol carried in the

TABLE 9.3   Classification of Total Blood Cholesterol, Lipoproteins, Triglycerides, and Glucose

Total cholesterol
<200	Desirable
200–239	Borderline high
≥240	High

LDL cholesterol
<100	Optimal
100–129	Near optimal/above optimal
130–159	Borderline high
160–189	High
≥190	Very high

HDL cholesterol
<40	Low
≥60	High (good)

Triglycerides
<150	Normal
150–199	Borderline high
200–499	High
≥500	Very high

Glucose
<100 mg/dl	Normal fasting glucose
100 to 125 mg/dl	Pre-diabetes (impaired fasting glucose)
≥126 mg/dl	Diagnosis of diabetes (after confirmation on a separate day)

Source: National Cholesterol Education Program (NCEP). http://www.nhlbi.nih.gov/.

FIGURE 9.10

Trends in serum total cholesterol.

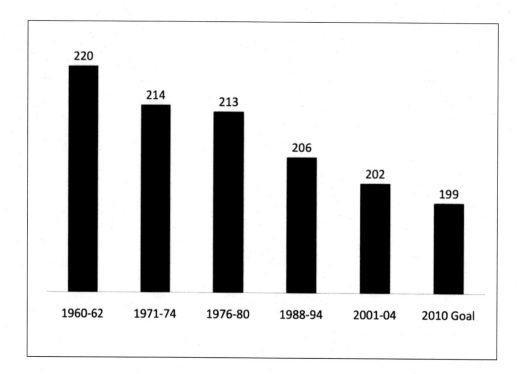

LDL (called LDL-cholesterol) is called "bad" cholesterol because it contributes to the buildup of atherosclerosis, increasing heart disease risk. Try to keep your LDL-cholesterol as low as possible (Table 9.3). For all age groups, a blood LDL-cholesterol under 100 mg/dl is optimal because heart disease is rare below this level. At the very least, children and adolescents should keep their blood LDL-cholesterol under 100 mg/dl, and adults under 130 mg/dl.

In contrast, HDL-cholesterol is called the "good" cholesterol. The HDL carrier acts as a type of shuttle as it takes up cholesterol from the blood and body cells and transfers it to the liver, where it is used to form bile acids. Bile acids pass from the liver to the intestine to aid in fat digestion. Eventually, some of the bile acids pass out of the body in the stool, providing the body with a major route for excretion of cholesterol.

HDLs have for this reason been called the "garbage trucks" of the body, collecting cholesterol and dumping it into the liver. Thus, if levels of HDL-cholesterol are high (i.e., 60 mg/dl or above), the risk of heart disease is decreased. An HDL-cholesterol level of less than 40 mg/dl is considered low or undesirable.

Triglycerides or blood fats are carried in LDL and HDL lipoproteins, but predominate in VLDLs (very low density lipoproteins). Triglycerides can be kept below 150 mg/dl by staying lean and fit.

How to Keep Your Blood Lipoproteins and Lipids Desirable

How can you ensure a good blood lipoprotein profile—low total cholesterol and LDL-cholesterol, and high HDL-cholesterol? Several lifestyle factors have a strong influence. In order of importance, the factors that increase HDL-cholesterol are:

- Vigorous aerobic exercise, at least 80 to 90 minutes per week.
- Maintaining a lean body weight and avoiding weight gain.
- Smoking cessation.

The most important factors for lowering LDL-cholesterol and total cholesterol are:

- Reduction of dietary saturated fat intake to less than 10 percent of calories (found mainly in meats, dairy products, and some tropical oils like palm and coconut oil), with a greater emphasis on most plant oils and fish which are high in unsaturated fats. (See figure 9.11, and review Chapter 8).

FIGURE 9.11

Percent saturated and unsaturated fats found in common dietary fats. Notice that all foods contain both saturated and unsaturated fats, but typically one type of fat predominates.

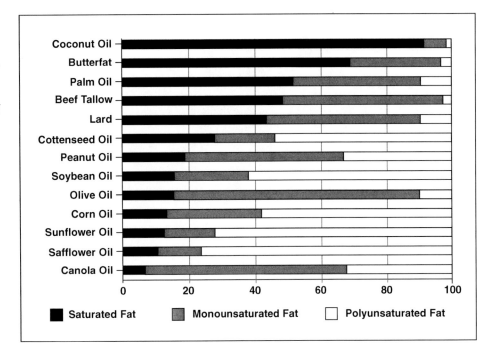

- Reduction in body weight (if high).
- Reduction in dietary cholesterol intake to less than 300 mg/day (found in foods of animal origin).
- Increase in carbohydrates to more than 55 percent of calories and dietary fiber to more than 20 grams/day (especially fruits and vegetables, beans and oat products).

These guidelines can be met by following the DASH diet outlined in Box 9.4. See Health and Fitness Activities 9.1 and 9.3 for more information on heart-healthy diets.

Obesity

Many of the risk factors for heart disease—high blood pressure, high blood cholesterol and LDL-cholesterol, low HDL-cholesterol, and diabetes—can be linked to obesity. As a result, obese people are at a high risk for heart disease.

Obese people most vulnerable to heart disease tend to have large amounts of fat in the abdominal region. (Review Chapters 5 and 10). Thus a high waist circumference—above 35 inches for women and 40 inches for men—predicts a high risk for heart disease.

Diabetes

Diabetes strongly increases the risk for CVD. The most common cause of death for a diabetic is CVD. Heart disease and stroke are two to four times more common among diabetics, and are present in 75 percent of diabetes-related deaths. Diabetics often have several risk factors for cardiovascular disease, including high blood pressure, elevated blood cholesterol, and low HDL-cholesterol. See Box 9.5 for more information on diabetes.

Physical Inactivity

Physical inactivity doubles the risk for CHD, while regular activity cuts the risk in half (figure 9.12). This is similar to the effect of high blood pressure, high blood cholesterol, and cigarette smoking on CHD risk. Physical activity must be a current and regular lifestyle habit in order for CHD risk to be lowered, however. In other words, you cannot "rest on

BOX 9.5

Diabetes: A Major Risk Factor for Heart Disease

Diabetes is a group of diseases, all of which cause the blood glucose or sugar to be unusually high, leading to a host of health problems and damage to the eyes, kidneys, nerves, heart, and blood vessels. The major cause of death among individuals with diabetes is heart disease. More than 24 million people in the United States (11 percent of adults) have diabetes now, three times more than had the disease in 1990. Another 50 million have prediabetes, a major risk factor for developing diabetes later on in life.

High blood glucose can occur because the cells of the pancreas that make insulin are mostly or entirely destroyed by the body's own immune system (for reasons that are not fully understood). The patient, typically a child or adolescent, then needs insulin injections to survive, and is diagnosed with Type 1 diabetes.

Far more common is Type 2 diabetes, in which the pancreas does make insulin, but the person's tissues aren't sensitive enough to the hormone and use it inefficiently. Type 2 diabetes is often diagnosed in obese adults.

Measuring glucose levels in samples of the patient's blood is key to the diagnosis of both types of diabetes. Here are the standards for blood glucose in the fasted state (i.e., at least nine hours of avoiding all caloric intake through food or beverages):

- less than 100 mg/dl = normal fasting glucose
- 100 to 125 mg/dl = prediabetes
- greater than or equal to 126 mg/dl = diagnosis of diabetes

Obesity, especially upper-body or abdominal obesity, is the strongest predictor of the development of Type 2 diabetes. In the United States, approximately 85 percent of patients with Type 2 are obese at the time of diagnosis. In severely obese populations, such as the Pima Indians, the prevalence of Type 2 diabetes is the highest worldwide.

Obesity causes insulin resistance, or a decreased ability of the body to respond to the action of insulin, and a reduced number of insulin receptors. A growing number of studies have shown that the risk of Type 2 diabetes climbs in direct proportion to the increase in the waist circumference. When the accumulation of abdominal fat is lost, insulin resistance is reduced, and blood glucose levels often return to normal.

Physical inactivity also causes Type 2 diabetes, but ranks behind obesity. The estimated reduction in the risk of Type 2 diabetes associated with maintaining desirable body weight compared with being obese is 50 to 75 percent, considerably higher than the 30 to 50 percent reduction in risk associated with regular moderate or vigorous exercise versus a sedentary lifestyle.

Few studies have been conducted on the role of diet in the development of Type 2 diabetes. Diet is regarded as an important component of treatment, but whether low-fat, high-fiber diets help *prevent* Type 2 diabetes is largely unknown. In one six-year study of over 65,000 nurses, researchers from the Harvard School of Public Health showed that the risk of developing diabetes was 2.5 times greater in those using refined and processed grain products (e.g., white bagels and bread, refined breakfast cereals) compared to those using grains in a minimally refined form (whole grain breads and cereals).

Rates for Type 2 diabetes rise dramatically as the westernized lifestyle is adopted by people from developing societies. The bottom line is that risk for Type 2 diabetes can be minimized by staying lean and physically active throughout adulthood.

FIGURE 9.12

Regular aerobic physical activity like running cuts the risk of CHD in half.

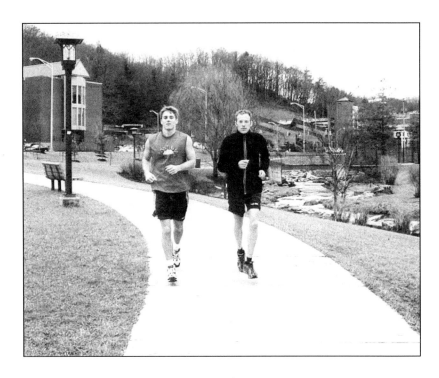

your laurels" or let "the grass grow under your feet," and hope that your exercise habits of years gone by are sufficient for today.

How Physical Activity Lowers CHD Risk   Physically active people have less CHD because they typically have other risk factors under good control. For example, few active people smoke cigarettes, are obese or diabetic, or have high blood cholesterol or high blood pressure. Active people have more HDL-cholesterol, and generally experience less anxiety and depression than those who are physically inactive.

There are other important reasons why regular exercise is identified with lower CHD risk. The coronary arteries of aerobically fit people are less stiff, can expand more, and are larger than those who avoid exercise. As explained earlier, most heart attacks are triggered by clots. Although the issue is not yet settled, regular exercise appears to decrease the potential for clot formation. In other words, regular physical activity will lower your CHD risk by giving you larger, more compliant coronary arteries, and a diminished likelihood to form clots.

How Much Physical Activity Is Necessary to Lower CHD Risk?   About 150 to 300 minutes of moderate-intensity physical activity per week is sufficient, with CHD risk lowered even further when greater amounts of more vigorous exercise are engaged in. In other words, while moderate exercise is a "sufficient threshold" for lowering CHD risk, additional benefit is gained when people are willing to exercise more vigorously for longer periods of time.

As little as two to three miles of brisk walking on most days of the week will lower CHD risk. The physical activity does not have to be structured or vigorous. Thus, you should set a long-term goal to accumulate at least 150 minutes or more of moderate-intensity physical activity during each week. If you are motivated to push harder or exercise longer, go ahead, and even greater benefits to your heart will be experienced.

Can Physical Activity Be Used to Treat CHD?   Yes, especially when combined with other lifestyle changes such as smoking cessation, weight control, and dietary improvement. CHD patients should participate in supervised exercise programs led by certified professionals to achieve optimal physical and emotional health.

FIGURE 9.13

Exercise is generally safe, but high-intensity exercise can cause heart attacks in those at high CHD risk.

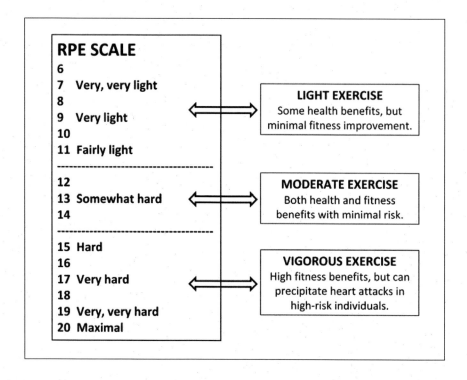

Each year, more than one million Americans have a heart attack. Although one third die soon after, the majority live to face an uncertain future. Cardiac rehabilitation programs were first developed in the 1950s in response to the growing epidemic of heart disease. The goal is to help cardiac patients return to productive, active, and satisfying lives with a reduced risk of recurring health problems. The emphasis in cardiac rehabilitation programs is on lifestyle change, appropriate drug therapy, and group and family therapy. Patients in cardiac rehabilitation programs typically experience an improved quality of life.

Is There a Risk of Dying of a Heart Attack During Exercise? Yes, a small risk does exist. But most people over age 30 who suffer a heart attack during or after vigorous exercise are at high risk for CHD, and then exercise too hard for their fitness level, triggering the final heart attack event. If an individual is at low risk for heart disease, has not experienced any symptoms, and exercises moderately, risk is extremely low, and overall, heart disease risk should be lowered because of the regular exercise program.

The risk of a heart attack during exercise is a rare event. In any given year, about 6 out of 100,000 men will have a heart attack during exercise. These victims tend to be men who were sedentary, already had heart disease or were at high risk for it, and then exercised too hard for their fitness level. These people should avoid heavy exertion until being cleared by their physicians. Even after clearance, intense exercise should be avoided until fitness has been gradually improved, and heart disease risk factors have been brought under control.

Certain physical activities should be approached cautiously by those at high CHD risk. For example, heavy snow shoveling causes a marked increase in heart rate and blood pressure, which may explain the common press reports of excess heart attacks after heavy snowfalls. Figure 9.13 outlines recommendations for intensity of exercise using the rating of perceived exertion scale.

Summary

1. Heart and blood vessels disease, or cardiovascular disease, is most often caused by deposits of material called plaque or atherosclerosis that block the coronary arteries and the arteries that supply blood to the brain.

2. Coronary heart disease is the narrowing of coronary arteries from atherosclerosis. Most heart attacks are caused when a blood clot forms in the narrowed coronary artery, blocking the blood flow to that part of the heart.

3. Stroke or cerebrovascular disease is usually caused by clots that plug brain arteries already narrowed by atherosclerosis. Hemorrhagic strokes occur when a blood vessel in the brain or on its surface ruptures and bleeds.

4. Risk factors are defined as personal habits or characteristics that medical research has shown to be associated with an increased risk of disease. Increasing age, male sex, ethnicity (African American), and family history of stroke are important risk factors for stroke that you cannot change. Other major risk factors for stroke can be changed, and include high blood pressure, cigarette smoking, physical inactivity, obesity, excessive alcohol intake, elevated blood cholesterol, diabetes mellitus, and illicit drug use.

5. CVD death rates are now 64 percent lower than what they used to be in 1950. Medical treatment has improved, but the majority of the decline is because of improvements in lifestyle by Americans.

6. There are 13 heart disease risk factors. Heredity, gender (being a male), race, and increasing age are major risk factors that you cannot change. You can change six risk factors: cigarette/tobacco smoke, high blood pressure, high blood cholesterol, physical inactivity, obesity, and diabetes. Your response to stress is listed as a "contributing factor."

7. High blood pressure can be prevented and treated by following these recommendations: Lose weight if overweight, reduce sodium intake to less than 2,400 mg per day, maintain adequate dietary potassium intake (fruits and vegetables), limit alcohol intake, and exercise regularly.

8. For all age groups, a blood cholesterol under 160 mg/dl is optimal, because heart disease is rare below this level. At the very least, children and adolescents should keep their blood cholesterol under 170 mg/dl, and adults under 200 mg/dl.

9. Two specific types of cholesterol carriers are LDL and HDL. LDL-cholesterol is called "bad" cholesterol because it contributes to the buildup of atherosclerosis. HDL-cholesterol is called the "good" cholesterol because it helps remove cholesterol from the body.

10. To lower LDL-cholesterol and total cholesterol, reduce dietary saturated fat and cholesterol intake, reduce body weight (if high), and increase intake of carbohydrates and dietary fiber. HDL-cholesterol can be increased by vigorous aerobic exercise, maintaining a lean body weight and avoiding weight gain, and quitting smoking.

11. Physical inactivity doubles the risk for CHD. Physically active people have less CHD because they typically have other risk factors under good control. The coronary arteries of aerobically fit people are less stiff, can expand more, and are larger than those who avoid exercise. About 150 minutes of moderate-intensity physical activity per week is sufficient, with CHD risk lowered even further when greater amounts of more vigorous exercise are engaged in.

Name _____   Date _____

HEALTH AND FITNESS ACTIVITY 9.1
Are You Ready to Adopt a Heart-Healthy Diet?

As emphasized in this chapter, the "heart-healthy" diet is rich in fruits, vegetables, and whole-grain products, and low in fatty meats and dairy products. Listed below are several practical ways to improve your diet and lower your risk of heart disease. Indicate by checking the appropriate box whether or not you are ready to make the diet change.

I do not intend to make this change in the next 6 months.
  I am thinking about making this change in the next 6 months.
    I am currently eating this way, but not regularly.
      I am currently eating this way, but have only done so within the last 6 months.
        I am currently eating this way, and have done so for longer than 6 months.

❑ ❑ ❑ ❑ ❑ When I buy chicken and turkey, I'll get the skinless kind—or take the skin off myself.

❑ ❑ ❑ ❑ ❑ I'll limit my daily meat servings to the size of two decks of cards.

❑ ❑ ❑ ❑ ❑ I will bake, roast, or broil meat instead of frying most of the time.

❑ ❑ ❑ ❑ ❑ I will select lean cuts of meat and trim away visible meat fat most of the time.

❑ ❑ ❑ ❑ ❑ I'll use fresh or plain frozen fish each week.

❑ ❑ ❑ ❑ ❑ I'll use cholesterol-free egg substitute instead of whole eggs at least once a week.

❑ ❑ ❑ ❑ ❑ I will limit the number of egg yolks in my diet to four or less per week.

❑ ❑ ❑ ❑ ❑ For breakfast, instead of doughnuts and muffins, I'll use a hot or cold cereal with skim milk.

❑ ❑ ❑ ❑ ❑ Most of the time, I'll top my spaghetti or other pasta with lightly stir-fried vegetables instead of meat or a creamy sauce.

❑ ❑ ❑ ❑ ❑ I will drink 1% or skim milk instead of whole or 2% milk.

❑ ❑ ❑ ❑ ❑ I will use low- and fat-free cookies most of the time.

❑ ❑ ❑ ❑ ❑ I will use low- and fat-free frozen yogurt or ice cream instead of regular ice cream most of the time.

❑ ❑ ❑ ❑ ❑ I will use pretzels or butter-free air popped popcorn instead of regular chips most of the time.

❑ ❑ ❑ ❑ ❑ Instead of using butter or lard, I will use oil or soft tub margarine in cooking or with my food.

❑ ❑ ❑ ❑ ❑ I will eat at least five servings of fruits and vegetables each and every day.

❑ ❑ ❑ ❑ ❑ I will select whole-grain breads and cereals most of the time.

❑ ❑ ❑ ❑ ❑ I will go meatless at least one day per week, and use more beans, lentils, seeds, and nuts.

❑ ❑ ❑ ❑ ❑ I will check cholesterol and saturated fat information on food labels on a regular basis.

235

HEALTH AND FITNESS ACTIVITY 9.2
What's Your Heart Disease Risk?

The American Heart Association recommends that everyone should become aware of their risk factors—the personal characteristics and habits that may increase one's chances of having a heart attack or stroke. In this Health and Fitness Activity, you will visit the American Heart Association's Internet site and assess your heart disease risk. The Internet site is: *http://www.heart.org/*. At the home page, click on "Healthy Lifestyle" and then "Health Tools." Next click on "My Life Check." Answer the questions in this assessment to estimate your "heart score." Answer the questions to the best of your ability. When finished, print the summary. Summarize the results below, and provide comment on what you learned (and turn in your printouts).

_____

_____

_____

_____

_____

_____

_____

_____

_____

_____

_____

_____

_____

_____

_____

_____

_____

_____

_____

_____

_____

HEALTH AND FITNESS ACTIVITY 9.3
Create Your Own Heart-Healthy Diet

The National Heart, Lung, and Blood Institute (NHLBI) has created an interactive Internet site to help you become more aware of how you can prevent heart disease. Go to this site: *http://www.nhlbi.nih.gov/*. At this site, click on "Interactive Tools." Next click on "Menu Planner." Follow the instructions, create your personal diet, and then print out the results. Summarize what you learned in this Health and Fitness Activity below (and turn in your printouts).

_____

_____

_____

_____

_____

_____

_____

_____

_____

_____

_____

_____

_____

_____

_____

_____

_____

_____

_____

_____

_____

_____

_____

HEALTH AND FITNESS ACTIVITY 9.4
Your Mother's Risk of Diabetes

Go to *www.diabetes.org/risk-test.jsp* and answer questions for your mother from the Diabetes Risk Test from the American Diabetes Association. Print out the results, and also print out information from this site that you can use in explaining the results to your mother. Summarize your counseling notes below (this can be conducted over the phone):

_____

_____

_____

_____

_____

_____

_____

_____

_____

_____

_____

_____

_____

_____

_____

_____

_____

_____

_____

HEALTH AND FITNESS ACTIVITY 9.5
Living Long and Healthfully—A Self-Test

This self-test will help you understand just how closely you adhere to a wide variety of recommended health practices. The choices you make now to improve your personal health habits will have much to do with the quality of the rest of your life.

Directions: Circle one number at the far right of each category that best represents your personal lifestyle. When finished, total all the numbers circled, and apply the result to the norms listed at the end.

1. Cigarette Smoking

A. Never smoked or quit more than 15 years ago	0
B. Ex-smoker, quit 5 to 15 years ago	3
C. Ex-smoker, quit within last 5 years	5
D. Current smoker, less than 20 cigarettes per day	9
E. Current smoker, 20 to 40 cigarettes per day	12
F. Current smoker, more than 40 cigarettes per day	15

2. Beverage Consumption (Alcohol, Coffee, Water)

Alcohol: How many alcoholic drinks do you consume? (A standard alcoholic drink contains .5 oz. of ethanol which is found in a 12 fl. oz. can of beer, a 4–5 fl. oz. glass of wine, or one ounce of 100-proof distilled spirits or whiskey.)

A. Never use alcohol	0
B. Less than once per week	2
C. 1 to 6 times per week	4
D. Once per day	7
E. 2 to 3 per day	9
F. More than 3 per day	13

Coffee: How many cups (6 fl. oz.) of coffee (do not include decaffeinated) do you drink?

A. Never use coffee	0
B. Less than once per week	1
C. 1 to 6 times per week	2
D. Once per day	3
E. 2 to 4 per day	4
F. More than 4 per day	6

Water: How many glasses (8 fl. oz.) of water do you drink per day?

A. More than 6 glasses per day	0
B. 4 to 6 glasses per day	1
C. Less than 3 per day	4

3. Diet

Note: Carefully note the portions sizes as you answer the questions. In addition, remember to include amounts used in cooking and mixed dishes.

Fruits and Vegetables (1/2 to 1 cup)
5 or more servings each day	0
2 to 4 servings each day	2
1 or less servings each day	3

Grain products (breads, cereals, pasta, rice) 1 slice/1/2 cup
6 or more servings each day	0
3 to 5 servings each day	2
2 or less servings each day	3

Red meats (beef, pork, lamb, veal; not fish or poultry) 3 oz.
Seldom or never use	0
Less than once per week	2
1 to 4 per week	3
5 to 6 per week	5
Daily	7

Cheeses (do not include cottage or low-fat cheese), 1 oz.
Seldom or never use	0
Less than once per day	1
More than once per day	2

Whole milk (not low-fat/skim), 1 cup
Seldom or never use	0
Less than once per day	1
More than once per day	2

Eggs (including yolk) 1 whole
Seldom or never use	0
1 or 2 per week	1
3 or 4 per week	2
More than 4 per week	3

4. Exercise/Fitness

Outside of your normal work or daily responsibilities, how often do you engage in exercise which moderately increases your breathing and heart rate, and makes you sweat, for at least 20 continuous minutes such as in brisk walking, cycling, swimming, jogging, aerobic dance, etc.?

A. 5 or more times per week	0
B. 3 to 4 times per week	1
C. 1 to 2 times per week	3
D. Less than 1 time per week	5
E. Seldom or never	7

5. Desirable Weight

How would you rate your body weight?

A. Very close to ideal	0
B. About 10% too high	2
C. About 11 to 25% too high	5
D. About 26 to 40% too high	7
E. More than 40% too high	10

6. Mental/Social/Spiritual Well-Being

A. In general, how satisfied are you with your life?

Mostly satisfied	0
Partly satisfied	1
Mostly disappointed	3

B. How often do you get insufficient rest so that you are unable to function efficiently?

Less than weekly	0
Usually one night per week	1
2 or 3 nights per week	2
4 or more nights per week	3

C. How would you describe the emotional stress you experience: *On the job (which includes being a student):*

Experience average or low levels of stress	0
Experience much stress but am able to cope with it	1
Experience much stress and often feel unable to cope	3

At home:

Experience average or low levels of stress	0
Experience much stress but am able to cope with it	1
Experience much stress and often feel unable to cope	3

D. Have you suffered a serious personal loss or misfortune in the past year? (For example, divorce, separation, jail term, death of a close person, job loss, disability)?

No	0
Yes, one serious loss	2
Yes, two or more serious losses	4

E. How many friends and relatives (including your spouse) do you feel close to? (People that you feel at ease with, can talk to about private matters, and can call on for help).

10 or more	0
5 to 9	1
1 to 4	2
None	3

F. How would you describe your spiritual health?

Good to Excellent	0
Fair to Poor	2
Very Poor	4

"Optimal spiritual health is defined as the ability to develop one's spiritual nature to its fullest potential. This includes our ability: to discover, articulate and act on our own basic purpose in life; to learn how to give and receive love, joy and peace; to pursue a fulfilling life; and to contribute to the improvement of the spiritual health of others."

[Am J Health Promotion 1(2):12–17, 1987.]

7. Personal Factors

A. Among your close relatives (parents, grandparents, aunts, uncles), how many deaths from heart disease or cancer have occurred before age 60:

None	0
1	2
2 or more	5

B. What percent of the time do you use seat belts while driving or riding?

100%	0
50–99%	2
25–49%	4
Less than 25% of the time	6

C. How often do you see your physician for a physical check-up?

At least once per year	0
Only once every three years	2
Only once every last five years	4

D. Your blood pressure is:

Low or normal (less than 120/80 mm Hg)	0
Borderline high (120/80 to 139/89)	3
Moderately high (140/90 to 159/94)	8
Very high (160/95 and higher)	12

E. Your serum cholesterol is:

Low (less than 180 mg/dl)	0
Borderline high (180–199 mg/dl)	3
Moderately high (200–239 mg/dl)	8
Very high (240 mg/dl and higher)	12

---

*If you do not know your blood pressure, we highly recommend that you get it measured very soon. To complete the self-scoring test, you can estimate your blood pressure ranking by evaluating two lifestyle factors: body weight and sale intake. If your body weight and sodium intake are optimal, your risk of high blood pressure is greatly lowered.

**If you do not know your serum cholesterol, we highly recommend that you get it measured very soon. To complete the self-scoring test, you can estimate your serum cholesterol ranking by evaluating several lifestyle factors: saturated fat, dietary cholesterol, and dietary fiber intakes, body weight, and regular exercise. If your dietary intake of meats and dairy products (which are high in saturated fat and cholesterol) is low, while your intake of whole grains, fruits, and vegetables (rich in dietary fiber) is high, and your body weight and physical activity levels are at desirable levels, there is a good chance your serum cholesterol level is low.

What Does Your Score Mean?

Score	Rating	Explanation
0 to 20	Excellent	Congratulations! You adhere very well to the recommended lifestyle. Your potential for increased longevity and decreased risk of both heart disease and cancer are very high.
21 to 40	Very Good	If you find yourself in this category, you are probably only one or two lifestyle habits away from earning an excellent rating. You've already made wonderful progress—keep up the good work.
41 to 70	Fair	Many Americans will find themselves in this category. To fall in this category, you may not have but one or two outstanding health problems. However, due to several less than optimal health practices in a wide variety of areas, your point total has reached an undesirable level. By gradually working on selected areas, improving health practices that you are presently motivated to act on, you can steadily progress to the "excellent" rating. Improved longevity and quality of life will be your reward.
71 to 95	Poor	Your risk of heart disease, cancer, and early death is high. Now is the time to sit down with your spouse or close friends and establish health behavior change goals, following the principles outlined in this book. There are many case histories of people who have turned their health lifestyles completely around, reaping abundant health benefits. The human body responds fruitfully to an improved lifestyle, often repairing some of the damage already experienced.
96 to 140	Very Poor	Unusually high risk of early death due to heart disease and/or cancer. You are urged to make an appointment with your physician to have a thorough check-up, and to seek counseling for an improved lifestyle.

CHAPTER 9 QUIZ
Prevention of Heart Disease

Note: Answers are given at the end of the quiz.

1. Which subgroup listed below has the highest smoking prevalence?
   A. people with a college education
   B. American Indian/Alaskan Native
   C. Blacks
   D. the elderly
   E. Asians

2. Smoking kills over 443,000 Americans each year; what is the #2 ranked killer of smokers?
   A. cancer
   B. respiratory disease
   C. CVD
   D. other

3. The Year 2020 goal for smoking prevalence among adults is _____ %.
   A. 25
   B. 33
   C. 5
   D. 18
   E. 12

4. Chest pain that radiates to the neck and arms because of CHD is called:
   A. cerebrovascular accident (CVA).
   B. myocardial infarction.
   C. angina pectoris.
   D. thrombus.
   E. endarterectomy.

5. Which one of the following risk factors is considered by the American Heart Association to be a contributing (but not major) factor that can be changed?
   A. stress
   B. cigarette smoking
   C. physical inactivity
   D. high blood pressure
   E. high blood cholesterol

6. Which one of the following risk factors is not used by the American Heart Association (AHA)?
   A. obesity
   B. high blood pressure
   C. high homocysteine
   D. stress
   E. high total serum cholesterol

7. Which term is defined as the formation of a clot in one of the arteries that conduct blood to the heart muscle?
   A. coronary thrombosis
   B. cerebrovascular accident
   C. cerebral embolism
   D. congestive heart failure
   E. bradycardia

8. Excessive alcohol intake tends to increase risk of what type of stroke?
   A. cerebral hemorrhage
   B. cerebral thrombosis
   C. cerebral embolism
   D. TIA
   E. CHD

9. When the systolic blood pressure is greater than a threshold of _____ mm Hg, this is an indication of high blood pressure (when based on two or more readings).
   A. 160
   B. 170
   C. 80
   D. 140
   E. 90

10. A heart attack is also called a:
    A. stroke.
    B. myocardial infarction.
    C. angina pectoris.
    D. cerebral thrombus.

11. Sudden temporary weakness or numbness on one side of the face is a sign of a:
    A. heart attack.
    B. myocardial infarction.
    C. stroke.
    D. angina pectoris.

12. All Americans are urged to consume no more than ____ grams of sodium a day.
    A. 1
    B. 1.5
    C. 2.4
    D. 3.5
    E. 4

13. More than a threshold of _____ alcoholic drinks a day can lead to high blood pressure.
    A. 1
    B. 2
    C. 3
    D. 5

14. Aerobic exercise, weight reduction, and _____ help to increase the HDL-C.
    A. smoking cessation
    B. low-fat diet
    C. low-cholesterol diet
    D. high-fiber diet

15. The single most important lifestyle-change measure to reduce high blood pressure is:
    A. cigarette smoking cessation.
    B. reduction of body weight.
    C. control of high blood cholesterol levels.
    D. sodium restriction.
    E. alcohol restriction.

16. An optimal LDL-C level (according to the NCEP) is less than a threshold of ____ mg/dl.
    A. 100
    B. 130
    C. 160
    D. 200

17. Which factor listed below is most important in decreasing LDL-C and total serum cholesterol?
   A. control of stress
   B. decrease in coffee consumption
   C. decrease in dietary cholesterol intake
   D. decrease in dietary saturated fat intake
   E. increase in water soluble fiber intake

18. HDL-C is considered "too low" by the National Cholesterol Education Program (NCEP) when under a threshold of _____ mg/dL.
   A. 25
   B. 40
   C. 45
   D. 65
   E. 55

19. The National Cholesterol Education program has established that total serum cholesterol levels of _____ – _____ mg/dL indicate "borderline-high" levels.
   A. 180–200
   B. 200–239
   C. 220–279
   D. 240–299
   E. 130–160

20. Another name for stroke is:
   A. coronary thrombosis.
   B. cerebrovascular accident.
   C. cerebral embolism.
   D. congestive heart failure.
   E. arteriosclerosis.

chapter ten

Prevention and Treatment of Obesity

"If a company came up with a drug that would help burn fat, allow you to eat more and not gain weight, and had no major side effects, you would probably buy stock. But we already have this in physical activity"
—Dr. James Hill, obesity researcher

Introduction

This is the "era of caloric anxiety," a time in which we stand torn between our thin standards of beauty and fat ways of living. Thin is in, but so are triple cheese burgers, drive-through banking, golf carts, and the Internet.

Is it any wonder that our waistlines are growing as rapidly as our rich food supply and technology? The consequence is a preoccupation with weight loss. The Centers for Disease Control and Prevention (CDC) estimates that four in 10 adults try to lose weight within a given year. Among adults attempting to lose or maintain weight, only one in five follows the two key recommendations to eat fewer calories and to increase physical activity.

In our drive to lose weight, we use many methods, including exercise, low-fat foods, low-calorie beverages, fasting, weight-loss classes, medication, herbs, and meal substitutes. A *Consumer Reports* survey of 95,000 people showed that although most had tried to lose weight on their own, 24 percent had used meal-replacement products such as Slim-Fast and DynaTrim, 20 percent had joined a commercial weight-loss program (e.g., Jenny Craig, Inc.), and 6 percent had tried over-the-counter appetite suppressants such as Acutrim and Dexatrim. Concerns about health, fitness, and appearance are cited most frequently by Americans for their repeated attempts to lose weight.

Widespread Problem

Despite our nationwide obsession with weight loss, government studies over the past 50 years have shown that we are losing the war. **Overweight,** defined as a Body Mass Index (BMI) of 25 and higher, now afflicts two thirds of the population, with the highest rates found among the poor and minority groups. (Review figure 10.1 and Chapter 5 for information on BMI and other methods for determining body composition). And 33 percent of adults are **obese,** defined as a BMI of 30 and higher.

FIGURE 10.1

How to estimate overweight and obesity using the Body Mass Index.

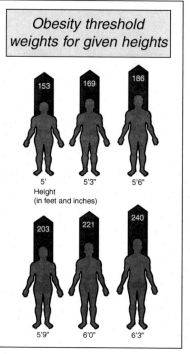

How to Estimate Obesity

Obesity can be estimated by using a mathematical formula called the body mass index (BMI)—weight in kilograms divided by height in meters squared (BMI = kg/m².)

⇨ A BMI of 18.5 to 24.9 is considered a "nomal" weight.

⇨ A BMI of 25 to 29.9 is considered overweight.

⇨ A BMI of 30 or above is considered obese.

Obesity threshold weights for given heights

FIGURE 10.2

The percent of overweight adults has increased strongly since the 1960s.

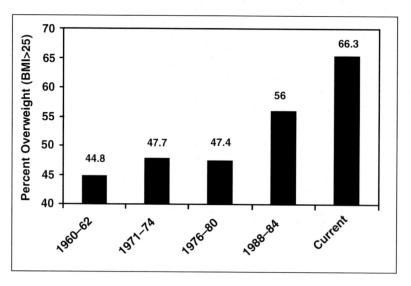

We failed to achieve the federal government's year 2010 goal to reduce the prevalence of obesity among adults to no more than 15 percent (figure 10.2). Data collected since the 1960s show significant increases in overweight and obesity prevalence for all segments of the American society. Among children and adolescents, nearly one in five is rated as overweight, up substantially from the 1960s (figure 10.3). Several international comparisons have shown that Americans are among the heaviest people in the world.

Health Hazards of Obesity

There are many health hazards associated with obesity, now regarded as one of the most important medical and public health problems of our era. About 400,000 deaths each year can be traced to obesity, physical inactivity, and poor diet. Only smoking exceeds obesity in its contribution to early death. In general, people enjoying the best health weigh

FIGURE 10.3

The percent of overweight children and adolescents has more than tripled since the 1960s.

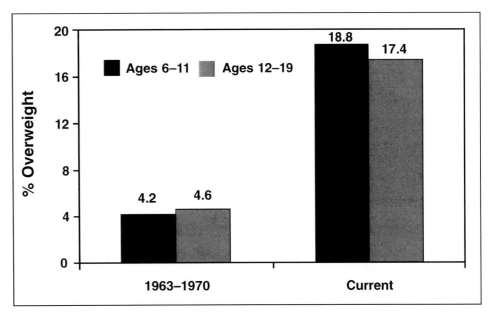

15 percent to 20 percent less than the average American. In contrast, those gaining weight suffer a loss in quality of life and vitality, and an increase in bodily pain.

There are at least nine major health problems of obesity. Eight in 10 obese persons have one of the health problems listed below, with 25 percent having two or more. Obese people most vulnerable to these health problems tend to have more of their fat in the abdomen rather than the hip and thigh areas (as reviewed in Chapter 5).

- *A psychological burden:* Because of strong pressures from society to be thin, obese people often suffer feelings of guilt, depression, anxiety, and low self-esteem.
- *Increased high blood pressure:* High blood pressure is much more common among the overweight, and the risk climbs strongly with increase in body weight (see Chapter 9).
- *Increased levels of cholesterol and blood fats:* Overweight individuals are more likely than normal weight persons to have high blood cholesterol and triglycerides, and lower HDL-cholesterol (see Chapter 9).
- *Increased heart disease and stroke:* Obese people not only have more of the risk factors for heart disease and stroke, they also die from these two types of cardiovascular disease at a much higher rate (see Chapter 9).
- *Increased diabetes:* Obesity is the strongest of all lifestyle risk factors for diabetes.
- *Increased cancer:* Obese men and women have higher cancer death rates for most of the major cancers when compared to the nonobese (see Box 10.1).
- *Increased osteoarthritis:* Overweight persons are at high risk of osteoarthritis in the knee and hips.
- *Increased gallbladder disease:* The risk for gallstones rises sharply with increase in Body Mass Index.
- *Increased early death:* Death rates from all causes are higher among the obese, while men and women of normal weight have the lowest death rates. The odds are most dismal in the heaviest people, who are at least two times more likely to die early than slimmer folks (figure 10.4).

Why Are So Many Overweight?

Explaining why so many Americans weigh more than they should has been a source of confusion to researchers and the public alike. Many changes have occurred in U.S. society during the past century that encourage obesity including the growth of the fast food industry, the availability of more high-calorie snacks, greater time spent viewing television

BOX 10.1

Obesity and Cancer

Obese compared to nonobese males have higher death rates for several types of cancers, including colon and prostate. For obese females, risk of death is greater for breast, uterine, ovarian, and gallbladder cancer. Although obesity is a risk factor for certain types of cancer, poor diets and tobacco use account for the majority of cancer.

There are many types of cancers, but they can all be characterized by uncontrolled growth and spread of abnormal cells. If the spread is not controlled, it can result in death, as vital passageways are blocked and the body's oxygen and nutrient supply is diverted to support the rapidly growing cancer.

The lifetime risk of developing cancer is 44 percent for men and 38 percent for women. About 1.3 million Americans are diagnosed with cancer each year (not including the more than 1 million cases of skin cancer). Just under one in four deaths each year in the United States are from cancer. The leading cancer killer for both men and women is lung cancer, followed by prostate or breast cancer, and colorectal cancer.

About 75 percent of cancers are preventable and are linked to lifestyle. Here are the chief risk factors for cancer:

- Dietary factors (33% of all cancers)
- Tobacco use (31% of all cancers)
- Physical inactivity and obesity
- Alcohol use
- Reproductive factors (primarily for breast cancer)
- Unsafe sex (exposure to certain types of cancer promoting viruses)
- Environmental factors (especially sunlight, radiation and radon exposure, and air pollution)
- Family history

Overall, to reduce cancer risk, people should avoid all tobacco use, consume low-fat, high-fiber diets containing plenty of whole grains, fruits, and vegetables, be physically active and maintain a healthy weight, limit consumption of alcoholic beverages, practice safe sex, and limit exposure to ultraviolet radiation.

With regular screening and self-exams, cancer can often be detected early, greatly enhancing the success of treatment. More than half of all new cancer cases occur in screening-accessible cancer sites. If the cancer is detected early, it can often be successfully treated by surgery, radiation, chemotherapy, hormones, and immunotherapy.

Regular physical activity helps protect against three common cancer killers: colon, breast, and prostate cancer. The strongest evidence comes from research on colon cancer, where physical activity has been shown to reduce the risk by up to 50 percent. Physical activity may alter the concentration of hormones in the body, which are related to breast and prostate cancer, help keep people lean, and have a fiber-like effect in accelerating the movement of fecal matter through the colon. An international cancer panel recommends that to optimize cancer prevention, people should take a brisk walk for about an hour daily (or the equivalent) and exercise vigorously at least one hour total a week.

FIGURE 10.4

Deaths rates climb strongly with increase in body mass index.

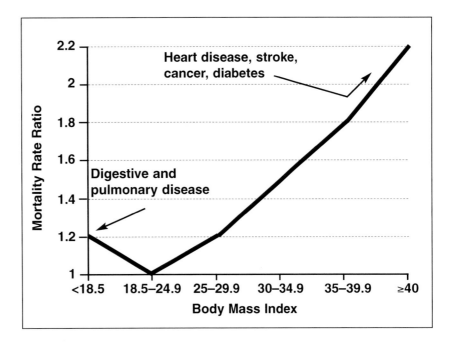

and the Internet, a lack of physical education in our schools, an automated workplace and household, and the use of the automobile for short-distance travel instead of through walking or bicycling. One study, for example, showed that when needing to travel distances shorter than one mile, three out of four times, people use the car.

In general, three factors are most responsible for weight gain leading to obesity: (1) genetic and parental influences, (2) high calorie and high fat diets, and (3) insufficient physical activity.

Genetic and Parental Influences

We have numerous genes that have the potential to interact with each other, and the lifestyle to promote obesity. A certain genetic makeup can favor the development of obesity, especially when diet and exercise habits are less than desirable. For example, the Pima Indians in Arizona were once of normal weight, living as hardy farmers near the Gila River. Today the majority of Pima Indians are obese and physically inactive, and consume a high-fat diet. Although modern Pima Indians have the same genetic makeup of their forebearers, their lifestyles have been drastically altered, allowing the expression of certain genes that favor obesity.

Genetic factors do have a strong effect on body weight and shape as we grow older. Studies show, for example, that even when reared apart as infants and children, the body weights of identical twins by middle age are much closer than those of fraternal twins or siblings. A study of adults who had been adopted before the age of one revealed that despite being brought up by their adoptive parents, their body weights were still more similar to those of their real parents.

Despite genetic influences, personal lifestyle choices for most people are more powerful in explaining body weight. In other words, diet and exercise habits have more to do with the way we look than our genes. Some people, however, especially those with obese parents and siblings, are more prone to obesity than others because of genetic factors, and will have to be unusually careful in their lifestyle habits to counteract these influences.

High-Calorie, High-Fat Diets

There is good reason to believe that the abundance of tasty, calorically rich foods, especially those high in fats, is a major factor explaining the widespread problem of obesity in western societies. When dietary intake of fat is high, most people tend to gain weight rather easily and quickly. When intake of dietary fats is low, and most calories are in the form of carbohydrate, desirable body weight is more readily achieved.

Obese compared to lean people tend to eat faster, choosing more high-fat and energy-rich foods. It is difficult to control body weight when eating high-fat foods because they are high in calories and taste good, prompting people to eat a surplus of energy that is easily converted to body fat. See Health and Fitness Activity 10.2 to estimate how many calories you should be eating based on your body size, age, gender, and physical activity.

A significant proportion of obese people, about 25 percent to 50 percent according to some estimates, suffer from binge eating, defined as consuming large amounts of food at one sitting while feeling out of control. Binge eating disorder is diagnosed by health professionals using these criteria:

- During a binge eating episode, large amounts of food are eaten rapidly until feeling uncomfortably full, often while alone because of embarrassment.
- The amount of food eaten is definitely larger than most people would eat in a similar period of time, and there is a feeling that one cannot stop eating or control what or how much one is eating.
- The binge eater experiences feelings of disgust, depression, and extreme guilt after overeating.
- The binge eating occurs, on average, at least two days a week for six months.

Insufficient Physical Activity

Are overweight children and adults less active than normal-weight people? As you might have suspected, the answer is "yes." Obese men, for example, have been found to walk about 3.7 miles during the normal course of their day, compared to 6 miles for normal weight men. Obese people tend to stay in bed longer, spend less time on their feet, and when given the choice of an escalator or stairs, are more likely than the lean to take the escalator. Obese compared to lean adolescents and adults also tend to watch television and play video games more. Obese children spend 40 percent less time in general physical activity than lean children. During an average day, lean individuals burn about 20 calories for each pound of body weight in physical activity, compared to only 8 calories per pound for the obese.

Even when playing sports, obese individuals are less active. For example, obese compared to lean teenage girls spend less time moving their arms and legs and more time standing and floating while in the swimming pool.

Does the inactivity cause obesity or is it the other way around, with obesity leading to inactivity? It is both—lack of activity promotes a gain in body weight, and then a vicious cycle sets in as physical activity becomes more onerous.

How to Lose Weight: The Basics

As you may have experienced (or seen in others), losing weight and then keeping it off is a difficult challenge. According to weight management experts, many overweight people will not stay in treatment. Of those who do, most will not achieve ideal body weight, and of those who lose weight, most will regain it. People find it somewhat easy to lose weight in the short term, but after completing the weight-loss scheme, tend to quickly regain the weight back.

Obesity has typically been treated as if it is an acute illness like the flu, when it is more appropriately viewed as a chronic condition (e.g., like heart disease or diabetes). Since the ultimate goal of a weight-reduction program is to lose weight and then maintain the loss, a healthy but low-calorie diet that fits into one's lifestyle is best.

A comprehensive weight-loss program that incorporates diet, exercise, and behavior modification is more likely to lead to long-term weight control.

- **Diet** The caloric intake should be reduced, preferably by reducing the fat content of the diet, while increasing intake of carbohydrates and dietary fiber (e.g., whole grains, fruits, and vegetables).
- **Exercise** Energy expenditure should be increased by at least 200 to 400 calories per day. This can be accomplished by including a 30 to 45 minute exercise session on most days of the week, and also by adding physical activity throughout the normal routine of each day (e.g., taking the stairs instead of the elevator, or walking during work breaks). An hour a day or more of physical activity is best for losing weight.
- **Behavior modification** Behavior modification is defined as the development of skills to extinguish undesirable behaviors. Several techniques can be employed to increase awareness of caloric intake, with rewards provided for good behavior and achieving personal goals.

Role of Diet

The CDC estimates that more than two thirds of U.S. adults are trying to lose or maintain weight. However, only a fifth of those trying to lose weight are following the recommended combination of eating fewer calories and engaging in 150 minutes or more of physical activity each week. The typical American is bewildered, confused, and misguided by the onslaught of conflicting information on weight loss methods.

In 1998, the first federal guidelines for the treatment of overweight and obesity in adults were released by the National Heart, Lung, and Blood Institute (NHLBI) as a part of their nationwide Obesity Education Initiative. With millions of overweight Americans, the NHLBI has made education about overweight and obesity a major priority. Key diet recommendations from this initiative include the following:

- The initial goal of a weight loss regimen should be to reduce body weight by about 10 percent. With success, further weight loss can be attempted, if needed.
- Weight loss should be about 1 to 2 pounds per week for a period of six months, with additional plans based on the amount of weight loss. Seek to create a deficit of 500 to 1,000 calories per day through a combination of decreased caloric intake and increased physical activity.
- Reducing dietary fat intake is a practical way to reduce calories, but reducing dietary fat alone without reducing calories is not sufficient for weight loss.

Each pound of body fat represents about 3,500 calories. To follow the NHLBI for weight loss, one must expend 500 to 1000 calories more than the amount taken in through the diet. This can be accomplished by increasing energy expenditure 200 to 400 calories a day through physical activity, and reducing dietary fat intake by 300 to 600 calories. Each tablespoon of fat represents about 100 calories, so an emphasis on low-fat dairy products and lean meats, and a low intake of visible fats (oils, butter, margarine, salad dressings, sour cream, etc.) is the easiest way to reduce caloric intake without reducing the volume of food eaten.

The NHLBI recommends this diet for weight loss:

- Eat 500 to 1,000 calories a day below usual intake.
- Keep total dietary fat intake below 30 percent of calories, and carbohydrate at 55 percent or more of total calories.
- Emphasize a heart-healthy diet by keeping saturated fats under 10 percent of total calories, cholesterol under 300 mg per day, and sodium less than 2,400 mg per day.
- Choose foods high in dietary fiber (20–30 grams per day).

This diet starts in the grocery store, by learning to read food labels and choosing healthy foods. Another challenge is eating healthfully when dining out. Learn to ask for salad dressing on the side and to leave all butter, gravy, or sauces off the dish. Select foods that are steamed, garden fresh, broiled, baked, roasted, poached, or lightly sautéed or stir-fried. See Health and Fitness Activity 10.3 to learn more about the calorie and fat content of fast foods.

BOX 10.2

Weight Loss Claims Are No Joke for Dieters

Are you one of the millions of Americans who will go on a diet this year? If so, you may be tempted by advertisements for products promising easy, quick ways to lose weight. You should know that when it comes to losing weight, gimmicks usually don't deliver on their promises.

While some dieters succeed in taking off weight, perhaps as few as 5 percent manage to keep it off in the long run. Most experts agree that the best way to lose weight is to eat fewer calories and burn more energy by increasing physical activity. Experts suggest aiming for a goal loss of about a pound a week. This usually means cutting about 500 calories a day from your diet, eating healthy, low-fat foods, finding a regular exercise activity you enjoy, and sticking to it.

When it comes to evaluating claims for weight loss products, the Federal Trade Commission recommends a healthy portion of skepticism. Before you spend money on products or programs that promise fast or easy weight loss, weigh the claims and consider these tips:

Deceptive Claims versus the Truth

- *"Lose 30 Pounds in Just 30 Days."* As a rule, the faster you lose weight, the more likely you are to gain it back. Also, fast weight loss could harm your health. Don't look for programs that promise quick weight loss.
- *"Lose All the Weight You Can For Just $39.99."* Some weight loss programs have hidden costs. For example, some don't advertise the fact that you must buy their prepackaged meals that cost more than the program fees. Before you sign up for any weight loss program, ask for all the costs. Get them in writing.
- *"Lose Weight While You Sleep."* Claims for diet products and programs that promise weight loss without effort are phony.
- *"Lose Weight And Keep It Off For Good."* Be suspicious about products promising long-term or permanent weight loss. To lose weight and keep it off, you must change how you eat and how much you exercise for the rest of your life.
- *"John Doe Lost 84 Pounds in Six Weeks."* Don't be misled by someone else's weight loss claims. Even if the claims are true, someone else's success may have little relation to your own chances of success. And their methods may have been unhealthy. A major objective is to lose body weight while keeping your health.
- *"Scientific Breakthrough . . . Medical Miracle."* There are no miracle weight loss products. To lose weight, you have to reduce your intake of calories and increase your physical activity. Be skeptical about exaggerated claims.

For more information, visit the Federal Trade Commission's web site: http://www.ftc.gov.

Choosing a Safe and Successful Weight-Loss Program

Many overweight people lose weight on their own without entering a weight-loss program; others need the social and professional support that commercial weight-loss programs provide. Almost any of the commercial weight-loss programs can work on the short term, but they may not promote safe and healthy habits that can be followed over the long term. Avoid programs that make unbelievable claims, as summarized in Box 10.2 by the Federal Trade Commission. Box 10.3 lists several Internet sites that provide excellent information on weight management programs.

BOX 10.3

Internet Sites for Weight Management

National Heart, Lung, and Blood Institute (NHLBI)
http://www.nhlbi.nih.gov/
Includes consumer information on weight management, and clinical guidelines on overweight and obesity for professionals.

Weight-Control Information Network (WIN)
http://win.niddk.nih.gov/
A reliable source of weight control, obesity, and nutrition information for consumers and health professionals. A service of the National Institute of Diabetes and Digestive and Kidney Diseases, National Institutes of Health, U.S. Department of Health and Human Services.

Weightfocus.com
http://www.weightfocus.com/
Offers visitors a wide variety of webcast programming featuring weight management experts, complemented by in-depth articles on weight loss strategies, diet myths, and health issues.

Shape Up America!
http://www.shapeup.org/
Provides information on safe weight management, healthy eating, and physical fitness.

Diettalk
http://www.diettalk.com/
A comprehensive source of information on obesity, nutrition, physical activity, diets, and eating disorders.

Cyberdiet
http://www.cyberdiet.com/
A complete source of information on diet and nutrition, exercise and fitness, weight loss, and self-assessment of body fat distribution and disease risk.

American Anorexia Bulimia Association, Inc.
http://www.aabainc.org/
Gives complete information about eating disorders for sufferers, family and friends, and professionals.

What elements of a weight-loss program should you look for in judging its potential for safe and successful weight loss? Look for these features:

- *Provides or encourages food intake that exceeds 1,200 calories per day for a woman and 1,600 calories per day for a man.* Diets lower than this amount are not recommended for most overweight and obese individuals, because they are typically low in essential vitamins and minerals, and can lead to excess muscle loss and lower metabolism.
- *The diet is nutritionally safe.* It should include all of the vitamins and minerals at recommended intake levels. Although low in calories, it should be based on the Food Guide Pyramid, providing servings from all of the recommended food groups. High-protein diets are not recommended (see Box 10.4). Weight loss diets should promote your health, not harm it.

BOX 10.4

An Evaluation of Low-Carbohydrate, High-Protein Diets

Low-carbohydrate, high-protein diets are back in the news. These diets have been around since the 1930s, but were first popularized in the 1970s when liquid protein diets and Dr. Atkins' first book on the high protein diet hit the market. The liquid protein diets were made of poor-quality protein, and provided only 300 to 500 calories per day. By the late 1970s, 58 deaths were related to the liquid protein diet. Dr. Atkins promoted a low-carbohydrate, high-protein diet as the best way to lose weight quickly. Several studies refuted the usefulness and healthfulness of this diet and other similar plans, and the public moved on to other schemes.

Well, they're back. Of the top 10 diet books today, nearly all deal with carbohydrate restriction or "bad carbs" versus "good carbs." Today, best-selling books like *Dr. Atkins' New Diet Revolution* push low-carbohydrate, high-protein diets as the superior method to lose weight. These low-carbohydrate diets (less than 30% of calories) are higher in fat (30% to 80% of calories) and protein (30% to 40% of calories) than is recommended for health.

These books recommend building breakfast, lunch, and dinner around eggs, meat, or fish. High-carbohydrate foods such as pasta, bread, rice, potatoes, sugar-rich desserts, and most fruits are restricted. If you follow these rules, the authors say, you can eat what you like while losing body fat.

Do they work? Yes, most people lose weight when on these diets, at least for a while, because they eat fewer calories than normal. But any diet that prompts people to eat less than normal will promote weight loss. People lose weight, but not because of the misleading rationale provided by the diet authors. Most importantly, the diet plans are not healthy over the long term—high protein diets are also high in fat, and low in fruits, vegetables, and whole grains, a sure recipe for heart disease and cancer.

What about the research reports that the Atkins diet decreases blood cholesterol and levels of other heart disease risk factors? Subjects in these studies were only followed for a few months, and weight loss by just about any method will help counter disease risk factors. Over the long term, every major study has found that animal-saturated fat will increase both heart disease and cancer risk. In fact, the single most important diet factor behind high LDL-cholesterol (i.e., your "bad cholesterol") is saturated fat, the kind marbled in and coating that steak people eat on the Atkins diet. Concerns have also been raised regarding the low dietary fiber and calcium content of the Atkins diet, which increase risk for colon cancer and osteoporosis.

The bottom line is that those successful at weight loss have "caloric awareness." In other words, those who lose weight and keep it off over the long term are aware of the calories they eat relative to those expended through exercise. These individuals know how to balance the calories coming in with those going out. No gimmick diets or hocus pocus—they just work at keeping under caloric control.

We are in the midst of an obesity epidemic. Nearly two in three Americans are overweight or obese, and most of our major disease killers are related to carrying extra fat. The cause is simple—Americans are eating too much and exercising too little. Fad diets such as the Atkins diet are not the solution, because they postpone the ultimate decision to get one's diet and exercise habits under control. You can't live on the Atkins diet for the rest of your life, because your heart can't take it. You may lose weight in the short term with this diet, but in the end, you're facing the same habits that got you into trouble in the first place.

- *Promotes a safe and realistic weight loss of 1 to 2 pounds per week.* Good weight management programs don't promise or imply dramatic, rapid weight loss. Don't seek a "quick fix," because the quicker the weight comes off, the quicker it goes back on. Although not as appealing, slow and gradual weight loss is more effective.
- *Does not attempt to make you dependent on special products that are sold for a profit.* The best programs emphasize wise choices from the traditional food supply, and feature supermarket and restaurant tours and cooking schools to teach you how to improve food selection and meal preparation. Learn how to improve eating habits within the context of your own sociocultural and income background.
- *Do not promote or sell products that are unproven or spurious.* Companies sell a wide array of weight loss products that have little if any value, including starch blockers, grapefruit pills, sauna belts, body wraps, ear staples, and hormone releasers.
- *Is led by a qualified instructor.* Health promotion professionals, registered dietitians, and physicians specializing in weight control are qualified to direct weight control programs. Check out the experience and credentials of the weight control program leaders before signing up.
- *Includes a maintenance phase.* It is difficult to change behaviors that you have formed over many years. Relapse often occurs during stressful life events. Weight control programs should provide support on a regular basis for at least one year after you have lost weight.
- *Emphasizes a lifestyle approach.* Good programs include guidance on exercise, diet, and behavior change that are continued for a lifetime, not just the duration of the program.

If you want or need to lose weight, try to reduce on your own, or through a free hospital-based program, before spending money on a commercial weight loss center. Focus first on exercising and eating a healthful diet, and see how successful you can be on your own.

Do not be tempted by advertisements for products promising easy, quick ways to lose weight (Box 10.2). In general, if the weight loss product seems to good to be true, it usually is. Weight loss is hard work, and there is no magic. A lifelong commitment to a change in lifestyle is necessary. For most obese people, modest goals and a slow course will maximize the probability of both losing the weight and keeping it off.

The whole concept of dieting can be criticized on psychological grounds, for going *on* a diet implies going *off* it, and the resumption of old eating habits. For this reason, one can argue that the most effective diet is not a diet at all but rather a gradual change in eating patterns and a shift to foods that the person can continue to eat indefinitely. This means increasing the intake of complex carbohydrates such as fruits, vegetables, legumes, and cereals, and decreasing the intake of fats and refined sugars. In other words, the diet that is being recommended for the treatment and prevention of heart disease, cancer, and diabetes is the same diet that should be used in preventing and treating obesity. This course of action probably gives the best chance of maintaining the weight that is lost, and it is an eminently safe one. In general, one should not lose weight by any method that cannot be included permanently within a healthy lifestyle.

Role of Physical Activity

Physical activity is a critical strategy in the "battle of the bulge." It makes sense that if one pound of fat contains 3,500 surplus calories, you have to burn these calories through extra activity to lose the fat. See Health and Fitness Activity 10.4 to learn more about the role of physical activity in weight management.

Physical activity can influence body weight three different ways (figure 10.5):

- Prevent weight gain in the first place.
- Help you lose weight if overweight or obese.
- Maintain a good body weight after the excess weight is lost.

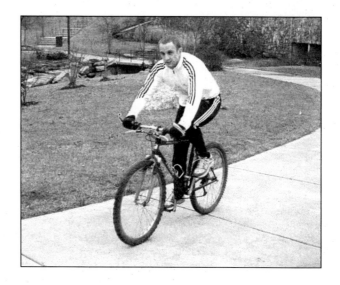

FIGURE 10.5

Physical activity is important for preventing and treating overweight, and maintaining a good body weight after the excess weight is lost.

Physical Activity and Prevention of Weight Gain

Near-daily physical activity that is continued month after month, year after year, lowers the risk of gaining weight as we grow older. In fact, one of the strongest predictors of leanness during adulthood is regular physical activity. In one study, researchers from the American Cancer Institute followed over 79,000 people for 10 years and found that those engaging in vigorous exercise one to three hours a week, or walking for more than four hours a week, were better able to ward off weight gain than their more sedentary counterparts.

Most adults gain weight slowly, about one pound a year on average, according to most estimates. At the same time, muscle mass is slowly lost while body fat increases. This slow change in the quality and quantity of body weight is countered by regular physical activity if the diet is also kept under good control. In other words, one of the chief benefits of near-daily physical activity is the capacity to fight off the "creeping obesity" that most adults experience from ages 25 to 65.

Exercise in the Treatment of Obesity

Does aerobic exercise accelerate weight loss significantly when combined with a reducing diet? The answer is "yes," but for most overweight and obese people, the extra weight lost is small when compared to that caused by the diet.

Because most overweight people can only exercise moderately, the actual amount of energy expended tends to be lower than expected, and has a rather small impact on weight loss during a two- to four-month reducing diet. For example, one analysis of nearly 500 studies showed that diet alone helps the average person lose about 23 pounds over 15 weeks, and 24 pounds when a moderate exercise program is added.

Brisk walking two to three miles a day increases energy expenditure about 125 to 250 calories above normal (depending on body size), a rather small amount when contrasted with the 3,500 calories stored in one pound of fat. If aerobic exercise is to have a major effect on weight loss during a two- to four-month weight loss program, daily exercise sessions need to be unusually long in duration (more than one hour) and high in intensity, something that most overweight people cannot do (or desire).

The practical advice is that exercise alone must not be seen as the one and only major weapon in the treatment of obesity. Instead, improvements in the quality and quantity of the diet should take the lead, with exercise relegated to an important supporting role. Regular exercise has many other more important benefits, especially those related to health. Over the long term, the calories expended during exercise do add up, helping to prevent weight gain or maintain weight loss, but during a short two- to four-month weight loss program, do not expect that moderate exercise will cut down your body fat significantly.

Exercise and the Resting Metabolic Rate

The resting metabolic rate (RMR) is the energy expended by the body to maintain life and normal body functions such as respiration and circulation. The RMR can be estimated using various formulas. See Health and Fitness Activity 10.1 to estimate the number of calories you burn each day through your RMR. The RMR of the average 154 pound person is about 1,700 calories per day, or 60 percent to 75 percent of all the energy expended in one day.

Does exercise cause the RMR to stay elevated for a long time after the bout, burning extra calories? There is a slight increase in RMR for a short time after moderate exercise, but the actual amount of extra energy expended is too small to have a meaningful effect on body weight. For example, jogging (12 minutes per mile), walking, or cycling at moderate intensities for about one half hour causes the RMR to stay elevated for 20 to 30 minutes, burning 10 to 12 extra calories. When the intensity is increased to higher levels, RMR is increased for about 35 to 45 minutes, with 15 to 30 extra calories expended.

For the obese individual who takes a 20 to 30 minute walk, about 10 extra calories will be burned during recovery, hardly enough to be meaningful when balanced against other factors.

Physical Activity and Maintenance of Weight Loss

More vigorous efforts should be put forth to maintain weight loss following programs. Losing weight and then keeping it off is hard work, and relapse occurs in 95 of 100 people attempting to achieve a healthy weight. In general, you should seek to redouble your efforts and obtain professional help whenever you regain 10 pounds.

Regular physical activity is one of the best predictors of those who are able to maintain weight loss over the long term. Researchers at the University of Pittsburgh and University of Colorado have formed a national registry of people who have lost more than 30 pounds and kept it off for more than a year. Several hundred people are now in this registry, and several interesting findings have emerged:

- 94 percent of successful losers increased their physical activity level to accomplish their weight loss, with walking the most common activity reported.
- 92 percent report that they are continuing to exercise to maintain weight loss. Those most successful in fighting back weight regain typically exercise for at least one hour a day, burning at least 400 calories each day.
- 98 percent decreased their food intake in some way.
- 57 percent received professional help from doctors, registered dietitians, Weight Watchers, and others.

In other words, there is no magic as to why people lose and keep it off. They just keep exercising and watching what they eat.

The Benefits of Physical Activity for the Overweight and Obese

As emphasized earlier, many health hazards are linked to being overweight and obese. Regular physical activity helps to counter many of these health problems. Long-term exercise is also a vital factor together with prudent dietary habits to keep body weight under good control and to build physical fitness. There are at least five health-related benefits of exercise for those who are overweight and obese:

- Improves aerobic fitness.
- Decreases blood fats and increases HDL-cholesterol (the "good" cholesterol).
- Improves psychological well-being and vigor, and decreases anxiety and depression.
- Decreases the risk of diseases that are common among the obese (e.g., diabetes, heart disease, cancer, and high blood pressure). Weight loss can also reduce symptoms of arthritis by lessening strain on the hip and knee joints, and it lowers the risk for low back pain by taking strain off the spine.
- Prevents future weight gain, and enhances long-term maintenance of weight loss.

Losing Weight by Changing Your Behavior

Any diet will help you lose weight, but to achieve permanent weight control, you should select a program that focuses on your eating and exercise behaviors. If your problem behaviors have not been addressed, the weight will likely return.

Eating habits lie at the very core of your being. Changing them is hard work, and means taking a look at every aspect of your lifestyle including food use during social and cultural events, family meal patterns, shopping and cooking techniques, and how you use food when stressed or depressed. Several useful behavior change principles can be followed:

- *Self-monitor your dietary habits:* Keep a diet diary, recording the amount of food consumed and circumstances surrounding each eating episode. For example, you may find that you tend to eat high-calorie snacks when studying, or overeat when dining out with your friends. Food records are valuable tools that can help you become aware of your eating behaviors. Once the problem areas are identified, seek support from friends, family, and professionals to make positive changes in these areas. See Health and Fitness Activity 10.5 for further instructions on how to monitor your dietary habits.
- *Control the events that precede eating:* Identify and control the circumstances that elicit eating and overeating (e.g., avoid reading or watching television while eating, or stay away from food when depressed or stressed); shop wisely (shop from a list, and avoid going to a store when hungry); plan meals (eat at scheduled times and according to an overall plan); reduce temptation (store food out of sight, eat all food in the same place, keep serving dishes off the table, and use smaller dishes); plan for parties (practice polite ways to decline food, and eat a low-calorie snack before parties).
- *Develop techniques to control the act of eating:* Slow down the eating process by putting the fork down between bites; keep serving sizes moderate, and don't go back for seconds; avoid unscheduled snacks; chew thoroughly before swallowing.
- *Be wise and think positively:* Avoid setting unreasonable goals; think about progress and not shortcomings; avoid imperatives like "always" and "never"; counter negative thoughts with reason.
- *Reinforce success with rewards:* A system of formal rewards facilitates progress. For example, close friends or family members could arrange for a special gift, trip, or award for meeting established goals.

Eating Disorders

Our food-laden, sedentary society equates thin with beautiful. Quite a paradox, isn't it? On the one hand, our magazine covers, movie stars, and athletic heroes advance the concept that thin is in. On the other hand, we are led through advertising to believe that technological labor-saving devices and sumptuous foods rich in fats and sugars are desirable rewards of a successful society.

Bulimia and Anorexia

It is not surprising that one sector of our population finds itself extremely disordered in its eating habits—those with bulimia nervosa and anorexia nervosa. **Bulimia nervosa** is described as a disorder in which frequent episodes of binge eating (rapid consumption of food in one sitting) are almost always followed by purging (ridding the body of food). Bulimics may consume 10,000 to 20,000 calories in eight hours, sometimes resorting to stealing food or money to support their obsession. Binging and purging are often accompanied by intense feelings of guilt and shame. The bulimic may not be visibly underweight, and may even be slightly overweight. The bulimic uses self-destructive eating behaviors to deal with psychological problems that may go much deeper than the obsession with food and weight. Usually the individual feels out of control, and recognizes that the behavior is not normal.

Health professionals use these criteria to diagnose bulimia nervosa:

- Engage in binge eating and purging behavior at least twice per week for three months.
- While binge eating, a large amount of food is eaten accompanied by a sense of lack of control.
- Purging behavior accompanies the binge eating to prevent weight gain, and includes self-induced vomiting; misuse of laxatives, diuretics, enemas, or other medications; fasting; or excessive exercise.

The salient feature of **anorexia nervosa** is a refusal to maintain normal body weight. Because of an intense fear of becoming fat, anorexics literally starve themselves to a very low body weight. Diagnostic criteria include the following:

- Refusal to maintain a normal body weight for age and height; body weight falls below 85 percent of that expected.
- Intense fear of gaining weight or becoming fat, even though underweight.
- Disturbance in body image, with denial of the seriousness of the current low body weight.
- Loss of at least three consecutive menstrual cycles due to undereating and low body fat.

Who Suffers from Eating Disorders?

More than five million American suffer from eating disorders. Five percent of females and one percent of males have anorexia nervosa, bulimia nervosa, or binge eating disorder. About 85 percent of eating disorders have their onset during the adolescent age period. Symptoms of bulimia and anorexia, such as binge eating, induced vomiting, and an extreme fear of gaining weight are present in significant numbers of college students and obese individuals.

Signs of Eating Disorders

Signs to watch for if someone is suspected of being bulimic and/or anorexic include:

- Change in personal weight goal to a much lower standard.
- Dieting accompanied by an increased criticism of one's body weight and shape.
- Social isolation, depressive moods, mood swings.
- Cessation of menstrual periods in women.
- Episodes of hiding food, vomiting, and misusing laxatives, diuretics, and diet pills.
- Dental problems; swollen glands in neck and face.
- Relentless, excessive exercise.
- Wearing baggy or layered clothing.
- Bathroom visits immediately after meals.
- Stomach and bowel problems including constipation, bloating, heartburn, and indigestion.

See Health and Fitness Activity 10.6 to determine if you or a friend is at risk for an eating disorder.

Risk Factors for Eating Disorders

Eating disorders are associated with multiple risk factors that represent a complex interplay among genetic, psychological, and social influences:

- Childhood obesity.
- Weight concern and social pressure about weight.
- Perfectionism.
- Low self-esteem.
- Eating disorders among family members.

- Parental discord.
- Childhood sexual abuse.
- Over-protective mother.
- High parental education and income.
- Personal illness such as asthma or diabetes; physical disability.

Health Problems of Eating Disorders

Binge eating and the various forms of purging (vomiting, laxative and diuretic use) can cause serious medical problems, including stomach dilation and rupture, infection of the lung from vomitus, infection and rupture of the esophagus (food tube), enlargement of the salivary glands, and tooth erosion and loss.

Stomach and intestinal complaints are the most common medical complaint of eating-disordered patients, and include slow stomach emptying, bloating, constipation, and abdominal discomfort. Death is possible among anorexics, who can suffer serious medical complications or literally starve themselves to death. Karen Carpenter, a famous pop singer of the 1970s, died from complications related to her battles with anorexia. She used syrup of ipecac to induce vomiting and died after buildup of the drug irreversibly damaged her heart. Each year in the United States, approximately 70 people die from anorexia.

What can be done to help the anorexic or bulimic? Generally, they find it difficult to stop on their own, and most experts feel they need specialized professional help. Eating disorder clinics have a staff of professionals including physicians, psychologists, dietitians, and nurses to meet the varied needs of people with eating disorders. Often, bulimics and anorexics have deep-seated emotional problems at the foundation of their eating problems. Long-term professional care is necessary. The American Anorexia Bulimia Association (www.aabainc.org) can provide referral to therapists, support groups, and other resources.

HEALTH AND FITNESS INSIGHT
"Supersize Me"

The popular documentary "Supersize Me," seems to serve up the message that restaurants or corporations are responsible for increased obesity in America. Is this a rational viewpoint for a person to consider? Is McDonald's really to blame?

No one doubts that each of us has primary control of our waistlines. Nonetheless, all of us could use some help. Would the obesity epidemic be expanding if every city and town had bike trails, walking paths, and easy access to recreational facilities, or if school cafeterias, fast food restaurants, and stores made healthy food choices as easy as finding a Big Mac? Probably not, but let's not carry this too far.

Some obesity experts argue that we have little choice about what we eat, and that we are captives in an environment in which food is too cheap, tasty, and available, with scant opportunities for physical activity. Little wonder, they claim, that two thirds of American adults are overweight, and obesity-related disorders such as arthritis, diabetes, and high blood pressure are on the rise.

Our course of action? The government, they say, must rescue children and adults from the environmental forces that make us fat, thereby protecting taxpayers from high healthcare costs. These obesity activists propose to accomplish this mission through taxes, censorship, and regulation. For example, some favor something similar to the

"Twinkie tax" that would require consumers to pay more for foods high in sugar and fat, thus pressuring families to reduce consumption of junk foods while at the same time providing tax funds for bike paths, running tracks, and nutrition education.

This mentality—that we are helpless victims in a fat society ruled by greasy, greedy food corporations—is also behind the recent upsurge in fast food lawsuits. New York City attorney Samuel Hirsch represented two overweight New York teenagers who claimed to have eaten at McDonald's on most days of the week for years. That lawsuit was dismissed twice, with U.S. District Judge Robert Sweet declaring that "any liability based on over-consumption is doomed if the consequences of such over-consumption are common knowledge. . . . If a person knows or should know that eating copious orders of super-sized McDonald's products is unhealthy and may result in weight gain . . . it is not the place of the law to protect them from their own excesses. Nobody is forced to eat at McDonald's. . . . Even more pertinent, nobody is forced to supersize their meal or choose less healthy options on the menu."

No one disputes that it is easy to overeat when food is good tasting, easy to find, inexpensive, full of fat and sugar, and provided in large portions. And this food easily turns into body fat because we no longer exercise at work or school, and find enjoyment in watching television, surfing the Internet, and playing video games. But the judge summarized the core issue well—each of us must assume personal responsibility for the unhappy consequences, because no one is forcing us to live this way.

Summary

1. Overweight, defined as a body mass index (BMI) of 25 and higher, now afflicts two thirds of the adult population. The federal government's year 2010 goal to reduce the prevalence of obesity among adults to no more than 15 percent was not achieved.
2. Health hazards of obesity include increased risk of depression, anxiety, and low self-esteem, high blood pressure, high blood cholesterol, heart disease and stroke, diabetes, cancer, osteoarthritis, gallbladder disease, and early death.
3. Three factors are most responsible for weight gain leading to obesity: (1) genetic and parental influences, (2) high calorie and high fat diets, and (3) insufficient physical activity. A certain genetic makeup can favor the development of obesity, especially when diet and exercise habits are less than desirable.
4. When dietary intake of fat is high, most people tend to gain weight rather easily and quickly. When intake of dietary fats is low, and most calories are in the form of carbohydrate, desirable body weight is more readily achieved.
5. Lack of activity promotes a gain in body weight, and then a vicious cycle sets in as physical activity becomes more onerous.
6. A comprehensive weight loss program incorporates diet, exercise, and behavior modification.
7. In a good weight loss diet, the caloric intake is reduced, preferably by reducing the fat content of the diet, while increasing intake of carbohydrates and dietary fiber.
8. Energy expenditure should be increased by at least 200 to 400 calories per day. This can be accomplished by including a 30- to 45-minute exercise session on most days of the week, and also by adding physical activity throughout the normal routine of each day.
9. Behavior modification is defined as the development of skills to extinguish undesirable behaviors. Several techniques can be employed to increase awareness of caloric intake, with rewards provided for good behavior and achieving personal goals.
10. The NHLBI Obesity Education Initiative recommends that the initial goal of a weight loss regimen should be to reduce body weight by about 10 percent. Weight loss should be about 1 to 2 pounds per week for a period of six months. Seek to create a deficit of 500 to 1,000 calories per day through a combination of decreased caloric intake and increased physical activity. The weight loss diet should be "heart-healthy."

11. Physical activity can influence body weight three different ways: (1) prevent weight gain in the first place, (2) help you lose weight if overweight or obese, and (3) maintain a good body weight after the excess weight is lost.

12. Regular physical activity helps to counter many obesity-related health problems.

13. Bulimia nervosa is described as a disorder in which frequent episodes of binge eating (rapid consumption of food in one sitting) are almost always followed by purging (ridding the body of food).

14. The salient feature of anorexia nervosa is a refusal to maintain normal body weight. Because of an intense fear of becoming fat, anorexics literally starve themselves to a very low body weight.

15. Eating disorders are associated with multiple symptoms and risk factors that represent a complex interplay among genetic, psychological, and social influences.

HEALTH AND FITNESS ACTIVITY 10.1

Estimating Your Resting Metabolic Rate

The resting metabolic rate (RMR) is the energy expended each day by the body to maintain life and normal body functions like respiration and circulation. In other words, if you sat or lay down all day, and did not move a muscle, the RMR is the energy expended by your body to keep you alive.

The RMR is slightly less than 1 calorie per minute in women (or 1,200 to 1,500 calories per day), and somewhat higher than this rate in men (1,600 to 1,900 calories per day). Your RMR equals the heat released by a burning candle or a 75-watt light bulb.

The RMR varies from person to another, but nearly all of this is due to differences in body size, with the greatest RMR found in big people with high amounts of muscle and bone. You may want to claim your slow metabolism is to blame for those extra pounds, but this seldom is the case. Actually, the metabolism increases as you gain weight, as the body fights to keep off the extra pounds.

Can exercise rev up a slow metabolism? For example, let's say you go out for a 30-minute jog. Will your RMR be higher than normal for hours afterwards, burning extra calories and helping you get slim? Unfortunately, no. It's true your metabolism will stay slightly elevated after this run for about 20 to 30 minutes, but you'll only burn about 10 to 12 extra calories, or the equivalent of one bite of an apple. If you push the pace, run hard, and sweat, the RMR stays elevated a bit longer than after the jog, but the extra calories burned is still small, about 15 to 30.

Will weight training boost your metabolism? It is true that weight lifting adds muscle, and every pound of muscle increases your metabolism 7 to 10 calories a day. However, most fitness enthusiasts who take up weight training only add 4 to 5 pounds of muscle, increasing RMR by 28 to 50 kcal/day, hardly an impressive gain.

A slow metabolism can make it difficult to keep slim, but for most people the issue is not metabolism but rather control of food intake. Moderate exercise is good for your health, but it will not rev up your metabolism.

What is your RMR? It varies according to age, sex, and weight. RMR falls about 1 to 2 percent per decade of life, with the lowest levels measured in the elderly. Heavy people have higher RMR rates than those with low body weight.

RMR can be measured by connecting people to a metabolic cart for 10 to 15 minutes while they are resting comfortably, but this method is expensive, and requires trained technicians. RMR can be estimated quite accurately through the use of these equations:

MALES: $(15.3 \times kg) + 679 = RMR$ (Calories/day)
FEMALES: $(14.7 \times kg) + 496 = RMR$ (Calories/day)

First, calculate your body weight in kilograms (kg). Take your weight in pounds and divide it by 2.2. For example, if you weigh 154 pounds, then your weight in kilograms is 154 pounds/2.2=70 kg. Finally, multiply your kilogram body weight by the appropriate number listed in the formula, and add the constant. For example, if you are a 20-year-old male weighing 70 kg, your RMR would be calculated as follows: $(15.3 \times 70) + 679 = 1750$ calories per day.

Your estimated RMR = _____   calories per day

HEALTH AND FITNESS ACTIVITY 10.2
How Many Calories Do You Burn at Rest (RMR)?

The number of calories you burn at rest each day depends on your body size, age, and gender. Use the Shape Up America metabolic calculator to estimate RMR. Go to: http://www.shapeup.org/interactive/rmr1.php. Enter your profile information and let the program determine your RMR. Write this below:

_____ calories/day from the diet

The program will also calculate the number of fat grams recommended for your diet.

_____ fat grams/day from the diet

Name _____   Date _____

HEALTH AND FITNESS ACTIVITY 10.3
Counting the Calories and Fat Grams from Fast Food

Most fast foods are high in calories and fat grams—more than you may think. Visit the Internet site "The Fast Food Explorer" *http://www.fatcalories.com/*. Use the search engine provided at this Internet site, and list the number of calories and fat grams given for each fast food below.

Food Description	Calories	Fat grams
McDonald's Big Mac (hamburger)		
McDonald's Quarter Pounder, with cheese		
Burger King BIG KING (hamburger)		
Burger King Bacon Double Cheeseburger		
Burger King DOUBLE WHOPPER		
Wendy's Big Bacon Classic (hamburger)		
Domino's Pizza, bacon topping, 14 inches		
Domino's Pizza, beef topping, 14 inches		
Papa John's Pizza, All the Meats		
Pizza Hut Cheese Personal		

What is your reaction to this information?

_____

_____

_____

_____

_____

_____

_____

_____

HEALTH AND FITNESS ACTIVITY 10.4
Physical Activity and Weight Management

As emphasized earlier, physical activity is especially useful for preventing weight gain and maintaining an ideal weight as the years pass by. Visit at least two Internet sites listed in Box 10.3, look for information on physical activity and weight management, and summarize five important guidelines that you gleaned from your search.

1. _____

_____

_____

2. _____

_____

_____

3. _____

_____

_____

4. _____

_____

_____

5. _____

_____

_____

HEALTH AND FITNESS ACTIVITY 10.5

Monitoring Your Dietary Habits

A key strategy in weight management is to know your personal dietary habits. When do you eat and where are you? How hungry are you when you eat? What else are you doing when you eat? Who do you eat with? What are your feelings before and during eating? This information will help you improve your eating habits, keeping caloric intake under control.

    Fill in the food diary for one day (the more typical the better). Fill in all of the blanks, using the instructions listed below. You will notice that keeping this food diary will make you unusually aware of everything you eat, and why.

Instructions	
Time	Record the starting time for a meal or snack.
Minutes spent eating	Record the length of each eating episode (no matter how short or long).
Food type and quantity	Describe the type of food eaten and how much.
Hunger scale	Record a "0" if you had no hunger, a "1" if you had some hunger, a "2" if you had much hunger, and a "3" if you had extreme hunger.
Activity while eating	Record any activity that accompanied eating such as watching television, reading, partying with friends, driving your car, walking to class, etc.
Location of eating	Record where you ate the meal or snack, such as your kitchen table, your car, the living room couch, your bed, a restaurant, etc.
Feelings	Record your feelings and mood before and during eating (e.g., bored, angry, confused, depressed, frustrated, sad, tense).

Time of Day	Minutes spent eating	Food type, quantity, and Calories (use NutriWellness^{Plus})	Hunger scale (0 to 3)	Activity while eating	Location of eating	Feelings

HEALTH AND FITNESS ACTIVITY 10.6
Do You Have An Eating Disorder?

Go to this Web site and take the Eating Attitudes Test: *www.river-centre.org* (Click on the Eating Attitudes Test.)

The Eating Attitudes Test (EAT) is the most widely used standardized measure of symptoms and concerns characteristic of eating disorders. Early identification of an eating disorder can lead to earlier treatment, thereby reducing serious physical and psychological complications or even death.

Record your score here and classification: _____

Norms: *20 or above = high probability of an eating disorder*
             Below 20 = low probability of an eating disorder

If you have a low score on the EAT-26 (below 20), you still could have an eating problem, so do not let the results deter you from seeking help if you think that you might need it. If you do have a high score, do not panic. It does not necessarily mean that you have a life-threatening condition or that you will have to immediately seek a form of treatment that may be uncomfortable. If you have a score of 20 or more, this simply means that you should seek the advice of a qualified mental health professional who has experience with treating eating disorders. If you score at or above 20, please contact your physician or an eating disorders treatment specialist for a follow-up evaluation.

CHAPTER 10 QUIZ
Prevention and Treatment of Obesity

Note: Answers are given at the end of the quiz.

1. There are many disadvantages associated with obesity. Which one of the following is NOT included?
   A. increased levels of serum cholesterol
   B. increased prevalence of high blood pressure
   C. increased diabetes
   D. increased HDL-C
   E. increased colon and breast cancer

2. When the Body Mass Index rises above the threshold of _____ kg/m^2, mortality from heart disease, cancer, and diabetes also increases.
   A. 15
   B. 20
   C. 25
   D. 35
   E. 40

3. There are three major theories of obesity. Which one of the following is NOT included?
   A. high energy intake
   B. low protein intake
   C. low energy expenditure
   D. genetic and parental influences

4. Which criteria listed below are used to determine if a person is anorexic?
   A. minimum average of 2 binge-eating episodes per week for at least 3 months
   B. regularly engages in self-induced vomiting, use of laxatives, or other purging techniques to counteract the effects of the binge-eating
   C. weight loss so severe that weight is more than 15 percent below normal

5. For bulimia nervosa to be diagnosed, the binge eating and inappropriate compensatory behaviors need to both occur, on average, at least two times a week for _____ months.
   A. 1
   B. 2
   C. 3
   D. 4
   E. 5

6. About _____ % of Americans are considered overweight/obese using government conservative criteria.
    A. 10
    B. 26
    C. 66
    D. 75
    E. 40

7. The initial weight loss goal for a 250-pound woman is to reduce body weight by _____ pounds during the first six months.
    A. 10
    B. 50
    C. 25
    D. 30
    E. 15

8. Moderate intensity aerobic exercise causes the RMR to stay elevated ___ minutes, burning 10–12 extra Calories.
    A. 100–200
    B. 50–100
    C. 35–40
    D. 20–30
    E. 2–5

9. Which statement below is true in regards to obesity trends in America?
    A. The percentage of obese children and teenagers has increased since the 1960s.
    B. Approximately 80% of adults are considered obese.
    C. Obesity is less prevalent among the poor and minority groups.
    D. Prevalence decreases between the ages of 25 and 55 years.

10. Which statement below is true in regards to the resting metabolic rate?
    A. For the average person amounts to one-third of daily energy expenditure.
    B. Is higher in obese people than lean people.
    C. Decreases as the body weight of an individual increases.
    D. Is the major factor explaining obesity in the U.S.

11. The NHLBI Obesity Education Initiative recommends that for most over-weight/obese clients, a decrease of 300–1,000 Calories per day will lead to weight losses of _____ pounds per week.
    A. 0.1–0.5
    B. 0.5–2.0
    C. 2.0–3.0
    D. 3.0–4.0
    E. 4.0–5.0

12. The NHLBI Obesity Education Initiative recommends that for most over-weight/obese clients, energy expenditure should be increased to at least _____ Calories per day.
    A. 100–200
    B. 200–400
    C. 400–500
    D. 500–600
    E. 600–1000

13. To follow the NHLBI Obesity Education Initiative plan for weight loss, one must expend 500 to 1000 calories more than the amount taken in through the diet. This can be accomplished by increasing energy expenditure 200–400 calories a day through physical activity, and reducing dietary fat intake by _____ calories.
    A. 100–20
    B. 200–300
    C. 300–600
    D. 600–1000
    E. 1000–2000

14. The NHLBI Obesity Education Initiative recommends keeping total dietary fat intake below 30% of calories, and carbohydrate at _____ % or more of total calories.
    A. 30
    B. 38
    C. 44
    D. 50
    E. 55

15. The Year 2010 goal was to reduce obesity prevalence to below _____ %.
    A. 10
    B. 15
    C. 20
    D. 30
    E. 40

16. Which one of the following diseases is not promoted by obesity?

    A. osteoporosis

    B. hypertension

    C. diabetes

    D. coronary heart disease

    E. cancer of the gallbladder

17. Which statement listed below would indicate to you that the weight loss program is probably fraudulent?

    A. Promotes a diet of 1250 calories a day.

    B. Promotes near daily activity.

    C. Promotes a plan that will lead to a weight loss of 1–2 pounds a week.

    D. Promotes a high-carbohydrate, high-fiber, low-fat dietary regimen.

    E. Attempts to make a client dependent on a special product.

18. _____ is considered by most experts to be the most important factor explaining the high prevalence of obesity in the United States.

    A. High sugar intake

    B. Genetic/parental influences

    C. High energy/fat content of the diet

    D. Low protein diets

    E. Physical inactivity

Answers: 1. D 2. C 3. B 4. C 5. C 6. C 7. C 8. D 9. A 10. B 11. B 12. B 13. C 14. E 15. B 16. A 17. E 18. C

chapter eleven

Stress Management and Mental Health

"My body must be set a-going if my mind is to work."
—Jean Jacques Rousseau

Introduction: Fact or Fancy?

John came home feeling tense, anxious, and irritable. He was a manager for a large business firm and had spent all day, unsuccessfully, trying to mend sharp differences between two of his key department heads. After fighting traffic for 45 minutes on the way home, he felt he needed to clear his mind. Slipping on his well-worn jogging shoes, John went out for a 30-minute jog through the dirt trails behind his house. By the time he returned home, he felt completely different. His mind felt relaxed, his mood was elevated, and all his built-up tension was erased. After stretching and showering, John enjoyed the evening with his family.

Donna felt depressed. She had just received a low C grade on her first biochemistry test, and as a freshman medical student, she was extremely worried about her chances of staying in the program. Pulling on her jacket, she went out for a 40-minute brisk walk on the hilly roads near her school. By the time Donna returned to her dorm room, her spirits were lifted, her depression was gone, and she sat down at her desk with renewed determination to keep pressing on with her studies.

Is this fact or fancy? Is it really true that exercise can help alleviate mental anxiety, depression, and other problems? Does the motion of the body influence the mind?

Defining the Magnitude of the Problem

As discussed in Chapter 1, the U.S. government and various health groups are urging Americans to adopt regular exercise habits. While directed primarily at the reduction of cardiovascular diseases, obesity, and other chronic diseases, this campaign could also have some beneficial effects on the population's mental health. Even a small effect could have a significant impact, because mental health problems and stress are so widespread in most Western countries.

Mental health is a general term used to refer to the absence of mental disorders like schizophrenia, depression, panic attacks, and phobias, but also to the ability of a person to negotiate the daily challenges and social interactions of the life successfully. See Box 11.1 for more facts on mental health.

In the United States, for example, one in four of the population (nearly 65 million Americans) is affected by one or more mental disorders during any given six-month period, and 32 percent within a lifetime (see figure 11.1). Depression is more than a case of the "blues." Major depression is characterized by a prolonged and unrelenting feeling of sadness, loss of interest in virtually all activities, changes in eating and sleeping patterns, and sometimes suicidal thoughts.

Anxiety disorders are the most prevalent of all mental illnesses, and affective disorders, including depression, are widespread. Critical life events, chronic work strain, accumulating everyday life hassles, and environmental pressures like urban overcrowding and noise pollution regularly contribute to stress overload.

About one half of U.S. adults report at least a moderate amount of stress during the past two weeks. Over 40 percent of Americans report experiencing adverse health effects from stress within the past year. The percentage of Americans experiencing "great stress" at least once per week is 64 percent. Nearly one third, especially women in their forties and those with a college education, feel "great stress" almost every day.

Despite this relatively high prevalence of stress, however, few adults seek help for a personal or emotional problem. Most people suffering from depression do not receive treatment. Americans report taking steps to control or reduce stress, but most do so unsuccessfully. Obviously a large percentage of the population could benefit by using various stress management techniques.

The Meaning of Stress

Stress has been defined as any action or situation (stressor) that places special physical or psychological demands on a person—in other words, anything that unbalances one's equilibrium. Dr. Hans Selye, one of the great pioneers of medicine and the originator of the concept of stress, wrote in his famous 1956 classic, *The Stress Life,* "In its medical sense, stress is essentially the rate of wear and tear in the body . . . the nonspecific response of the body to any demand."

In Dr. Seyle's view, there are both good and bad stressors producing stress reactions in the body. A divorce is stressful—but so is getting married. Both upset a person's equilibrium, and require adjustment and adaptation.

FIGURE 11.1
Mental disorder prevalence among American adults.

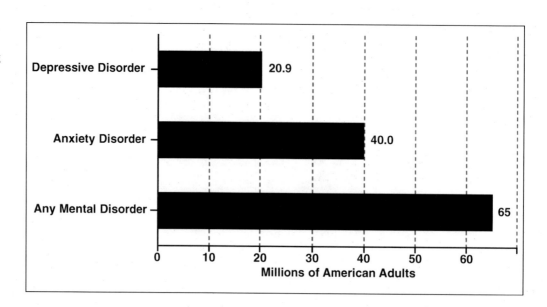

BOX 11.1

Facts on Mental Health and Disorders in America

- Mental health is defined as "the successful performance of mental function, resulting in productive activities, fulfilling relationships with other people, and the ability to adapt to change and to cope with adversity; from early childhood until late life, mental health is the springboard of thinking and communication skills, learning, emotional growth, resilience, and self-esteem."
- Mental illness refers collectively to all mental disorders, and are defined as "health conditions that are characterized by alterations in thinking, mood, or behavior (or some combination thereof) associated with distress and/or impaired functioning."
- 65 million (26.2% of American adults) suffer from a diagnosable mental disorder in a given year.
  - 40 million—anxiety disorder (18.1% of adults)
  - 20.9 million—depressive disorder (9.5% of adults)
- More than 90 percent of suicides involve people who have a diagnosable mental disorder.
- Anxiety is a condition characterized by apprehension, tension, or uneasiness, and stems from the anticipation of real or imagined danger. If the anxiety becomes excessive and unrealistic, it can interfere with normal functioning.
- Anxiety disorders are two times as prevalent in females as males.
- General Anxiety Disorder (GAD) is defined as the constant, exaggerated worrisome thoughts and tension about everyday routine life events and activities, lasting at least six months—almost always anticipating the worst even though there is little reason to expect it, accompanied by physical symptoms, such as fatigue, trembling, muscle tension, headache, or nausea.
- Anxiety disorders frequently co-occur with depressive disorders, eating disorders, or substance abuse. Many people have more than one anxiety disorder.
- Depression is a pernicious illness linked with episodes of long duration, relapse, and social and physical impairment. Most people with major depression are misdiagnosed, receive inappropriate or inadequate treatment, or are given no treatment at all.
- The lifetime estimate for major depression is 17 percent, and is most common among females, the elderly, young adults, and people with less than a college education.
- A depressive disorder is an illness that involves the body, mood, and thoughts. It affects the way a person eats and sleeps, the way one feels about oneself, and the way on thinks about things. Depression may range in severity from mild symptoms to more severe forms.
- Nearly twice as many women as men are affected by a depressive disorder.
- The average age at onset for major depressive disorder is the mid-20s.

Source: National Institute of Mental Health. *www.nimh.hih.gov*

But it is not the stressor itself that creates the response. Instead, it is the person's reaction to the stressor. Therefore people will respond in varying ways to the same stressor, based on their individual ways of reacting.

Medical research on stress dates back to the 1920s, when Walter Cannon began experimenting with the physiological effect of stress on cats and dogs. Studying the animals' reactions to danger, the Harvard physiologist noted a regular and common pattern, now known as the fight-or-flight response.

In this response, the muscles tense and tighten, breathing becomes deeper and faster, the heart rate rises and blood vessels constrict (raising the blood pressure), the stomach and intestines temporarily halt digestion, perspiration increases, the thyroid gland is stimulated, while the secretion of saliva and mucus slows, and sensory perception becomes sharper. Various stress hormones are released in the body, in particular epinephrine and cortisol, depressing immune function, and adversely affecting bodily functions in many other ways (see figure 11.2).

In the 1940s and 1950s, Dr. Selye extended Cannon's work and laid the foundation for much of today's work on stress. Experimenting with rats, he used various stressors, and found a regular pattern of responses, which he described as the General Adaptation Syndrome (alarm, resistance, exhaustion).

He discovered that if the stressor were maintained for a prolonged period of time, the body would first go through an alarm reaction (fight-or-flight response), followed by a stage of resistance where functions would return close to normal as the body strove to

FIGURE 11.2

The stress response affects the entire body through both hormonal and nerve pathways.

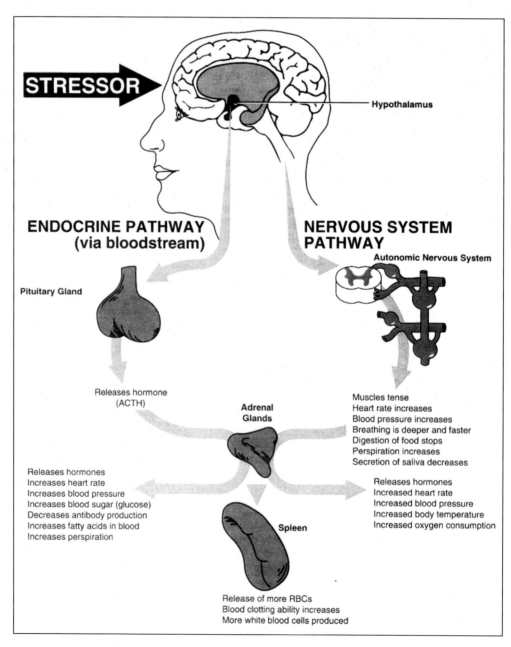

resist the stress. Finally, there would be a stage of exhaustion where the symptoms of the alarm reaction returned. In animal experiments, the animals would die.

The Ill Effects of High Stress

Stress can have a profound effect on one's physical health. If you are chronically anxious, depressed, or emotionally distressed, your health can suffer.

For example, in one study of 1,300 graduates of the Johns Hopkins Medical School, depression was found to be an important predictor of heart disease. In England, people who experienced chronic mild anxiety and depression were more likely to develop heart disease than those who did not. In a study of 10,000 Israeli men, anxiety over problems and conflicts about finance, family, and relationships with co-workers was associated with 2 to 3 times the risk of developing heart disease.

In a 17-year study of 2,000 middle-aged men, depression has been associated with twice the risk of death from cancer. A one-year study of 100 people found that flus and colds were four times as prevalent following stressful life events. An Australian study found that stressed people had twice as many days when they had flu and cold symptoms.

Dr. Donald Girard from the Oregon Health Sciences University has reviewed the literature on this subject and concluded that repressed feelings of loss, denial, depression, inflexibility, conformity, lack of social ties, high levels of anxiety and dissatisfaction, and an over-abundance of life-change events are associated with increased cancers, heart disease, and infection. Writes Dr. Guard, "It seems that the best advice the physician can offer patients is that good mental health is important for maintaining physical well-being."

National surveys suggest that marital happiness contributes far more to happiness in societies throughout the world than any other variable, including satisfaction with work and friendships. Divorced and separated people have poorer mental and physical health than those who remain married, or are widowed or single. Marital disruption has been found to be the single most powerful predictor of stress-related physical illness; separated partners have about 30 percent more acute illnesses and physician visits than those who remain married. It has been concluded that depression of immune function is associated with marital discord.

A number of other studies have found bereavement and a lack of social and community ties to be associated with an overall increase in mortality. A study of 95,647 widows found more than double the normal mortality rate during the first week following widowhood, primarily from cardiovascular disease, violent causes, and suicides. Dr. Ruberman of New York has reported that highly stressed and socially isolated heart disease patients (few contacts with friends, relatives, church or club groups) had more than four times the risk of dying from heart disease of men with tow levels of isolation and stress.

A statement made by William Harvey in 1628 applies today: "Every affection of the mind that is attended with either pain or pleasure, hope or fear, is the cause of an agitation whose influence extends to the heart."

Dr. George Vaillant of Harvard University tracked 204 men over 40 years and found that poor mental health was associated with increased disease and death, after allowance had been made for the effects of drug abuse, obesity, and family history of long life. Concluded Vaillant: "Good mental health facilitates our survival."

Stress Management Principles

Much has been written about controlling stress. It can all be summarized under five basic stress management principles.

1. Control Stressors

Stressors are everywhere. They can't all be avoided, but you can do a great deal in the way of reducing, modifying, or avoiding many of them in a way that will allow you to accomplish your goals. For example, if you are going to climb a tall mountain, you can make the trip miserable by hiking too fast with a heavy backpack, or satisfying and pleasurable by walking at a moderate pace with a lighter load. Same goal, same path, but a completely different experience.

Let's say that a college student is taking a heavy academic load in a subject area (e.g., biochemistry) that is too difficult for him at present, working 15 hours a week to help pay for expenses, living in a crowded and noisy apartment with an unbearable roommate, experiencing constant transportation problems because of a car that keeps breaking down, and dealing with crushing family problems due to the divorce of his parents. The first step would be for the student to sit down, make a list of all his major goals, in order of importance, and then catalog each of the stressors, along with plans to either eliminate or modify them (see sample form, figure 11.3).

For example, finishing biochemistry has a high priority because he must do so to have a chance to achieve his major life goal of becoming a physician. He should give it his first attention (he could increase his study time by quitting work and taking out a loan). He could move closer to campus, find more desirable living accommodations, and walk or bicycle for transportation until finances improve.

Just as in climbing a mountain, the stressors of life often can be managed by controlling the pace of life and the load carried, A key is to avoid crowding too much into the schedule, and learning to control circumstances to allow the pace of life to flow with one's psychological makeup. The important objective is to control your circumstances—don't let them control you.

2. Let the Mind Choose the Reaction

This strategy is also called "stress reaction management." As we've seen, a stress reaction (the fight-or-flight response) stimulates production of various stress hormones, depressing immune function, increasing blood pressure, and so on. In all, the response has negative health effects, so the goal is to head off the stress reaction before it can take place.

To understand how to do this, one needs to remember that events only cause stress when they are seen, heard, felt, or sensed by the brain. The mind interprets the event, and the type of interpretation governs the reaction. The good news is that when a stressor presents itself, you can decide what kind of reaction you will have. The bad news is that usually we have "knee-jerk" reactions to potentially stressful events, without taking the opportunity to calmly reason them out. In other words, we are largely responsible for creating our emotional reactions and we miss our opportunities to control them.

Once again, the principle is not new. Marcus Aurelius said long ago: "If you are distressed by anything external, the pain is not due to the thing itself but to your estimate of it. This you have the power to revoke at any time."

So when an event takes place (e.g., a flat tire on your way to work or school), you can choose how you will react. You can either react with the stress response of anger (as you kick the tire and blame the tire manufacturer), or you can choose a calm response by considering your practical options (I'll call at the first opportunity and work it out with the boss or professor).

3. Seek the Social Support of Others

A survey has shown that as many as one fourth of the American population feel extremely lonely at some time during any given month—especially divorced parents, single mothers, people who have never married, and housewives.

It is now clear that when people are socially isolated (few social contacts with family and friends, neighbors or the "society at large"), they are more vulnerable to sickness, mental stress, and even early death. One nine-year study (of 7,000 residents of Alameda County, California) found that people with few ties to other people had death rates from various diseases two to five times higher than those with more ties. The researchers measured social ties by looking at whether or not people were married, the number of close friends and relatives they had and how often they were in contact with them, church attendance, and involvement in Informal and formal group associations.

Step One   List top 5 major life goals, in order of importance.
Step Two   List stressors associated with each goal.
Step Three   Summarize plans to modify or eliminate stressors so that goals can be achieved.

Step One Top 5 Goals	**Step Two** Major stressors associated with each goal
Goal 1	
Goal 2	
Goal 3	
Goal 4	
Goal 5	

Step Three   Summarize plans to modify or eliminate stressors so that goals can be achieved.

1. _____

2. _____

3. _____

4. _____

5. _____

6. _____

7. _____

8. _____

9. _____

10. _____

FIGURE 11.3
Sample form for evaluating goals and stressor.

Social support means reaching out to other people, sharing emotional, social, physical, financial, and other types of comfort and assistance. The principle was summarized by the Government's Institute of Medicine (Division of Health Promotion and Disease Prevention) " . . . a lack of family and community supports plays an important role in the development of disease. An absence of social support weakens the body's defenses through psychological stress. Isolated individuals must be identified, and strategies for increasing social contact and diminishing feelings of loneliness must be developed. Clinicians, family, friends, and social institutions bear a responsibility for diminishing social isolation." (*The Second Fifty Years: Promoting Health and Preventing Disability*, Washington, D.C.: National Academy Press, 1990.)

4. Find Satisfaction in Work and Service

Dr. Albert Schweitzer once wrote, "I don't know what your destiny will be. But I do know that the only ones among you who will find true happiness are those who find a place to serve." Dr. Selye echoed this thought in his book, *Stress Without Distress* (New York: New American Library, 1974): "My own code is based on the view that to achieve peace of mind and fulfillment through self-expression, most men need a commitment to work in the service of some cause that they can respect."

5. Keep Healthy

It is far easier to handle stressors when the body is healthy from adequate exercise, sleep, good food and water, clean air and sunshine, and relaxation.

Problems with sleep have become a modern epidemic that is taking an enormous toll on our bodies and minds. Desperately trying to fit more into the hours of the day, many people are stealing extra hours from the night. The result, say sleep researchers, is a sleep deficit that undermines health, sabotages productivity, blackens mood, clouds judgment, and increases the risk of accidents. See the Health and Fitness Insight at the end of this chapter for more information on sleep.

Physical Activity and Stress

One of the most important habits one can acquire to improve mood state and manage stress is the habit of regular exercise. As Dr. John Farquhar of Stanford University says: "Through prudent, regular and systematic use of your body, you will discover a greater sense of well-being, far greater energy, and a calmer, more relaxed attitude toward the pressures you experience daily."

The rest of this chapter will describe how regular physical activity can reduce depression, anxiety, and mental stress, while enhancing psychological well-being and a vigorous attitude toward life.

Relationship Between Physical Activity and Psychological Health

We have seen that poor psychological health is associated with poor physical health. Is there proof for the converse association? Is a healthy and fit body positively associated with psychological health? Were the ancient Greeks right in their assertion that a physically fit and strong body would lead to a sound mind?

The part of the brain that enables us to exercise, the motor cortex, lies only a few millimeters away from the part of the brain that deals with thought and feeling. Might this proximity mean that when exercise stimulates the motor cortex, it has a parallel effect on cognition and emotion?

Since the beginning of time many have believed in the "cerebral satisfaction" of exercise. The Greeks maintained that exercise made the mind more lucid. Aristotle started his "Peripatetic School" in 335 B.C.—so named because of Aristotle's habit of walking up and down *(peripaton)* the paths of the Lyceum in Athens while thinking or lecturing to his students walking with him. Plato and Socrates had also practiced the art of peripatetics, as did the Roman *Ordo Vagorum* or walking scholars. Centuries later, Oliver Wendell Holmes explained that "in walking the will and the muscles are so accustomed to working together and perform their task with so little expenditure of force that the intellect is left comparatively free."

John F. Kennedy, echoed the Greek ideal when he said:

> Physical fitness is not only one of the most important keys to a healthy body, it is the basis of dynamic and creative intellectual activity. Intelligence and skill can only function at the peak of their capacity when the body is strong. Hardy spirits and tough minds usually inhabit sound bodies.

The highly acclaimed "Perrier Survey of Fitness in America," conducted by Louis Harris and Associates, showed that modern-day men and women strongly believe in the Greek concept of a "strong mind in a strong body." The survey found that those who have a deep commitment to exercise report feeling more relaxed, less tired, more disciplined, more attractive, more self-confident, more productive in work, and in general, more at one with themselves.

The Campbell's *Survey on Well-Being in Canada* revealed that physically active people have less depression and higher sense of positive well-being than inactive people. When active people are asked why they exercise, the most common response is "to feel better mentally and physically." A survey by *Runner's World* magazine discovered that although most people *start* running to "improve physical fitness," most *continue* to run to "improve mental fitness" and to "relieve stress."

There have been several national surveys in the United States and in Canada to study the relationship between physical activity and feelings of mental well-being. One of the questionnaires used in Canada studies was the "general well-being scale" (GWBS), used in the health and fitness activity at the end of this chapter. The GWBS is highly regarded as one of the best measures of stress and mental health that can be used by the general public. It consists of 18 questions, covering such areas as energy level, satisfaction, freedom from worry, and self-control. A high score on the GWBS reflects an absence of bad feelings, an expression of positive mood state, and low stress.

Figure 11.4 summarizes the findings from the four national studies. 'The inescapable conclusion from these four national studies," says Dr. Stephens, "is that physical activity is positively associated with good mental health, especially positive mood, general well-being, and less anxiety and depression." This relationship was found to be stronger for the older age group (+40 years of age) than for the younger, and for women than for men. When you take the same test in this chapter's "health and fitness activity," compare your score with those summarized in Figure 11.4.

Controlled Studies on Exercise and Stress

Dr. Hans Selye, the early pioneer of the concept of stress, conducted an interesting experiment to demonstrate the remarkable anti-stress benefits of walking. In one part of the study, he subjected 10 rats to a month-long program of electric shocks, blinding lights, and loud noises. At the end of the month all 10 of the animals were dead from general stress. In the second part of this experiment, he subjected 10 other rats to the same stress program, but before doing so he had them walk on treadmills until they were in good physical condition. At the end of the month of stress all 10 rats remained alive and reasonably well (if somewhat disoriented). Dr. Selye concluded that physical fitness "buffered" the rats against the health-destroying effects of stress.

Since Dr. Selye's original studies, many other researchers have investigated the relationship for humans between exercise and mental stress. The research has focused on five general subjects: cardiovascular reactivity to mental stress; stressful life events; psychological mood state; self-esteem; and mental cognition.

FIGURE 11.4
With increased exercise, scores from the General Well-Being test were higher for all age and gender subgroups measured. See the Health and Fitness Activity at the end of this chapter to see how you score.

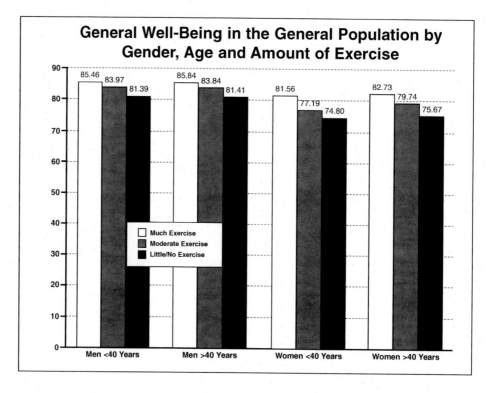

Cardiovascular Reactivity to Mental Stress

A considerable amount of recent research has indicated that aerobically unfit people show greater cardiovascular responses (in terms of elevated heart rates and blood pressure), to psychological stressors. When involved in stressful mental tasks, the less fit had heart rates nearly 30 beats per minute higher than the highly fit. And when originally unfit people participated in aerobic training programs, their heart rates were lower when they were subjected to psychological stressors.

In one study, subjects were randomly divided into a meditation group, a music appreciation class (the control groups), and an exercise group involving 30 minutes of calisthenics and jogging, four days per week for 10 weeks. In response to a battery of very stressful mental tasks, the exercise group at the end of 10 weeks demonstrated a faster recovery of the heart rate and autonomic system (skin electrical response) than the control groups. It was concluded that this faster recovery is very important in coping with stress. Since both exercise and mental stress increase the heart rate, blood pressure, adrenaline, and other biochemical measures. Strengthening the body to adapt to exercise stress apparently strengthens it to handle mental stress.

Stressful Life Events and Somatic Illness

During the past 25 years, a large number of studies have shown that life events of all types (marriage, divorce, buying a house, losing one's job, moving to a new location, surgery, etc.) are significant stressors that lead to predictable physical and psychological health problems. Several recent studies have shown, however, that such life stress has less impact on the health of physically active people.

For instance, a study of 112 students showed that the less physically fit were more susceptible to stress-related health problems. In a second study of college students who had reported a high number of negative life events over the preceding year, aerobic exercise and relaxation training were both found to be effective for reducing depression.

Psychological Mood State

As we discussed earlier, depression and fatigue are very common complaints of Americans. Adults who are physically inactive are at much higher risk for fatigue and depression than those who are physically active. Depression, anxiety, and mood state in general appear to be favorably affected by regular aerobic exercise.

A team of researchers at Duke University studied 32 middle-aged men and women, 16 of whom were placed in a 10-week program of walking and jogging, 45 minutes, three times per week. Compared to the 16 who did not exercise, the exercising group showed less anxiety and depression, less fatigue and confusion, and elevated vigor. A similar 12-week study of 36 policemen and firemen reported comparable results.

A study of people suffering from depression compared the effects of running with psychotherapy. Running was found to be at least as effective as psychotherapy in alleviating moderate depression in the short term, and even better on follow-up a year later.

In another study, 36 physically inactive women, most of them busy mothers with children, were divided into walking and sedentary groups. The walking group exercised at a brisk pace 45 minutes per day, 5 days per week for 15 weeks while the other group remained inactive. Psychological well-being was measured three times during the study using the General Well-Being Scale. (See questionnaire at the end of this chapter in the *Health and Fitness Activity*).

After just six weeks of exercise, the women walkers improved their psychological well-being scores from an average of 70 (which indicates a stress problem) to 81 (indicating a positive sense of well-being). The inactive group showed no significant change in their score. Other psychological tests revealed that the walkers over time had higher energy levels, felt more relaxed and less tense or anxious, and sensed that life was more satisfying and interesting.

Other types of aerobic exercises have also been proved to be mentally beneficial. A study comparing students in swimming classes with nonswimmers found the swimmers experienced less tension, depression, anger, and confusion, and more vigor. Other studies have found that mixed aerobic programs of swimming, soccer, running, and aquatic and land calisthenics that are more moderate in intensity and more fun are helpful in reducing anxiety. A study of 64 long-term unemployed women and men ages 25 to 45 showed that those exercising experienced a significant reduction in anxiety after three, months of regular (2 hours per week) recreational (volleyball and badminton) and low-aerobic intensity activity (calisthenics and swimming).

Self-Esteem

Exercise does more than reduce anxiety and depression and elevate mood. Self-esteem is also improved and has been strongly correlated with exercise in many studies. In a study of three groups of 40 college students, students were divided into a 10-week exercise group, a 10-week exercise group with supportive counseling, and a control group receiving no exercise or counseling. The combination of running and supportive counseling helped those with low self-esteem gain more positive views of themselves.

A study of women in a 12-week program of weight training showed an increase in both strength and self-esteem. So both aerobic and non-aerobic exercise may be helpful in improving self-esteem.

In a compelling study of young men in a juvenile detention center, two hours per week of running and hard basketball led to significant improvements in self-esteem and general psychological mood state. The researchers concluded that vigorous aerobic exercise can provide substantial psychological help for delinquent adolescents.

Mental Cognition and Reaction Time

Results from some studies have suggested that short-term memory and intellectual function may be improved during or shortly after an exercise session, but much more study is needed in this area. Several recent studies with elderly people have consistently shown that those who become physically active improve their ability to think and react mentally.

The theory is of course consistent with that of the Greeks, who walked while they discussed topics of importance and were believers in the ability of exercise to improve mental function.

Mechanisms: How Physical Activity Helps Psychological Health

So far we've seen that mounting evidence backs up the Greek ideal of a "strong mind in a strong body." Regular exercise such as walking, jogging, and swimming is associated with improved self-esteem, general mood elevation and increased vigor and reduced anxiety, depression, and fatigue (see Box 11.2 for a summary).

Explaining how and why exercise improves psychological health is at this time still in the speculation stage. However, several theories have received impressive research support.

Endogenous Opioids

The body has an amazing, recently discovered hormonal system of morphine-like chemicals called **endogenous opioids.** These are of interest because their receptors are found in the hypothalamus and limbic systems of the brain, areas associated with emotion and behavior. Endogenous opioids like ß-endorphin have been associated with reduced pain, enhanced memory, and improved regulation of appetite, sex, blood pressure, and ventilation.

During exercise, the pituitary gland increases its production of ß-endorphin, raising its concentration in the blood. A sharp rise requires very intense exercise (generally at levels of at least 80 to 90 percent $\dot{V}O_{2max}$). The increase in ß-endorphin does not differ significantly between athletes and nonathletes.

Although it is widely accepted by the exercising public that endorphins are responsible for the good feelings associated with exercise, scientists disagree in interpreting the evidence. Most have found that despite significant reduction in tension during exercise, the increase in blood ß-endorphin levels is unrelated to the improvement in mood.

Before any molecule from the blood can enter the brain cells, it must pass through what is called the blood brain barrier. Researchers have been unable to demonstrate convincingly that the endorphins secreted by the pituitary into the blood are able to gain entry into the brain. Unless they do enter, they cannot be responsible for the reduction in pain, elevation in mood, and reduced sense of fatigue.

Alpha Brain Waves

Research has shown that there is increased emission of alpha waves during exercise—brain waves associated with a relaxed, meditation-like state. These alpha waves appear approximately 20 minutes into a 30-minute jog, and are still measurable after the exercise is over. Researchers speculate that the increased alpha wave power could contribute to the psychological benefits of exercise, including reductions in anxiety and depression. Higher-intensity exercise has been associated with higher alpha brain wave activity.

Brain Neurotransmitters

Experiments with rats have shown that exercise may also raise levels of brain chemicals called neurotransmitters—norepinephrine, dopamine, and serotonin. More research is needed, but theoretically, the relief from depression felt by moderately depressed people following regular exercise may be due to altered levels of these neurotransmitters.

BOX 11.2

2008 Physical Activity Guidelines for Americans:
Conclusions Regarding Physical Activity and Mental Health

Does Physical Activity Protect Against the Onset of Depression Disorders or Treat Depression Symptoms?
Conclusions: Regular physical activity (both moderate and high levels) protects against developing depression symptoms and major depressive disorder. In people with depression, participation in physical activity programs reduces depression symptoms and is thus useful for treatment.

Does Physical Activity Protect Against the Onset of Anxiety Disorders or Treat Anxiety Symptoms?
Conclusions: Regular physical activity protects against the development of anxiety disorders and anxiety symptoms, and the odds of an anxiety disorder may be reduced by higher weekly frequency of exercise bouts. In people with anxiety disorders, participation in physical activity programs reduces symptoms and is useful for treatment.

Does Physical Activity Enhance Well-Being?
Conclusions: Yes, people who are physically active have enhanced feelings of well-being.

Does Physical Activity Protect Against the Onset of Age-Related Decline in Cognitive Function or Dementia?
Conclusions: Physical activity delays the incidence of dementia and the onset of cognitive decline associated with aging. Physical activity improves or maintains cognitive function among healthy older adults, more so than for young adults whose cognitive health is normally near peak function.

Does Physical Activity Protect Against the Onset of Insomnia or Other Sleep Problems?
Conclusions: Regular participation in physical activity lowers the odds of disrupted or insufficient sleep, including sleep apnea, and has favorable effects on sleep quality. Thus regular physical activity is a useful component of good sleep hygiene.

Overall Conclusions: The weight evidence supports the conclusion that physical activity has protective benefits for several aspects of mental health, especially for protection against symptoms of depression and cognitive decline associated with aging, including the onset of dementia. Substantial evidence also suggests that physical activity reduces symptoms of anxiety and poor sleep, as well as feelings of distress and fatigue, and enhances well-being. Thus regular participation in moderate-to-vigorous physical activity, consistent with current public health guidelines, confers mental health benefits when compared to participation in low levels of physical activity or a sedentary lifestyle.

Source: U.S. Department of Health and Human Services. *2008 Physical Activity Guidelines for Americans.* ODPHP Publication No. U0036, October, 2008. *www.health.gov/paguidelines.* Physical Activity Guidelines Advisory Committee. *Physical Activity Guidelines Advisory Committee Report, 2008.* Washington, DC: U.S. Department of Health and Human Services, 2008.

Other Theories

Some researchers feel the mental benefits of exercise may also be related to the social support most people get from exercising together. Exercise may also help because it is a distraction or a "time-out" session from the "real world" of work and responsibility.

Other researchers suggest that exercise reduces muscle electrical tension because of an increase in deep-body temperature. There is some evidence to suggest that fit people sleep better, and therefore feel better during the day. Some advance the idea that exercise increases blood and oxygen transport to the brain.

Whatever the real reasons for the positive impact of exercise on the brain—increase in ß-endorphin, increase in brain alpha power, or enhanced brain neurotransmission—the evidence is very compelling, and more research is certainly warranted.

Precautions: Running Addiction, Mood Disturbance, and Sleep Disruption

Dr. Morgan from the University of Wisconsin has described one type of exerciser as "running addicted." They are so committed to exercise that obligations to work, family, and interpersonal relationships, as well as ability to utilize medical advice, all suffer. Such people are also compulsive, use running for an escape, are overcompetitive, live in a state of chronic fatigue, are self-centered, and are preoccupied with fitness, diet, and body image. Certainly this is taking exercise too far, negating any psychological benefit that more moderate exercise may bring.

Dr. Morgan has also reported that mood disturbance can increase when training loads are increased too greatly. When swimmers increased their daily training distance from 4,000 to 9,000 meters per day during a 10-day period, there were significant increases in muscle soreness, depression, anger, fatigue, and overall mood disturbance, along with a reduced general sense of well-being. Intense physical exercise such as a competitive marathon has been shown to disrupt both rapid eye movement (REM) sleep and total sleep time.

Practical Implications

Although we are not sure why, the research presented in this chapter has shown that the same amount of exercise that helps the heart also helps the brain. The American College of Sports Medicine has established that three to five, 20 to 30 minute aerobic exercise sessions of moderate intensity per week, activities like logging, swimming, bicycling, or brisk walking, are necessary to fully develop the heart-lung blood vessel system. Most of the studies referred to in this article used these same exercise criteria, and thus showed that as the heart is strengthened, so is the brain.

We now can have confidence that in exercise we have a strong weapon to help counter the never-ending onslaught of stress, anxiety, and depression associated with our modern era. Exercise, acting as a buffer, does help reduce the strain of stressful events. Exercise can help to fortify the brain, alleviating anxiety and depression, while elevating mood.

Preliminary research is also indicating that the brain may function better cognitively during exercise. Though we need more research to evaluate the effect of regular exercise on overall mental function, there is evidence that it does more than just make people feel better. What this means for busy students and workers everywhere is that time spent in exercise may not be lost in terms of getting the job done. The half-hour exercise session may actually enhance mental functioning to the point of increasing overall effective use of time.

So the allocation of curricular time to physical education may not hamper academic achievement as some school boards have thought, and exercise breaks for normally sedentary office workers may actually enhance the productivity of a business.

In general, all of the evidence tends to support what we already strongly suspected and people like John and Donna at the beginning of the chapter have experienced. Exercise is good for both the body and the brain. Through regular, active use of the body, one can actually induce a sense of euphoria.

HEALTH AND FITNESS INSIGHT
Sleep and Exercise

The National Sleep Foundation reports that 74 percent of American adults are experiencing a sleeping problem a few nights a week or more, 39 percent get less than seven hours of sleep each weeknight, and 37 percent are so sleepy during the day that it interferes with daily activities. (See Box 11.3.)

According to a report issued by the National Commission on Sleep Disorders Research, 30–40% of Americans have insomnia within any given year, defined by the National Institutes of Health as "an experience of inadequate or poor quality sleep." Characteristics of insomnia include:

- difficulty falling asleep
- difficulty maintaining sleep
- waking up too early in the morning
- nonrefreshing sleep
- daytime tiredness, lack of energy, difficulty concentrating, and irritability

Lack of sleep leads to problems completing a task, concentrating, making decisions, working with and getting along with other people, and unsafe actions. Sleep duration is related to length of life, with death risk increased in those sleeping less than six hours a night. Sleep deprivation is linked to approximately 100,000 vehicle crashes and 1,500 deaths each year. Insomnia early in adult life is a risk factor for the development of clinical depression and mental health disorders. (See Health and Fitness Activity 11.2.)

A night's sleep consists of four or five cycles, each of which progresses through several stages. During each night a person alternates between non-rapid eye movement (NREM) sleep and rapid eye movement (REM) sleep. The entire cycle of NREM and REM sleep takes about 90 minutes. The average adult sleeps 7.5 hours (five full cycles), with 25 percent of that in REM. By age 70, total sleep time decreases to about six hours (four sleep cycles), but the proportion of REM stays at about 25 percent. Sleep efficiency is reduced in the elderly with an increased number of awakenings during the night.

In NREM sleep, brain activity, heart rate, respiration, blood pressure, and metabolism (vital signs) slow down, and body temperature falls, as a deep, restful state is reached. Slow wave sleep usually terminates with the sleeper's changing position. The brain waves now reverse their course as the sleeper heads for the active REM stage.

BOX 11.3

Facts on Sleep in America

- On average, adults sleep seven hours during the weekday, one hour less than recommended by sleep experts. Only 38 percent sleep eight hours or more on weekday nights, and 31 percent sleep less than seven hours.
- On weekends, adults sleep an average of 7.8 hours per night.
- One third of Americans say they get less sleep now than five years ago, and 69 percent say they experience frequent sleep problems, though most have not been diagnosed.
- A sizable proportion of adults (40%) report that they are so sleepy during the day this interferes with daily activities at least a few days a month or more. One in five (22%) experience this level of daytime sleepiness a few days per week or more. When they feel sleepy during the day, 65 percent say they are very likely to accept their sleepiness and keep going.
- More than one half of adults in the U.S. (53%) report that they have driven while drowsy in the past year, 19 percent have actually dozed off while driving, and 1 percent have had an accident because they dozed off or were too tired.
- About one half of adults (51%) report having experienced one or more symptoms of insomnia at least a few nights a week in the past year, and 29 percent have experienced insomnia nearly every night.
- Almost one-half of adults (46%) need an alarm clock to wake up four or more times a week.
- The most common activities within the hour before going to sleep are watching TV (87%), spending time with family and friends (73%), reading (53%), and taking a bath or shower (50%).
- More than one in ten adults (11%) report using prescription and/or over-the-counter medications

Source: National Sleep Foundation. *www.sleepfoundation.org*

In REM sleep, the eyes dart about under closed eyelids, and vivid dreams transpire that can often be remembered. The even breathing of NREM gives way to halting uncertainty, and the heart rhythm speeds or slows unaccountably. The brain is highly active during REM sleep, and overall brain metabolism may be increased above the level experienced when awake.

Getting a good night's sleep has proven to be a difficult goal for many people in this modern era. The National Sleep Foundation has published several guidelines for better sleep. Here are ten guidelines for better sleep:

- Maintain a regular bed and wake time schedule, including weekends.
- Establish a regular, relaxing bedtime routine such as soaking in a hot bath or hot tub and then reading a book or listening to soothing music.
- Create a sleep-conducive environment that is dark, quiet, comfortable and cool.
- Sleep on a comfortable mattress and pillows.
- Use your bedroom only for sleep and sex. It is best to take work materials, computers, and televisions out of the sleeping environment.
- Finish eating at least two to three hours before your regular bedtime.
- Avoid nicotine (e.g., cigarettes, tobacco products). Used close to bedtime, it can lead to poor sleep.

- Avoid caffeine (e.g., coffee, tea, soft drinks, chocolate) close to bedtime. It can keep you awake.
- Avoid alcohol close to bedtime. It can lead to disrupted sleep later in the night.
- Exercise regularly. It is best to complete your workout at least a few hours before bedtime.

Compared to those who avoid exercise, physically fit people claim that they fall asleep more rapidly, sleep better, and feel less tired during the day. These beliefs have been confirmed, and scientists have shown that people who exercise regularly do indeed spend more time in slow-wave sleep.

In a study conducted at Stanford University, physically inactive older adults were assigned to exercise or nonexercise groups for 16 weeks. Subjects in the exercise group engaged in low-impact aerobics and brisk walking for 30 to 40 minutes, 4 days per week. Exercise training led to improved sleep quality, longer sleep, and a shorter time to fall asleep. A year-long study of post-menopausal women showed that those exercising moderately in the morning for 3 to 4 hours per week had less trouble falling asleep compared to those exercising less.

In summary, in you exercise regularly, you should sleep better. There is some evidence, however, that exercising and sweating close to bedtime can have an adverse effect on sleep quality for both fit and sedentary subjects. This is why the National Sleep Foundation recommends avoiding heavy exercise late in the day.

Summary

1. Nearly one out of four Americans is affected by one or more mental disorders, and one half of U.S. adults experience at least a moderate amount of stress on a regular basis.
2. Many studies have shown that being chronically anxious, depressed, or emotionally distressed is associated with deterioration of health.
3. Stress has been defined as any action or situation (stressors) that places special physical or psychological demands upon a person—in other words, anything that unbalances one's equilibrium. It is not the stressor itself that creates the response. Instead, it is the person's reaction to the stressor. Five stress-management principles were reviewed: learn to control stressors, let the mind choose the reaction, seek the social support of others, find satisfaction in work and service, and keep healthy.
4. Studies of active people show them to have a better psychological profile than inactive people. However, a strong self-selection bias may be present when comparing active people with the general population. Controlled intervention studies are preferred when looking at the relationship between physical activity and psychological health.
5. A review of four national surveys has concluded that physical activity is positively associated with good mental health, defined as positive mood, general well-being, and relatively infrequent symptoms of anxiety and depression.
6. A considerable amount of research has indicated that less aerobically fit people show greater cardiovascular and subjective responses to psychological stressors than do those at high levels of aerobic fitness.
7. Stressful life events appear to cause fewer physical and psychological problems for physically active people than they do for inactive people.
8. Most studies support the proposition that depression, anxiety, and mood state in general are favorably affected by regular aerobic exercise.
9. Both aerobic and non-aerobic exercise have been shown to be helpful in improving self-concept.
10. Preliminary research suggests that short-term memory and intellectual function maybe improved during or shortly after an exercise session. More research is needed to study the long-term effects.

11. ß-endorphin rises in the blood during intense exercise, but not during low-intensity exercise. Most researchers have found that despite significant decreases in tension during exercise, the increase in ß-endorphin is unrelated to the improvement in mood. It appears that the complex ß-endorphin protein molecule is unable to cross the blood-brain barrier to gain access to the receptors located in the limbic system. However, exercise may trigger an increase in ß-endorphin levels within the brain itself.

12. During exercise, there is an increase in emission of alpha waves, brain waves associated with a relaxed, meditation-like state. These could contribute to the psychological benefits of exercise.

13. Exercise may enhance neurotransmitter activity in the brain, increasing the concentrations of brain norepinephrine and serotonin.

HEALTH AND FITNESS ACTIVITY 11.1
The General Well-Being Scale

As described earlier in this chapter, one measure of psychological status that has been used with good success in national surveys is the General Well-Being Scale (GWB). The GWB was designed by the National Center for Health Statistics, and consists of 18 questions covering such matters as energy level, satisfaction, freedom from worry, and self-control. A high score on the GWB reflects an absence of bad feelings and an expression of positive feelings. Results from national surveys have shown that higher scores for the GWB are significantly associated with increased amounts of physical activity for all age groups and for both men and women. (See: Stephens T. Physical Activity and Mental Health in the United States and Canada: Evidence from Four Population Surveys, *Prev Med* 17:35–47, 1988.)

The General Well-Being Scale

Instructions: The following questions ask how you feel and how things have been going for you *during the past month*. For each question, mark an "x" for the answer that most nearly applies to you. Since there are no right or wrong answers, it's best to answer each question quickly without pausing too long on any one of them.

1. How have you been feeling in general?
   - 5 ❏ In excellent spirits.
   - 4 ❏ In very good spirits.
   - 3 ❏ In good spirits mostly.
   - 2 ❏ I've been up and down in spirits a lot.
   - 1 ❏ In low spirits mostly.
   - 0 ❏ In very low spirits.

2. Have you been bothered by nervousness or your "nerves"?
   - 0 ❏ Extremely so—to the point where I could not work or take care of things.
   - 1 ❏ Very much so.
   - 2 ❏ Quite a bit.
   - 3 ❏ Some—enough to bother me.
   - 4 ❏ A little.
   - 5 ❏ Not at all.

3. Have you been in firm control of your behavior, thoughts, emotions, or feelings?
   - 5 ❏ Yes, definitely so.
   - 4 ❏ Yes, for the most part.
   - 3 ❏ Generally so.
   - 2 ❏ Not too well.
   - 1 ❏ No, and I am somewhat disturbed.
   - 0 ❏ No, and I am very disturbed.

4. Have you felt so sad, discouraged, or hopeless, or had so many problems that you wondered if anything was worthwhile?

    0 ❏ Extremely so—to the point I have just about given up.

    1 ❏ Very much so.

    2 ❏ Quite a bit.

    3 ❏ Some—enough to bother me.

    4 ❏ A little bit.

    5 ❏ Not at all.

5. Have you been under or felt you were under any strain, stress, or pressure?

    0 ❏ Yes—almost more than I could bear.

    1 ❏ Yes—quite a bit of pressure.

    2 ❏ Yes—some, more than usual.

    3 ❏ Yes—some, but about usual.

    4 ❏ Yes—a little.

    5 ❏ Not at all.

6. How happy, satisfied, or pleased have you been with your personal life?

    5 ❏ Extremely happy—couldn't have been more satisfied or pleased.

    4 ❏ Very happy.

    3 ❏ Fairly happy.

    2 ❏ Satisfied—pleased.

    1 ❏ Somewhat dissatisfied.

    0 ❏ Very dissatisfied.

7. Have you had reason to wonder if you were losing your mind, or losing control over the way you act, talk, think, feel, or of your memory?

    5 ❏ Not at all.

    4 ❏ Only a little.

    3 ❏ Some, but not enough to be concerned.

    2 ❏ Some, and I've been a little concerned.

    1 ❏ Some, and I am quite concerned.

    0 ❏ Much, and I'm very concerned.

8. Have you been anxious, worried, or upset?

    0 ❏ Extremely so—to the point of being sick, or almost sick.

    1 ❏ Very much so.

    2 ❏ Quite a bit.

    3 ❏ Some—enough to bother me.

    4 ❏ A little bit.

    5 ❏ Not at all.

9. Have you been waking up fresh and rested?

   5 ❏ Every day.
   4 ❏ Most every day.
   3 ❏ Fairly often.
   2 ❏ Less than half the time.
   1 ❏ Rarely.
   0 ❏ None of the time.

10. Have you been bothered by any illness, bodily disorder, pain, or fears about your health?

   0 ❏ All the time.
   1 ❏ Most of the time.
   2 ❏ A good bit of the time.
   3 ❏ Some of the time.
   4 ❏ A little of the time.
   5 ❏ None of the time.

11. Has your daily life been full of things that are interesting to you?

   5 ❏ All the time.
   4 ❏ Most of the time.
   3 ❏ A good bit of the time.
   2 ❏ Some of the time.
   1 ❏ A little of the time.
   0 ❏ None of the time.

12. Have you felt downhearted and blue?

   0 ❏ All the time.
   1 ❏ Most of the time.
   2 ❏ A good bit of the time.
   3 ❏ Some of the time.
   4 ❏ A little of the time.
   5 ❏ None of the time.

13. Have you been feeling emotionally stable and sure of yourself?

   5 ❏ All the time.
   4 ❏ Most of the time.
   3 ❏ A good bit of the time.
   2 ❏ Some of the time.
   1 ❏ A little of the time.
   0 ❏ None of the time.

14. Have you felt tired, worn out, used up or exhausted?

    0 ❑ All the time.

    1 ❑ Most of the time.

    2 ❑ A good bit of the time.

    3 ❑ Some of the time.

    4 ❑ A little of the time.

    5 ❑ None of the time.

Note: For each of the tour scales below, the words at each end describe opposite feelings. Circle any number along the bar that seems closest to how you have felt generally during the past month.

15. How concerned or worried about your health have you been?

    Not concerned at all   10   8   6   4   2   0   Very concerned

16. How relaxed or tense have you been?

    Very relaxed   10   8   6   4   2   0   Very tense

17. How much energy, pep, and vitality have you felt?

    No energy at all,   Very energetic,
    listless   0   2   4   6   8   10   dynamic

18. How depressed or cheerful have you been? Very depressed?

    Very depressed   0   2   4   6   8   10   Very cheerful

Directions: Add up all the points from the boxes you have checked for each question. Compare your total score with the norms listed below.

National Norms for the General Well-Being Scale

Stress State	Total Stress Score	% Distribution U.S. Population
Positive well-being	81–110	55%
Low positive	76–80	10%
Marginal	71–75	9%
Indicates stress problem	56–70	16%
Indicates distress	41–55	7%
Serious	26–40	2%
Severe	0–25	less than 1%

Note: Figure 11.4 gives the scores for the U.S. population by age, gender, and amount of exercise. Notice that all subgroups reporting "much exercise" fell within the "positive well-being" range of 81–110.

HEALTH AND FITNESS ACTIVITY 11.2
Determining Whether You Are Sleep-Deprived

If three or more of the following describe you, it's possible that you many need more sleep:

_____ I need an alarm clock in order to wake up at the appropriate time.

_____ It's a struggle for me to get out of bed in the morning.

_____ I feel tired, irritable, and stressed out during the week.

_____ I have trouble concentrating.

_____ I have trouble remembering.

_____ I feel slow with critical thinking, problem solving, being creative.

_____ I often fall asleep watching television.

_____ I find it hard to stay awake in boring meetings or lectures, or in warm rooms.

_____ I often nod off after heavy meals or after a low dose of alcohol.

_____ I often feel drowsy while driving.

_____ I often sleep extra hours on weekend mornings.

_____ I often need a nap to get through the day.

_____ I have dark circles under my eyes.

Source: National Sleep Foundation, 2005.

HEALTH AND FITNESS ACTIVITY 11.3
Depression

The National Institute of Mental Health has estimated that 20.9 million Americans suffer from depression. Only a minority of cases are diagnosed and treated, in part because many of the usual symptoms—feelings of hopelessness, despair, lethargy, self-loathing—tend to discourage the depressed individual from reaching out for help. The majority of cases of depression can be successfully treated, usually with medication, psychotherapy, or both. Nonetheless, the condition must first be identified. The Center for Epidemiologic Studies (CES) has developed a tool for measuring depression, known as the CES-D Scale. Take this test to see how you are feeling.

During the past week	<1 day	1-2 day	3-4 days	5-7 days
I was bothered by things that don't usually bother me	0	1	2	3
I did not feel like eating; my appetite was poor	0	1	2	3
I felt that I could not shake off the blues even with the help of my family or friends	0	1	2	3
I felt that I was just as good as other people	3	2	1	0
I had trouble keeping my mind on what I was doing	0	1	2	3
I felt depressed	0	1	2	3
I felt everything I did was an effort	0	1	2	3
I felt hopeful about the future	3	2	1	0
I thought my life had been a failure	0	1	2	3
I felt fearful	0	1	2	3
My sleep was restless	0	1	2	3
I was happy	3	2	1	0
I talked less than usual	0	1	2	3
I felt lonely	0	1	2	3
People were unfriendly	0	1	2	3
I enjoyed life	3	2	1	0
I had crying spells	0	1	2	3
I felt sad	0	1	2	3
I felt that people disliked me	0	1	2	3
I could not get "going"	0	1	2	3

Scoring: A score of 22 or higher indicates possible depression. In general, the higher the score, the greater the mood disturbance—even below that threshold.

Lenore Sawyer Radloff, *Applied Psychological Measurement,* June, 1977. Copyright © 1977 by Applied Psychological Measurement. Reprinted by permission of Sage Publications.

CHAPTER 11 QUIZ
Stress Management and Mental Health

Note: Answers are given at the end of the quiz.

1. The General Well-Being psychological stress test (the one you took in the health and fitness activity at the end of the chapter) has been used in several national surveys. In general,
   A. scores are highest for physically active people.
   B. scores are lowest for physically active people.
   C. no difference has been found in scores of active and inactive people.

2. Being chronically anxious, depressed, or emotionally distressed has been associated with various diseases, including;
   A. cancer.
   B. heart disease.
   C. infection.
   D. A + B only.
   E. all of the above.
   F. none of the above.

3. During any given six-month period, 26 percent of the U.S. population is affected by one or more mental disorders. The most prevalent of all is:
   A. schizophrenia.
   B. anxiety disorders.
   C. depression.
   D. Alzheimer's disease.

4. There are basic strategies for managing stress, with several recommendations included for each. Which recommendation for managing stress listed below is *not* included?
   A. Manage stressors by controlling the pace of life and daily schedules.
   B. Realize that when stressful events occur, the mind can choose the reaction.
   C. Good health and exercise can help the body deal with stress more easily.
   D. Limit the number of people in your social network so that you will not need to seek their support during stress.

5. Which one of the following does *not* occur during the fight-or-flight stress response?
   A. Blood pressure increases.
   B. Secretion of saliva diminishes.
   C. Immune system is suppressed.
   D. Perspiration increases.
   E. Digestion of food stops.
   F. Breathing is shallow and slow.

6. Regular physical exercise has been associated with:
   A. increased cardiovascular reactivity to mental stress.
   B. reduced anxiety.
   C. reduced depression.
   D. increased self-concept.
   E. all of the above.
   F. A + C.
   G. all but A.

7. T   F   Beta-endorphin is secreted into the blood from the pituitary during moderate forms of exercise (like walking), elevating mood and decreasing anxiety and depression.

8. T   F   The majority of people with depression do not receive treatment.

9. T   F   People with less education and income are more likely to report being stressed than those with more education and income.

10. T   F   Bad stressors such as divorce cause stress reactions, but good stressors such as marriage do not.

11. T   F   When people are socially isolated with few social contacts or interactions with others, sickness and mental stress are more likely.

Calisthenics for Development of Flexibility and Muscular Strength and Endurance

Flexibility Exercises

The key to developing good flexibility is to hold each of the following positions lust short of pain for 15 to 20 seconds. *Relax* totally, letting your muscles slowly go limp as the tension of the stretched muscle area slowly subsides. After the tension has subsided, it is a good idea to stretch just a bit farther to better develop your flexibility (hold this "developmental stretch" also for 15 to 30 seconds). Be sure that you do not stretch to the point of pain for flexibility cannot be developed white the stretched muscle is in pain.

Flexibility exercises should he conducted *following* the aerobic phase. Research has shown that stretching is safer and more effective when done with warm muscles and joints. You can stretch farther without injury more often following stimulating aerobics than before.

Do not be worried if you seem "tighter" than other people in many of the following stretches. Flexibility is an individual matter, and each person should "make the most" of what they have, realizing there are genetic differences.

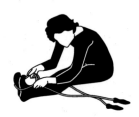

Flexibility #1

Lower Back, Hamstring Stretch (with Rope)

Start by sitting on the floor, one leg straight, the other relaxed off to the side (some people like the other leg bent at a 90° angle, foot against the other leg, some like it straight off to the side a bit, others slightly bent and loose). The rope should be doubled over the heel. (This exercise can also be done with both legs at one time.)

Stretch by reaching down the rope toward your foot with both hands until you feel a good tension in the back of your leg (some feel tension in the lower back also). Relax, breathe easily, letting the tension slowly subside, then reach a bit farther, holding this for 15 to 30 seconds also. Repeat with the other leg.

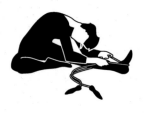

Benefits: This is perhaps the best stretch for the lower back and hamstrings (muscles on the back of your thigh). Your goal is to slowly work toward your foot as the weeks pass until you can at least hold on to your foot with one hand.

Flexibility #2

Calf Rope Stretch

Start just the same as the lower back, hamstring rope stretch, but put the rope on the ball of your foot.

Stretch by pulling your upper foot (easy does it) toward your body until you feel a good tension in the top of your calf muscle. Relax and hold this position for 15 to 30 seconds, then reach a bit farther down the rope for a second 15- to 30-second stretch. Repeat with the other leg.

Benefits: Stretches the calf muscle.

Flexibility #3

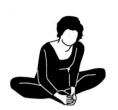

Groin Stretch

Start by sitting on the floor with the soles of your feet together, legs bent, knees up and out.

Stretch by pulling your feet with your hands to within a few inches of your crotch. Hold this position as you lean forward from the waist, keeping your chin up, and knees down as far as possible. Feel a good tension in the groin area and hold.

Benefits: Stretches the muscles in the groin area. Be careful that you do not overstretch.

Flexibility #4

Quad Stretch

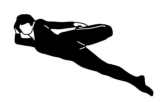

Start by lying on your right side, right hand supporting your head.

Stretch by bending your left leg, pulling the heel to your seat with the left hand grasping the ankle. Slowly move the entire left leg somewhat behind you until there is a good tension in front of the thigh, and hold. Repeat with the other leg.

Benefits: The muscles of the front of the thigh (quadriceps) are stretched in this exercise.

Flexibility #5

Spinal Twist

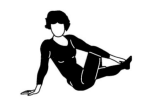

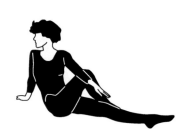

Start by sitting with your left leg straight out in front of you, your right leg bent, right foot crossed over the left knee.

Stretch by placing your left elbow on the outside of your right knee, pushing the right knee inward. At the same time, place your right hand on the ground behind you, and twist looking over your right shoulder. Keep pushing with your left elbow and twisting with your head over your right shoulder until you feel a good tension along your spine and hip, and hold for 15 to 30 seconds. Repeat on the other side.

Benefits: Stretches the muscles along the spine and side of the hips. Some people find this a hard stretch to coordinate. You may have to practice carefully with the pictures until you get used to all the important details.

Flexibility #6

Downward Dog

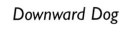

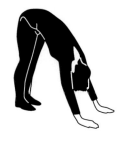

Start by getting on all fours.

Stretch by humping your seat straight up, with legs straight. Walk in with your hands toward your feet until you are about 3 feet from your feet. Then try to keep your heels on the ground as you lean somewhat backward, keeping your legs straight, hands on the floor, and head down. You should feel a good tension all along your posterior leg. Hold for 15 to 30 seconds until the tension slowly subsides.

Benefits: This is an excellent stretch for the hamstrings and calves of your legs as well as the lower back. Running tends to tighten the posterior leg muscles, and this exercise helps to counter this. The key is to keep the heels on the ground, but be careful not to hold a painful position as this could injure your legs.

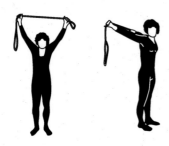

Flexibility #7

Upper Body Stretch

Start by grasping a rope or towel with your hands 2 to 4 feet apart.

Stretch by keeping your arms perfectly straight, and slowly circling them up and behind you. Move slowly, feeling the tension in the front of your chest and shoulders. If you cannot keep your arms straight, or if the pain is too intense, put your hands farther apart. Repeat several times.

Benefits: Running tends to tighten the muscles in the front of the chest. This exercise helps to stretch those muscles, improving your posture.

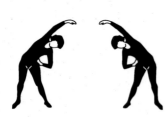

Flexibility #8

Standing Side Stretch

Start by standing with your feet 3 feet apart, hands on your hips.

Stretch by raising your right hand up and over your head as you lean way over to the left side. Keep your legs straight and lean straight to the side. Hold the position, feeling the stretch along your right side and inner left thigh. Repeat with the other side.

Benefits: This exercise stretches the muscles along both sides and inner thighs. If you do not feel a stretch in your thighs, put your feet farther apart.

Muscle Endurance and Strength Exercises

The following exercises localize movement to specific muscle groups, developing the strength and muscle endurance in each of these areas. Do 5 to 15 reps of each (remembering that a rep = one-one, two, three, two-one, two, three, etc.).

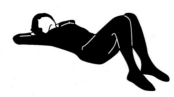

Abdomen #1

Bent Knee Sit-Ups

Start by lying on the ground, knees bent at a 90° angle. Most people need to tuck their feet under either another person or an object. If you are in good shape, you can put your hands behind your head. If your abdominal muscles are not in good shape, you can put your arms straight out in front of you (and even pull on your knees if you need to).

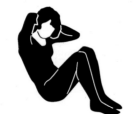

1—Sit up by flexing your abdominal muscles, and touch your elbows to your knees. If you need to, keep your arms out in front of you.
2—Lie back down, keeping your knees bent.
3 & 4—Repeat.

Continue for 5 to 10 counts (10 to 20 total sit-ups, or two every full repetition).

Benefits: The bent knee sit-up is an excellent exercise for toning up the abdominal muscles. The knees are bent so that the strong hip flexors will have minimal action, allowing the abdominal muscles to act.

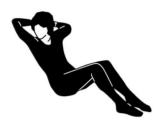

Abdomen #2

Ab-Curl Twisters

Start in the same basic position as the sit-up, except that you should have your torso two-thirds the way up toward your knees.

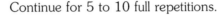

1—Keeping your body in a two-thirds sit-up position, twist to your left.
2—Next twist to your right.
3 & 4—Keep twisting back and forth, right and left, while leaning back, feeling a good tension in your abdominal area. If the movement becomes too hard, move closer to your knees.

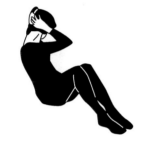

Continue for 5 to 10 full repetitions.

Benefits: The sides of the abdomen are given a great workout as well as the middle abdominal muscles.

Abdomen #3

Straight Leg Ab-Twisters

Start by sitting with your legs together, straight out in front of you, arms crossed over your chest.

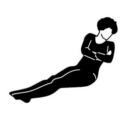

1—Lean back at least one-third of the way to the floor, hold this position throughout, and twist to the left, looking to the ground on the left side.
2—Next do the same to the right side.
3 & 4—Repeat, twisting left and right while leaning back, legs straight.
Continue for 5 to 10 repetitions.

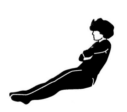

Benefits: This exercise also gives the sides of the abdomen a good workout while developing the muscle endurance of the middle abdominals as well.

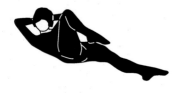

Abdomen #4

Steam Engine

Start by lying on your back, hands behind the head. Then lift the head off the ground and touch your left elbow to your right knee. The right leg is bent, foot off the ground, while the left leg is straight, off the ground as well.

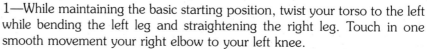

1—While maintaining the basic starting position, twist your torso to the left while bending the left leg and straightening the right leg. Touch in one smooth movement your right elbow to your left knee.
2—Return to the starting position, twisting your torso to the right.
3 & 4—Repeat, twisting right and left, touching the elbow on each side to the knee of the opposite bent leg. The alternating leg should be straight and off the ground.

Continue for 5 to 20 repetitions.

> *Benefits:* This is probably the best abdominal exercise because the entire abdominal area is given a great workout. The abdominal muscles are best developed when the trunk is curled and twisted, as in the steam engine exercise.

Abdomen #5

Wringer

Start by lying on the ground, legs straight and together, but arms straight and out to the sides.

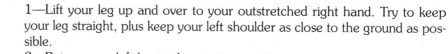

1—Lift your leg up and over to your outstretched right hand. Try to keep your leg straight, plus keep your left shoulder as close to the ground as possible.
2—Return your left leg to the starting position.
3—Repeat with your right leg, once again lifting it up and over to your left hand which is straight out perpendicular from your body.
4—Return your right leg to the starting position.

Continue for 10 to 15 full repetitions.

> *Benefits:* This exercise will not only develop the muscular endurance of the hip flexors and abdominal muscles, but also stretch the muscles along the sides of the body.

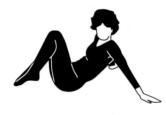

Abdomen #6

Gut Tucks

Start by sitting in a tuck position, with your legs drawn up close to your body, and hands on the floor slightly behind you for balance and support.

1—Lift your feet several inches off the ground as you straighten your legs halfway. It is important not to straighten the legs all the way because this places too great a strain on the lower back.

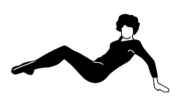

2—Return your legs to the tuck position, with your legs drawn up close to your body, and hands on the floor slightly behind you for balance and support.

3 & 4—Repeat, half straightening your legs and then tucking them back in, keeping the feet off the ground as you support yourself with your hands, leaning back slightly.

Continue for 5 to 10 repetitions.

> *Benefits:* This is an excellent abdominal exercise, firming up the muscles in the lower abdominal area especially.

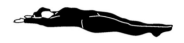

Abdomen #7

Half Pike Sit-Ups

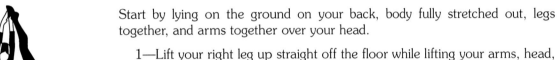

Start by lying on the ground on your back, body fully stretched out, legs together, and arms together over your head.

1—Lift your right leg up straight off the floor while lifting your arms, head, and shoulders up until you can touch your hands to your ankle or foot.

2—Return to the starting position.

3 & 4—Repeat with your left leg.

Continue for 10 repetitions.

> *Benefits:* The hip flexors are given a good workout, while the abdominals are developed to a lesser extent because there is little abdominal curling going on.

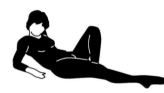

Abdomen #8

Single Leg Lifts

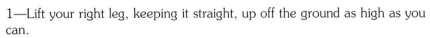

Start by supporting yourself on your elbows and seat, with your left leg bent, right leg straight.

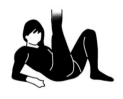

1—Lift your right leg, keeping it straight, up off the ground as high as you can.

2—Return your right leg to the starting position, but keep it several inches off the ground.

3 & 4—Repeat for 5 to 10 repetitions, then do the same with your left leg.

Continue lifting the straight leg up and down while keeping the other leg bent, supporting yourself with your elbows. It is important to stay in this position to prevent lower back strain from lifting the straight leg.

> *Benefits:* This exercise is especially good for the hip flexors, and secondarily for lower abdominal muscles.

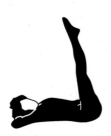

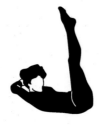

Abdomen #9

Extended Leg Sit-Ups

Start by lying on your back, legs straight up in a "pike" position, with your hands joined together behind your head, elbows out.

1—Lift your head, arms and shoulders up as high as you can off the ground making sure to keep the elbows out.
2—Return to the starting position.
3 & 4—Repeat, curling your upper body up and then down while keeping the legs straight up off the ground.

Continue for 5 to 10 repetitions.

Benefits: This is one of the best abdominal exercises you can do to develop a "flat tummy." The hip flexors are not involved because of the straight-leg-pike position which forces the abdominal muscles to curl your head and shoulders up.

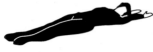

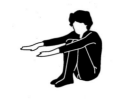

Abdomen #10

Rowing

Start by lying on your back, arms and legs fully stretched and together.

1—Draw your legs up to your body in a tuck position as you lift your upper body forward, reaching past your bent knees with your straight arms.
2—Return to the starting position.
3 & 4—Repeat, tucking your body into a tight ball, then returning to the starting position.

Continue for 5 to 10 repetitions.

Benefits: This is another excellent exercise for the abdominals and hip flexors. The tighter the ball you draw yourself into, the better.

Arms-Shoulders #1

Push-Ups

Start by supporting yourself on your knees and hands. It is important that your back be straight, seat not humped up. Your shoulders should be over your hands, arms straight. You should feel that you are supporting a good part of your weight on your hands. *Note:* If you are strong enough, support yourself between your feet and hands, keeping the trunk of your body perfectly straight and rigid. This can strain the lower back, so be certain that you possess sufficient strength.

1—Lower yourself down to within a few inches off the ground, keeping your back rigid and straight, weight equally distributed between knees and hands.
2—Straighten your arms up, once again keeping the back rigid and straight. Avoid sagging or humping.

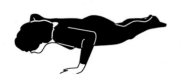

3 & 4—Repeat, lowering your body down and then pushing up, while the trunk is straight, and weight well felt on your arms and hands.

Continue for 5 to 15 repetitions (10 to 30 single push-ups).

> *Benefits:* This exercise develops muscular strength and endurance of the muscles of the front of the chest (pectorals) and back of the upper arm (triceps). The muscles of the trunk are also developed as the body is kept in a straight and rigid position throughout the exercise.

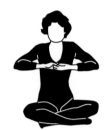

Arms-Shoulders #2

Sitting Hand Pull Raises

Start by sitting with your legs crossed, hands clasped together in the "Indian grip" (fingers hooked, hands opposite). Elbows should be out.

1—Pull hands apart, keeping them together with hooked fingers as you lift your hands and arms above your head. Keep pulling the hands hard the entire time.
2—Return the hands and arms to the starting position, still pulling hard.
3 & 4—Repeat, lifting the hands up and down as you try to pull them apart.

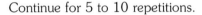

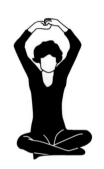

Continue for 5 to 10 repetitions.

> *Benefits:* This calisthenic especially develops the muscles between the shoulder blades, the rhomboids. The muscles of the upper back and neck, the trapezius in particular, are also developed. The overall benefit is to improve back posture.

Arms-Shoulders #3

Isometric Rope Curls

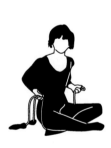

Start by sitting with legs crossed. Sit on top of your jumping rope and grasp the rope with both hands, palms up, arms at a 90° angle.

1—Forcefully lift up, contracting your arm muscles as tightly as possible. Hold for 5 seconds and then relax. Isometric means that there is muscle contraction without movement.

Repeat 3 to 5 times, contracting as forcefully as you can each time.

> *Benefits:* This develops the biceps, the muscles on the front of your upper arms, plus other muscles of the forearm. This simple exercise has been scientifically proven to increase the strength of your arms.

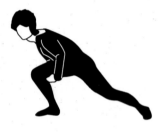

Hips-Thighs-Lower Back #1

Bear Hugs

Start by standing in a normal position, feet together.

1—Keeping your left foot in the same spot, step out straight to your right side, pointing your right foot in that direction. Reach out far enough so that your left leg remains straight, but your right leg is well bent. Wrap your arms around your right thigh as you finish stepping out to the right.
2—Return to the starting position.
3 & 4—Repeat with the left side. Continue stepping out to each side, hugging your thigh, and then returning back to the starting position.

Continue for 5 to 10 repetitions.

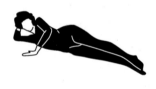

Benefits: The hamstrings and gluteus maximus (back of upper thigh and buttock muscles) are well developed in this exercise. Be careful not to overdo the first several times, for several people experience quite a bit of soreness. This exercise also develops the quadricep muscles in the front of your thigh.

Hips-Thighs-Lower Back #2

Lateral Leg Raises

Start by lying on your right side, your head held propped up with your right hand, your left leg lying on top of your right leg.

1—Lift your left leg up as high as you can. Keep the leg straight.
2—Return the leg to the down position.
3 & 4—Repeat. Keep lifting the leg up, then down, concentrating on a full range of motion. Repeat with the other leg.

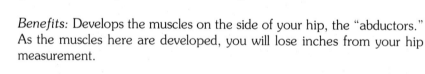

Benefits: Develops the muscles on the side of your hip, the "abductors." As the muscles here are developed, you will lose inches from your hip measurement.

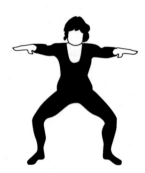

Hips-Thighs-Lower Back #3

Ballet Squats

Start by standing with your feet three feet apart, toes pointing out at a 45° angle. The arms should be straight, parallel to the ground, and out to the sides or angled forward.

1—Squat down until the thighs are parallel to the ground.
2—Straighten your legs only halfway. Do not stand all the way up, but keep the knees well bent.

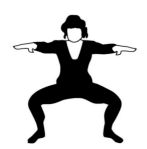

3 & 4—Repeat, moving up and down between a half squat and three-quarters squat position. The arms should be straight the entire time. The movement should be quick and almost bouncy.

Continue for 5 to 10 repetitions.

> *Benefits:* The quadriceps, the muscles on the front of the thigh, are highly developed in this exercise. The buttock muscles also get a good workout.

Hips-Thighs-Lower Back #4

Kneeling Leg Raises

Start by kneeling down on all fours.

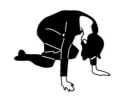

1—Lift your right leg slightly up and move it forward as you curl your head down, ending up with one-half of your body curled up. Your right knee should be close to your head.
2—Next lift your head up high as you also straighten and lift your right leg up high, arching your back.
3 & 4—Repeat, alternating curling and arching on one side of your body and then the other.

Continue for 5 to 10 repetitions.

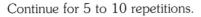

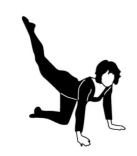

> *Benefits:* The major benefit is to the muscles of your back, especially near the neck and hip areas. Be careful not to strain your lower hack by lifting your leg too high.

Hips-Thighs-Lower Back #5

Kneeling Leg Swings

Start by kneeling on all fours.

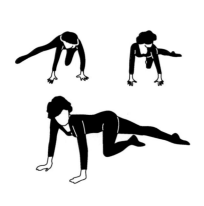

1—Straighten your leg and swing it out to the right side. Keep your leg straight, about 6 to 12 inches off the ground. Move your head and look right.
2—Next swing your leg behind you and cross over to the left side as far as you can while looking left. Your right leg should still be straight and off the ground 6 to 12 inches.
3 & 4—Repeat, swinging the leg back and forth, far to the right, and then crossing behind, while moving your head right, then left. Repeat with the other leg.

Continue for 5 to 10 repetitions.

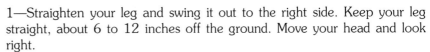

> *Benefits:* This is an excellent exercise for developing the muscles along the sides of the abdomen and in the lower back. In addition, the muscles along the sides of the trunk are given a good stretch each time the head and leg curl to the opposite side.

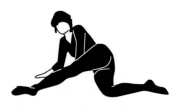

Hips-Thighs-Lower Back #6

Leg Pumps

Start by supporting yourself on your right side, right elbow, right hand, and bent right leg. Also put your left hand on the ground in front of you for support and balance. Your left leg should be straight, on top of the right.

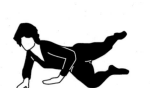

1—Forcefully swing your straight left leg forward, keeping it several inches off the ground,
2—Next swing your leg way back behind you (keep it straight off the ground several inches).
3 & 4—Repeat, swinging your leg forward and back over your bent right leg. Keep the top leg straight. Repeat with the other leg.
Continue for 5 to 10 repetitions.

Benefits: This calisthenic develops the muscles on the side of the hip, the "abductors" which will help to reduce the measurement of the hips. The muscles of the abdomen and lower back are also developed.

Hips-Thighs-Lower Back #7

Kneeling Bent Leg Raises

Start by supporting yourself on all fours.

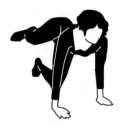

1—Lift your right leg, keeping it bent at a 90° angle, straight up to your side until it is parallel to the ground. Look at your leg with your head turned to the right side.
2—Return to the starting position.
3 & 4—Repeat, raising the bent leg up while looking right and then returning to the starting position. Do the same on the other side.
Continue for 5 repetitions on each leg.

Benefits: The muscles on the sides of the hips, the "abductors" are developed in this exercise.

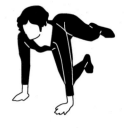

Hips-Thighs-Lower Back #8

Knee Leans

Start by kneeling, keeping your upper body straight, arms straight and reaching forward.

1—Keeping your body rigid and straight, lean back over your heels.
2—Return to the starting position.

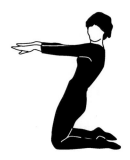

3 & 4—Repeat, leaning back and then going forward, keeping the trunk rigid. To get the lull effect, it is important that you do not bend at the waist.

Continue for 5 to 10 repetitions.

> *Benefits:* This is an excellent exercise for developing the quadricep muscles, the big muscles on the front of your thighs. Be careful that you do not overdo the first several times, for these muscles can get very sore with this movement.

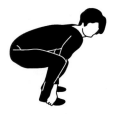

Hips-Thighs-Lower Back #9

Bent Over Squats

Start by squatting down, hands holding your feet (or if you are a stiff person, your ankles).

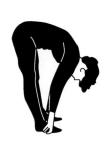

1—While holding your feet or ankles, straighten your legs so that your seat humps up above you. You should feel a good stretch as you straighten your legs.
2—Return to the starting position.
3 & 4—Repeat, straightening and bending the legs as you keep gripping your feet or ankles.

Continue for 5 to 10 repetitions.

> *Benefits:* This exercise does two things well—it develops the muscle endurance and strength of the quadricep muscles (front of the thigh), plus helps to stretch the muscles in the lower back and posterior leg. Be careful that you do not overstretch. The movement should be slow and methodical.

Major Bones, Muscles, and Arteries of the Human Body

Ulna
Radius
Cranium
Maxilla   Skull
Mandible

Phalanges
Metacarpals
Carpals

Clavical
and
Scapula
(pelvic girdle)

Sternum
Humerus
Ribs

Vertebral column

Cervical
vertebrae (7)

Thoracic
vertebrae (12)

Intervertebral disk
Radius
Ulna
Coxa
(hip bone)

Lumbar
vertebrae (5)

Sacrum
Coccyx

Femur

Patella

Tibia
Fibula

Tarsals
Metatarsals
Phalanges

☐ Axial skeleton   ☐ Appendicular skeleton

© Kendall/Hunt Publishing Company

B.1
Major Bones of Skeleton

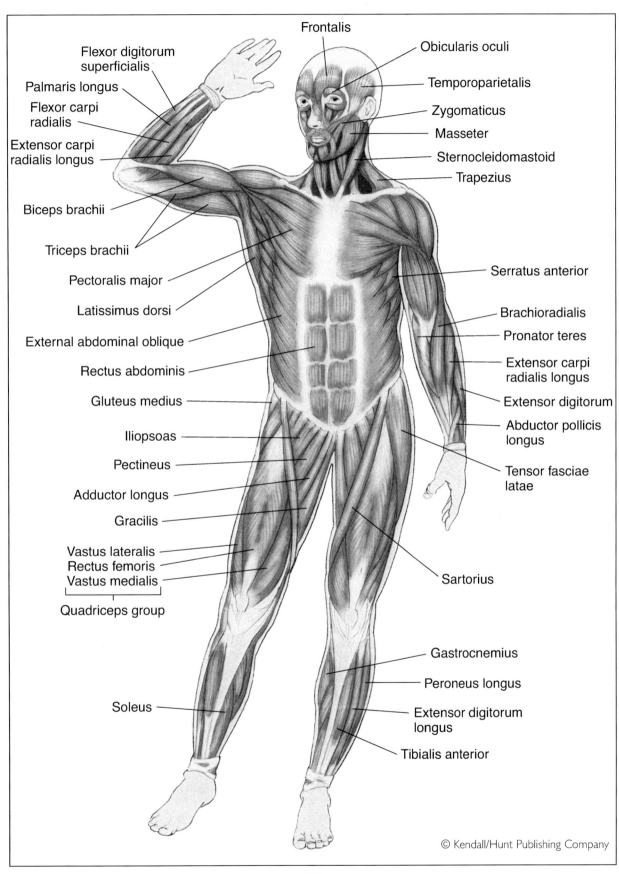

Flexor digitorum superficialis
Palmaris longus
Flexor carpi radialis
Extensor carpi radialis longus
Biceps brachii
Triceps brachii
Pectoralis major
Latissimus dorsi
External abdominal oblique
Rectus abdominis
Gluteus medius
Iliopsoas
Pectineus
Adductor longus
Gracilis
Vastus lateralis
Rectus femoris
Vastus medialis
Quadriceps group
Soleus

Frontalis
Obicularis oculi
Temporoparietalis
Zygomaticus
Masseter
Sternocleidomastoid
Trapezius
Serratus anterior
Brachioradialis
Pronator teres
Extensor carpi radialis longus
Extensor digitorum
Abductor pollicis longus
Tensor fasciae latae
Sartorius
Gastrocnemius
Peroneus longus
Extensor digitorum longus
Tibialis anterior

B.2
Major Muscles of Body (Anterior)

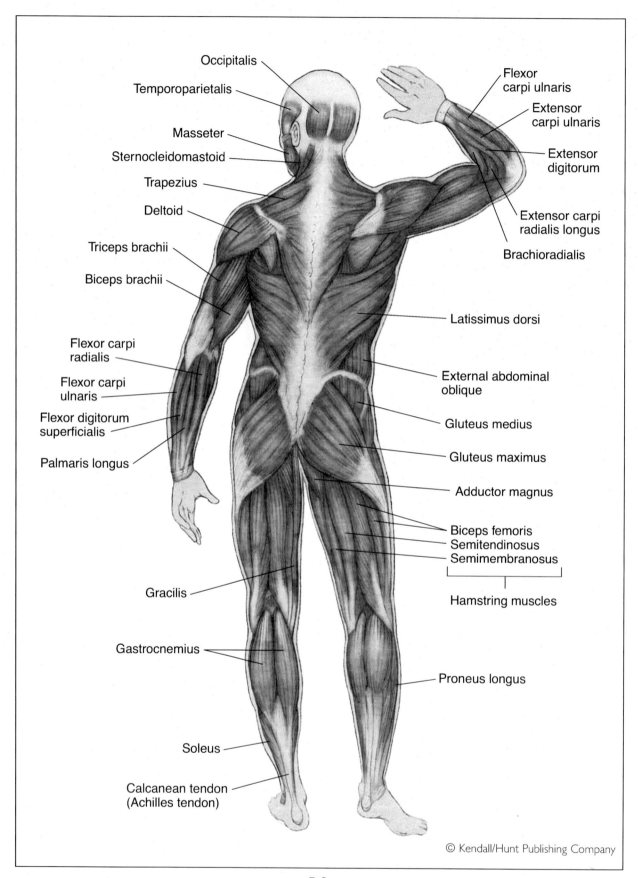

Occipitalis

Temporoparietalis

Masseter

Sternocleidomastoid

Trapezius

Deltoid

Triceps brachii

Biceps brachii

Flexor carpi radialis

Flexor carpi ulnaris

Flexor digitorum superficialis

Palmaris longus

Gracilis

Gastrocnemius

Soleus

Calcanean tendon (Achilles tendon)

Flexor carpi ulnaris

Extensor carpi ulnaris

Extensor digitorum

Extensor carpi radialis longus

Brachioradialis

Latissimus dorsi

External abdominal oblique

Gluteus medius

Gluteus maximus

Adductor magnus

Biceps femoris
Semitendinosus
Semimembranosus

Hamstring muscles

Proneus longus

© Kendall/Hunt Publishing Company

B.3
Major Muscles of Body (Posterior)

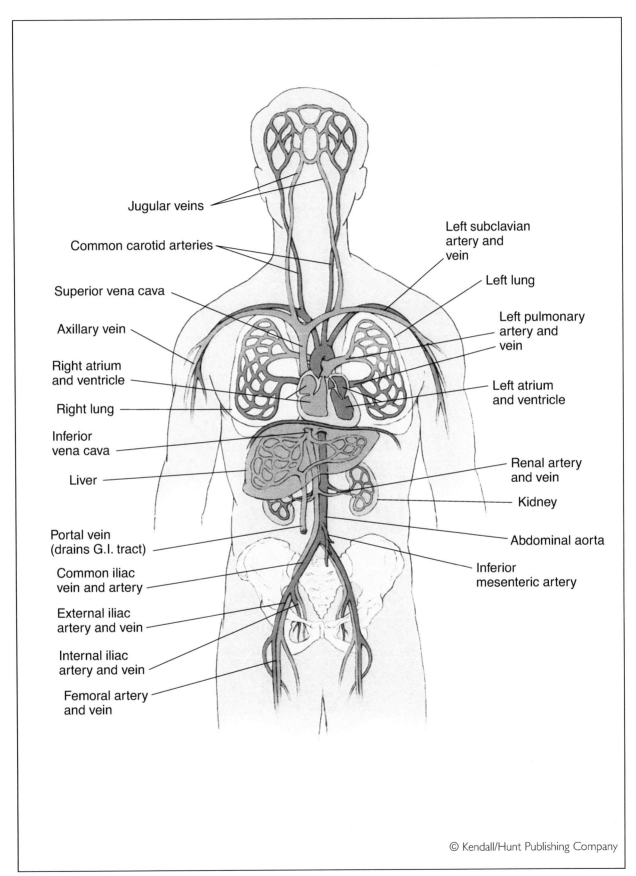

Jugular veins

Common carotid arteries

Superior vena cava

Axillary vein

Right atrium
and ventricle

Right lung

Inferior
vena cava

Liver

Portal vein
(drains G.I. tract)

Common iliac
vein and artery

External iliac
artery and vein

Internal iliac
artery and vein

Femoral artery
and vein

Left subclavian
artery and
vein

Left lung

Left pulmonary
artery and
vein

Left atrium
and ventricle

Renal artery
and vein

Kidney

Abdominal aorta

Inferior
mesenteric artery

© Kendall/Hunt Publishing Company

B.4
Major Arteries of Circulatory System

Glossary

A

Acclimatization The body's gradual adaptation to a changed environment, such as higher temperatures.

Acromegaly A chronic disease caused by excess production of growth hormone leading to elongation and enlargement of bones of the extremities and certain head bones.

Acute Sudden, short-term.

Acute muscle soreness Occurs during and immediately following the exercise. The muscular tension developed during the exercise reduces blood flow to the active muscles, causing lactic add and potassium to build up, stimulating pain receptors.

Adenosine triphosphate (ATP) Energy released from the separation of high energy phosphate bonds from is the immediate energy source for muscular contraction.

Adherence Sticking to something. Used to describe a person's continuation in an exercise program.

Adipose tissue Fat tissue.

Aerobic Using oxygen.

Aerobic activities Activities using large muscle groups at moderate intensities that permit the body to use oxygen to supply energy and to maintain a steady state for more than a few minutes.

Aerobic dance The original aerobic dance programs consisted of an eclectic combination of various dance forms including ballet, modern jazz, disco, and folk, as well as calisthenic-type exercises. More recent innovations include water aerobics (done in a swimming pool), non-impact or low-impact aerobics (one foot on the ground at all times), specific dance aerobics, and "assisted" aerobics whereby weights are worn on the wrists and/or ankles.

Aerobic power See maximal oxygen uptake.

Agility Relates to the ability to rapidly change the position of the entire body in space, with speed and accuracy.

Aging Refers to the normal yet irreversible biological changes that occur during the total years that a person lives.

Alcohol dependent Dependency on alcohol that leads to negative consequences such as arrest, accident, or impairment of health or job performance.

Alcoholism Alcoholism is a chronic, progressive, and potentially fatal disease. It is characterized by tolerance (brain adaptation to the presence of alcohol) and physical dependency (withdrawal symptoms occur when consumption of alcohol is decreased). Alcohol-related problems may include symptoms of alcohol dependence such as memory loss, inability to stop drinking until intoxicated, inability to cut down on drinking, binge drinking, and withdrawal symptoms.

Alveoli Air sacs of the lung.

Alzheimer's disease This disease progresses from short-term memory loss to a final stage requiring total care. It is a form of senile dementia, associated with atrophy of parts of the brain.

Amino acid An organic compound that makes up protein. Twenty amino acids are necessary for metabolism and growth, but only 11 are "essential" in that they must be provided from the food eaten. Some proteins contain all safe and adequate dietary intake is 0.05–0.20 mg per day. Peanuts, probes, oils, various vegetables, whole wheat bread, and chicken are good sources of chromium.

Amenorrhea Absence of menstruation.

Anabolic The building up of a body substance.

Anabolic steroids A group of synthetic, testosterone-like hormones that promote anabolism, including muscle hypertrophy. Their use in athletics is considered unethical and carries numerous serious health risks.

Anaerobic Not using oxygen.

Anaerobic activities Activities using muscle groups at high intensities that exceed the body's capacity to use oxygen to supply energy and which create an oxygen debt by using energy produced without oxygen. See oxygen debt.

Anaerobic threshold The point at which blood lactate concentrations start to rise above resting values. The anaerobic threshold can be expressed as a percent of VO_{2max}.

Androgenic Causing masculinization.

Android A type of obesity is characterized by the predominance of body fat in the upper half of the body.

Anemia Low hemoglobin concentration in the blood.

Aneurysm   Localized abnormal dilatation of a blood vessel due to weakness of the wall.

Angina   A gripping, choking or suffocating pain in the chest (angina pectoris) caused most often by insufficient flow of oxygen to the heart muscle during exercise or excitement.

Anorexia   Lack of appetite. Anorexia nervosa is a psychological and physiological condition characterized by inability or refusal to eat, leading to severe weight loss, malnutrition, hormone imbalances and other potentially life-threatening biological changes.

Anthropometry   The science dealing with the measurement (size, weight, proportions) of the human body.

Anticipatory response   Prior to exercise, heart rates can rise due to anticipation of the exercise bout.

Apoprotein   The protein part of the lipoprotein. They are important in activating or inhibiting certain enzymes involved in the metabolism of fats.

Aquasize   Aerobic dance in the water.

Arrhythmia   Any abnormal rate or rhythm of the heart beat.

Arteriosclerosis   Commonly called hardening of the arteries, this includes a variety of conditions that cause the artery walls to thicken and lose elasticity.

Arteriovenous oxygen difference ($\bar{a} - \bar{v}O_2$ difference)   The difference between the oxygen content of arterial and venous blood.

Artery   Vessel which carries blood away from the heart to the tissues of the body.

Asthma   A disease characterized by wheezing caused by a spasm of the bronchial tubes or by swelling of their mucous membranes.

Atherosclerosis   A very common form of arteriosclerosis, in which the arteries are narrowed by deposits of cholesterol and other material in the inner walls of the artery.

Atrioventricular (AV) Node   A small mass of specialized conducting tissue at the bottom of the right atrium through which the electrical impulse stimulating the heart to contract must pass to reach the ventricles.

Auscultation   Process of listening for sounds within the body with the stethoscope.

B

Balance   Relates to the maintenance of equilibrium while stationary or moving.

Ballistic movement   An flexibility exercise movement in which a part of the body is sharply moved against the resistance of antagonist muscles or against the limits of a joint.

Basal metabolic rate   The minimum energy required to maintain the body's life functions at rest. Usually expressed in calories per day.

Bee pollen   A substance gleaned from honey that is claimed by some to have unusual nutritional qualities enhancing performance. Double blind placebo studies do not support this claim.

Behavior modification   Behavior modification considers in great detail the eating behavior to be changed, events which trigger the eating, and its consequences.

Binge eating   The consumption of large quantities of rich foods within short periods of time.

Blood doping   An ergogenic procedure wherein an athlete's own blood or transfusion of type matched donor's blood is infused to enhance endurance performance.

Blood pressure   The pressure exerted by the blood on the wall of the arteries. Measures are in millimeters of mercury (as 120/80 mm Hg).

Bodybuilding   A unique activity in which competitors work to develop the mass, definition, and symmetry of their muscles, rather than the strength, skill, or endurance required for more common athletic events.

Body composition   The proportions of fat, muscle and bone making up the body. Usually expressed as percent of body fat and percent of lean body mass.

Body density   The specific gravity of the body, which can be tested by underwater weighing. Compares the weight of the body to the weight of the same volume of water. Result can be used to estimate the percentage of body fat.

Body mass index (BMI)   Body weight and height indices for determining degree of obesity.

Bradycardia   Slow heart beat of less than 60 beats per minute at rest.

Branched chain amino acids   Valine, isoleucine, leucine.

BTPS   The volume of air at the temperature and pressure of the body, and 100 percent saturated with water vapor.

Bundle of His   A bundle of fibers of the impulse-conducting system of the heart. From its origin in the A = V node it enters the interventricular septum where it divides into two branches (bundle branches) whose fibers pass to the right and left ventricles, becoming continuous with the Purkinje fibers of the ventricles.

C

Caffeine   A methylxanthine found in many plants. Caffeine has unpredictable effects on endurance performance, but may increase muscle utilization of free fatty acids, sparing muscle glycogen stores.

Calisthenics   A system of exercise movements, without equipment, for the building of muscular strength and endurance, and flexibility. The Greeks formed the word from "kalos" (beautiful) and "sthenos" (strength).

Caloric cost   The number of Calories burned to produce the energy for a task. Usually measured in Calories (kilocalories) per minute.

Calorie   The Calorie used as a unit of metabolism (as in diet and energy expenditure) equals 1,000 small calories, and is often spelled with a capital C to make that distinction. It is the energy required to raise the temperature of one kilogram of water one degree Celsius. Also called a kilocalorie (kcal).

Cancer   A large group of diseases characterized by uncontrolled growth and spread of abnormal cells.

Carbohydrate   Chemical compound of carbon, oxygen and hydrogen, usually with the hydrogen and oxygen in the right proportions to form water. Common forms are starches, sugars, and dietary fibers.

Carbohydrate loading   A dietary scheme emphasizing high amounts of carbohydrate to increase muscle glycogen stores before long endurance events.

Carbon dioxide   A colorless, odorless gas that is formed in the tissues by the oxidation of carbon, and is eliminated by the lungs.

Carbon monoxide   Produced mainly during combustion of fossil fuels such as coal and gasoline. Carbon monoxide is a tasteless, odorless, colorless gas.

Cardiac output   The volume of blood pumped out by the heart in a given unit of time. It equals the stroke volume times the heart rate.

Cardiac rehabilitation   A program to prepare cardiac patients to return to productive lives with a reduced risk of recurring health problems.

Cardiopulmonary resuscitation (CPR)   A first-aid method to restore breathing and heart action through mouth-to-mouth breathing and rhythmic chest compressions. CPR instruction is offered by local American Heart Association and American Red Cross units, and is a minimum requirement for most fitness instruction certifications.

Cardiorespiratory endurance   The same as aerobic endurance. Can be defined as the ability to continue or persist in strenuous tasks involving large muscle groups for extended periods of time. It is the ability of the circulatory and respiratory systems to adjust to and recover from the effects of whole-body exercise or work.

Cardiovascular   Pertaining to the heart and blood vessels.

Carotid artery   The principal artery in both sides of the neck. A convenient place to detect a pulse.

Catecholamine   Epinephrine and norepinephrine hormones.

Celluilte   A commercially created name for lumpy fat deposits. Actually this fat behaves no differently from other fat; it is just straining against irregular bands of connective tissue.

Cerebral thrombosis   Clot that forms inside the cerebral artery.

Cholesterol   An alcohol steroid found in animal fats. This pearly, fat-like substance is implicated in the narrowing of the arteries in atherosclerosis. All Americans are being urged to decrease their serum cholesterol levels to less than 200 mg/dl.

Chronic   Continuing over time.

Chronic diseases   Lifestyle related diseases, such as heart disease, cancer, and stroke, and also accidents, which together account for 75 percent of all deaths in America.

Circuit training   A series of exercises, performed one after the other, with little rest between.

Circuit weight training programs   Involve 8–12 repetitions with various weight machines at 7 to 14 stations, while moving quickly from one station to the next.

Citric acid cycle   See Krebs cycle.

Collateral circulation   Blood circulation through small side branches that can supplement (or substitute for) the main vessel's delivery of blood to certain tissues.

Compliance   Staying with a prescribed exercise program.

Concentric action   Muscle action in which the muscle is shortening under its own power. This action is commonly called "positive" work, or, redundantly, "concentric contraction."

Contraindication   Any condition which indicates that a particular course of action (or exercise) would be inadvisable.

Cool down   A gradual reduction of the intensity of exercise to allow physiological processes to return to normal. Also called warm-down.

Continuous passive motion (CPM)   Motorized machines that continuously move isolated muscle groups through their range of motion without requiring any effort by the user.

Coordination Relates to the ability to use the senses, such as sight and hearing, together with body parts in performing motor tasks smoothly and accurately.

Coronary arteries The arteries, circling the heart like a crown, that supply blood to the heart muscle. There are three major branches.

Coronary heart disease (CHD) Atherosclerosis of the coronary arteries.

Cortical bone Compact outer shaft bone.

Creatine phosphokinase (CPK) A muscle enzyme that can rise dramatically in the blood after unaccustomed exercise, indicating considerable muscle cell damage.

Cross-sectional study A study made at one point in time.

Cryokinetics A treatment that alternates cold and exercise for rehabilitation of traumatic musculoskeletal injuries in athletes.

D

Dehydration The condition resulting from the excessive loss of body water.

Delayed-onset muscle soreness (DOMS) Occurs from 1 to 5 days following unaccustomed or severe exercise, and involves actual damage to the muscle cell.

Detraining The process of losing the benefits of training by returning to a sedentary life.

Diastolic blood pressure The blood pressure when the heart is resting between beats.

DHEA This unapproved drug (dehydroepiandrosterone or dehydroandrosterone) is derived from human urine and other sources. Manufacturers tout DHEA as a "natural" weight-loss product, but this has not been substantiated.

Diabetes Mellitus A group of disorders that share glucose intolerance (high serum levels of glucose) in common. There are two common types: Type I, Insulin-Dependent Diabetes Mellitus (IDDM), and Type II, Non-Insulin-Dependent Diabetes Mellitus (IDUM). IDDM can occur at any age, but especially in the young, and is characterized by an abrupt onset of symptoms, and a need for insulin to sustain life. NIDDM is most common, usually occurring in people who are obese and over age 40.

Dietary fiber Complex plant cell wall materials that cannot be digested by the enzymes in the human small intestine. Examples from plants include cellulose, hemicellulose, pectin, mucilages, and lignin.

Diuretic Any agent which increases the flow of urine, ridding the body of water.

Drug dependence Criteria are: highly controlled or compulsive use, psychoactive effects, and drug-reinforced behavior.

Dry-bulb thermometer An ordinary instrument for indication temperature. Does not take into account humidity and other factors that combine to determine the heat stress experienced by the body.

Duration The time spent in a single exercise session. Duration, along with frequency and intensity, are factors called the F.I.T. which are related to improvement of cardiorespiratory endurance.

Dynamometer A device for measuring force. Common dynamometers include devices to test hand strength, and leg and back strength.

Dyspnea Difficult or labored breathing.

E

Eccentric action Muscle action in which the muscle resists while it is forced to lengthen. This action is commonly called "negative" work, or "eccentric contraction," but, since the muscle is lengthening, the word "contraction" is misapplied.

Economy Refers to ease of administration, the use of inexpensive equipment, the need for little time, and the simplicity of the test so that the person taking it can easily understand the purpose and results.

Ectomorphic A lean, thin, and linear body type.

Efficiency The ratio of energy consumed to the work accomplished.

EKG lead A pair of electrodes placed on the body and connected to an EKG recorder.

Elderly Individuals who reach of pass the age of 65. This group of Americans now represents the fastest growing minority in the United States.

Electrical muscle stimulators (EMS) EMS devices give a painless electrical stimulation to the muscle. Manufacturers claim that muscles are toned without exercise. Other benefits include face lifts without surgery, slimming and trimming, weight loss, bust development, spot reducing, and removal of cellulite. The Food and Drug Administration considers claims for EMS devices promoted for such purposes to be misbranded and fraudulent.

Electrolyte Scientists call minerals like sodium, chloride, and potassium "electrolytes" because in water they can conduct electrical currents. Sodium and potassium ions carry positive charges while chloride ions are negatively charged.

Electron transport system An additional metabolic pathway from which the products of Krebs cycle enter and yield ATP. This cycle requires oxygen.

Electrocardiogram (EKG, ECG) A graph of the electrical activity caused by the stimulation of the heart muscle. The millivolts of electricity are detected by electrodes on the body surface and recorded by an electrocardiograph.

Embolus A blood clot that breaks loose and travels to smaller arterial vessels where it may lodge and block the blood flow.

Endurance The capacity to continue a physical performance over a period of time.

Enzyme Complex proteins that induce and accelerate the speed of chemical reactions without being changed themselves. Enzymes are present in digestive juices, where they act on food substances, causing them to break down into simpler molecules.

Epidemiological studies Statistical study of the relationships between various factors that determine the frequency and distribution of disease in human populations.

Epinephrine A hormone primarily excreted from the adrenal medulla. This hormone is also called a catecholamine, and is involved in many important body functions, including the elevation of blood glucose levels during exercise or stress.

Ergogenic aids A physical, mechanical, nutritional, psychological, or pharmacological substance or treatment that either directly improves physiological variables associated with exercise performance or removes subjective restrains which may limit physiological capacity.

Ergometer A device that can measure work consistently and reliably. Stationary exercise cycles were the first widely available devices equipped with ergometers.

Estrogen replacement One of the major mainstays of prevention and management of osteoporosis is estrogen replacement. Women who are past menopause, and who are at high risk for osteoporosis, are often given estrogen replacements by physicians, and is highly effective.

Ethyl alcohol (ethanol) Grain alcohol. Ethyl alcohol is a social drug that is called a "sedative-hypnotic" because of its dramatic effects on the brain. Ethanol (CH_3CH_2OH) is a small water soluble molecule that is absorbed rapidly and completely from the stomach and small intestine.

Exercise Physical exertion of sufficient intensity, duration and frequency to achieve or maintain fitness, or other health or athletic, objectives.

Exercise-Induced Bronchospasm (EIB) EIB is defined as a diffuse bronchospastic response in both large and small airways following heavy exercise. Postexercise symptoms include difficulty in breathing, coughing, shortness of breath, and wheezing.

Exercise oxygen economy The oxygen cost of exercise, usually expressed as VO_2 at a certain running or exercise pace.

Exercise prescription A recommendation for a course of exercise to meet desirable individual objectives for fitness. Includes activity types; duration, intensity, and frequency of exercise.

Exercise program director Certification as exercise program director by the American College of Sports Medicine indicates the competency to design, implement and administer preventive and rehabilitative exercise programs, to educate staff in conducting tests and leading physical activity and to educate the community about such programs. Must have all the competencies of the certified fitness instructor, exercise test technologist and exercise specialist.

Exercise specialist A person certified by the American College of Sports Medicine as having the competency and skill to supervise preventive and rehabilitative exercise programs and prescribe activities for patients. Must also pass the ACSM standards for Exercise Test Technologist.

Exercise technologist A person certified by the American College of Sports Medicine as competent to administer graded exercise tests, calculate the data and implement any needed emergency procedures. Must have current CPR certification.

Expiratory reserve volume (ERV) The amount of air that can be pushed out of the lung following an expired resting tidal volume.

Extension A movement which moves the two ends of a jointed body part away from each other, as in straightening the arm.

Extensor A muscle that extends a jointed body part.

Extracellular Outside of the body cell.

F

Fartlek training Similar to interval training. Is a free form of training done out on trails or roads.

Fast-twitch fibers   Muscle fiber type that contracts quickly and is used most in intensive, short-duration exercises, such as weightlifting or sprints. Also called Type II fibers.

Fats   Fats serve as a source of energy. In food, the fat molecule is formed from one molecule of glycerol and is combined with three of fatty acids. Fats have a high caloric value yielding about 9 Calories per gram as compared with 4 Calories for carbohydrate and proteins. Saturated fats have no double bonds, are generally hard at room temperature, and have been associated with increased risk of heart disease.

Monounsaturated fats and polyunsaturated fats have one and two double bonds respectively, are generally liquid at room temperature, and have been associated with decreased risk of heart disease.

Fat cell theory   One of the many theories explaining obesity. Fat cell number can increase two to three times normal if an individual ingests too many Calories. And once formed, the extra fat cells cannot be removed by the body. This can happen anytime during the life-span of an individual, but appears to be particularly important during infancy when fat cells are still dividing.

Fat-free weight   Lean body mass or bone, muscle, and water.

Fatigue   A loss of power to continue a given level of physical performance.

Fitness   See physical fitness.

Fitness instructor   A person who directs classes or individuals in the performance of exercise. Certification by the American College of Sports Medicine indicates the competency to identify risk factors, conduct submaximal exercise tests, recommend exercise programs, lead classes and counsel with exercisers. Works with persons without known disease. CPR certification is required.

Flexibility   The range of motion around a joint.

Flexion   A movement which moves the two ends of a jointed body part closer to each other, as in bending the arm.

Food supplements   Food supplements are substances or pills that are added to the diet. Most reputable nutritionists state that vitamin or mineral supplementation is unwarranted for people eating a balanced diet.

Forced vital capacity (FVC)   The total amount of air that can be breathed into the lung on top of the residual volume.

Frame size   Elbow breadth measurement for determination of small, medium, or large skeletal mass.

Frequency   How often a person repeats a complete exercise session (e.g., 3 times per week). Frequency, along with duration and intensity affect the cardiorespiratory response to exercise.

Functional capacity   See maximal oxygen uptake.

Functional residual capacity (FRC)   The combined expiratory reserve volume and residual volume.

G

Gastric stapling   Surgery to radically reduce the volume of the stomach to less than 50 ml.

Genetic factors   One of the several theories advanced to explain the high prevalence of obesity in Western countries. Some studies have demonstrated that certain people are more prone to obesity than others due to genetic factors. Such people have to be unusually careful in their dietary and exercise habits to counteract these inherited tendencies.

Gluconeogenesis   The formation of glucose and glycogen from noncarbohydrate sources such as amino acids, glycerol, and lactate.

Glucose   Blood sugar. The transportable form of carbohydrate, which reaches the cells.

Glucose polymers   Four to six glucose units produced by partial breakdown of corn starch.

Glycogen   The storage form of carbohydrate. Glycogen is used in the muscles for the production of energy.

Glucagon   A hormone that is secreted by the pancreas, and helps to raise blood glucose levels by stimulating the breakdown of liver glycogen.

Glycolysis   A metabolic pathway that converts glucose to lactic acid to produce energy in the form of ATP.

Glycosuria   Glucose in the urine.

Golgi tendon organ   Organs at the junction of muscle and tendon that send inhibitory impulses to the muscle when the muscle's contraction reaches certain levels. The purpose may be to protect against separating the tendon from bone when a contraction is too great.

Graded exercise test (GXT)   A treadmill, or cycle-ergometer test with the workload gradually increased until exhaustion or a predetermined endpoint.

Grapefruit pills   For several decades, grapefruit has been promoted by various people as having special fat burning properties. This myth has been spread far and wide. Grapefruit pills contain grapefruit extract, diuretics, and bulk-forming agents. Some contain phenyl-propanolamine (PPA), along with herbs or other ingredients.

Growth hormone   A hormone released from the pituitary that elevates blood glucose. As its name indicates, this hormone also helps in the regulation of growth.

Growth hormone releasers   Various products such as Lipogene-GH, Nite Diet, Dream Away, Nite Time Diet, and HGH-3X are all sold with the claim that if they are taken before retiring, weight loss will occur overnight due to the increased release of growth hormone from the amino acids arginine and ornithine contained in the products. This is an erroneous concept.

Gynold   A form of obesity is characterized by excess body fat in the lower half of the body, especially the hips, buttocks, and thighs.

H

Haptoglobin   A mucoprotein to which hemoglobin released into plasma is bound. It is increased in certain Inflammatory conditions, and decreased during hemolysis.

HDL-C/TC   The ratio of HDL-C to total cholesterol, which has been found to be highly predictive of heart disease.

Health   The World Health Organization has defined health as a state of complete physical, mental, and social well-being, and not merely the absence of disease.

Health fraud   Defined as the promotion, for financial gain, of fraudulent or unproven devices, treatments, services, plans or products (including; but not limited to, diets and nutritional supplements) that alter or claim to alter the human condition.

Health promotion   The science and art of helping people change their lifestyle to move toward optimal health.

Health-related Fitness   Elements of fitness such as cardiorespiratory fitness, muscular strength and endurance, flexibility, and body composition that are related to improvement of health.

Heart attack   Also called myocardial infarction. Often occurs when a clot blocks an atherosclerotic coronary blood vessel.

Heart rate   Number of heart beats per minute.

Heart rate reserve   The difference between the resting heart rate and the maximal heart rate.

Heat cramps   Muscle twitching or painful cramping, usually following heavy exercise with profuse sweating. The legs, arms and abdominal muscles are the most often affected.

Heat exhaustion   Caused by dehydration. Symptoms include a dry mouth, excessive thirst, loss of coordination, dizziness, headaches, paleness, shakiness and cool and clammy skin.

Heatstroke   A life-threatening illness when the body's temperature-regulating mechanisms fail. Body temperature may rise to over 104 degrees F, skin appears red, dry and warm to the touch. The victim has chills, sometimes nausea and dizziness, and may be confused or irrational. Seizures and coma may follow unless temperature is brought down to 102 degrees within an hour.

Hegsted formula   A formula to predict change in serum cholesterol from saturated fats (S) and polyunsaturated fats (P) and cholesterol in the diet. Change in serum cholesterol = (2.16 × change in S) – (1.65 × change in P) + (0.097 × change in dietary cholesterol).

Hematocrit   Expressed as the percentage of total blood volume which consists of red blood cells and other solids.

Heme iron   Forty percent of the iron in animal products is called heme iron. The remaining 60 percent of the iron in animal products and all the iron in vegetable products are called non-heme iron. Heme iron is more easily absorbed by the body.

Hemoconcentration   Increase in the thickness of blood due to loss of plasma volume.

Hemorrhage   Abnormal internal or external discharge of blood.

Hemoglobin   The iron-containing pigment of the red blood cells. Its function is to carry oxygen from the lungs to the tissues. Low levels of hemoglobin is called anemia.

Hemolysis   Breakdown of red blood cells, with liberation of hemoglobin, and loss through the kidneys.

Hepatic lipase (HL)   An enzyme of the liver that removes HDL from circulation.

Herbalife   Herbalife sells items described as "herbal-based" health, nutrition, weight-control, and skin-care products, marketing them through a multilevel program. Herbalife International has been sued for misrepresentation.

High blood pressure   See hypertension.

High density lipoprotein cholesterol (HDL-C)   Cholesterol is carried by the high density lipoprotein to the liver. The liver then uses the cholesterol to form bile acids which are finally excreted in the stool. Thus high levels of HDL-C have been associated with low cardiovascular disease risk.

Homeostasis   State of equilibrium of the internal environment of the body.

Hormone   A substance secreted from an organ or gland which is transported by the blood to another part of the body.

Human growth hormone   Hormone which is liberated by the anterior pituitary and is important for regulating growth.

Hypercholesterolemia   High blood cholesterol levels.

Hypertension   A condition in which the blood pressure is chronically elevated above optimal levels. The diagnosis of hypertension in adults is confirmed when the average of two or more diastolic measurements on at least two separate visits is 90 mm Hg or higher. If the diastolic blood pressure is below 90 mm Hg, systolic hypertension is diagnosed when the average of multiple systolic blood pressure measurements on two or more separate visits is consistently greater than 140 mm Hg.

Hyperglycemia   Excessive levels of glucose in the blood.

Hyperplastic obesity   A high number of fat cells, two to three times normal.

Hyperthermia   Body temperatures exceeding normal.

Hypertonic   Describes a solution concentrated enough to draw water out of body cells.

Hypertriglyceridemia   High blood triglyceride levels.

Hypertrophy   An enlargement of a muscle by the increase in size of the cells.

Hypochromic   Condition of the red blond cell in which they have a reduced hemoglobin content.

Hypoglycemia   Blood sugar levels below 50 mg/dl accompanied by symptoms of dizziness, nausea, trembling, irritation, etc.

Hyponatremia   Low sodium levels in the blood stream which can be caused by excessive sweating and inadequate electrolyte replacement during ultramarathons.

Hypothalamus   A portion of the brain lying below the thalamus. Secretions from the hypothalamus are important in the control of important body functions, including the regulation of water balance, appetite, and body temperature.

Hypothermia   Body temperature below normal. Usually due to exposure to cold temperatures, especially after exhausting ready energy supplies.

Hypotonic   Describes a solution dilute enough to allow its water to be absorbed by body cells.

Hypoxia   Insufficient oxygen flow to the tissues.

I

IDEA   The International Dance-Exercise Association.

Iliac crest   The upper, wide portion of the hip bone.

Impaired glucose tolerance   Borderline hyperglycemia (between 115 and 140 mg/dl.

Indirect calorimetry   Measurement of energy expenditure by analysis of expired air.

Infarction   Death of a section of tissue from the obstruction of blood flow (ischemia) to the area.

Informed consent   A procedure for obtaining a client's signed consent to a fitness center's testing and exercise program. Includes a description of the objectives and procedures, with associated benefits and risks, stated in plain language, with a consent statement and signature line in a single document.

Inspiration   Breathing air into the lungs.

Inspiratory reserve volume (IRV)   The amount of air that can be breathed into the lung on top of a resting inspired tidal volume.

Insulin   A hormone secreted by special cells (beta cells) in the pancreas. Insulin is essential for the maintenance of blood glucose levels.

Insulin-Dependent Diabetes Mellitus (IDDM)   The form of diabetes mellitus in which the pancreas does not make or secrete insulin. The patient must use an external source of insulin to sustain life. This type of diabetes mellitus is also called Type I or juvenile-onset diabetes.

Intima   The inner layer of arteries.

Intracellular   Inside the cell.

Intensity   The level of exertion during exercise. Intensity, along with duration and frequency, are important for improving the cardiorespiratory endurance.

Interval training   An exercise session in which the intensity and duration of exercise are consciously alternated between harder and easier work. Often used to improve aerobic capacity and/or anaerobic endurance in exercisers who already have a base of endurance in training.

Iron deficiency   Iron deficiency is the most common single nutritional deficiency in the world today and is characterized by low iron stores in the body. Severe iron deficiency or anemia is characterized by low blood hemoglobin.

Iron deficient erythropoiesis   Stage 2 of iron deficiency, following the exhaustion of bone marrow iron stores, and characterized by a diminishing iron supply to the developing red cell. Iron deficient erythropoiesis (formation of red blood cells) occurs and is measured by increased total iron binding capacity and reduced serum iron and percent saturation (<16 percent is abnormal).

Ischemia   Inadequate blood flow to a body part, caused by constriction or obstruction of a blood vessel, leading to insufficient oxygen supply.

Isokinetic contraction   A muscle contraction against a resistance that moves at a constant velocity, so that the maximum force of which the muscle is capable throughout the range of motion may be applied.

Isometric action   Muscle action in which the muscle attempts to contract against an immovable object. This is sometimes called "isometric contraction," although there is not appreciable shortening of the muscle.

Isotonic contraction   A muscle contraction against a constant resistance, as in lifting a weight.

K

Karvonen formula   A method to calculate the training heart rate using a percentage of the "heart rate reserve" which is the difference between the maximum and resting heart rates.

Ketosis   An elevated level of ketone bodies in the tissues. Seen in sufferers of starvation or diabetes, and a symptom brought about in dieters on very low carbohydrate diets.

Kilocalorie (kcal)   A measure of the heat required to raise the temperature of one kilogram of water one degree Celsius. A large Calorie, used in diet and metabolism measures, that equals 1,000 small calories.

Kilogram (kg)   A unit of weight equal to 2.204623 pounds; 1,000 grams (g).

Kilogram-meters (kgm)   The amount of work required to lift one kilogram one meter.

Kilopond-meters (kpm)   Equivalent to kilogrammeters, in normal gravity.

Korotkoff sounds   Blood pressure sounds.

Krebs cycle   Final common metabolic pathway for fats, proteins, and carbohydrates that yields additional ATP. Carbon dioxide and water are produced.

L

L-Carnitine   An amine responsible for transporting fatty acids into the mitochondria for oxidation. Some have urged that L-carnitine supplements may increase the amount of fatty acid oxidation during exercise, sparing the glycogen. However, L-carnitine supplements have never been shown in reputable, double-blind, controlled studies to improve the athletic

performance of a healthy individual.

Lactate   Lactic acid.

Lactate dehydrogenase (LDH)   A muscle enzyme that can leak out of ruptured muscle cells into the blood.

Lactic acid   The end product of the metabolism of glucose (glycolysis) for the anaerobic production of energy.

Lactate system   Exercise of 1 to 3 minutes duration depends on the lactate system or anaerobic glycolysis for ATP.

Late-onset (PEL) hypoglycemia   Typically, PEL hypoglycemia happens during the night and occurs 6–15 hours after the completion of unusually strenuous exercise or play in diabetics.

Law of diminishing returns   There appears to be a certain amount of training that most humans will respond quickly and fruitfully to. But every step beyond that level brings less return for the time and effort invested.

Lean body weight   The weight of the body, less the weight of its fat.

Lecithin: cholesterol acyltransferase (LCAT)   An enzyme from the liver that "matures" the incomplete HDL's by connecting fatty acids to the free cholesterol in the HDL particle. The incomplete HDL (HDL_3) swells into a mature sphere (HDL_3). The LCAT enzyme then grabs more cholesterol from the tissues and other circulating lipoproteins to form even bigger HDL particles (HDL_2).

Life expectancy   The average number of years of life expected in a population at a specific age, usually at birth.

Life-span   The maximal obtainable age by a particular member of the species, which is primarily related to one's genetic makeup.

Lipid   A general term used for several different compounds which include both solid fats and liquid oils. There are three major classes of lipids: triglycerides, phospholipids, and sterols.

Lipid Research Center Program (LRCP)   A study providing information on food and nutrient intake and blood lipid profiles of Americans. The LRCP is a program of the National Health, Lung, and Blood Institute (NHLBI) of the National Institutes of Health (NIH).

Lipoprotein   A soluble aggregate of cholesterol, phospholipids, triglycerides, and protein. This package allows for easy transport through the blood. There are four types of lipoproteins: chylomicrons, low density lipoprotein (LDL), very low density lipoprotein (VLDL), and high density lipoprotein (HDL).

Lipoprotein lipase (LPL)   An enzyme that breaks down VLDL, providing fatty adds for the muscle or adipose tissue.

Longitudinal study   A study which observes the same subjects over a period of time.

Lordosis   Forward pelvis tilt, often caused from weak abdominals and inflexible posterior thigh muscles allow the pelvis to tilt forward, causing curvature in the lower back.

Low Density Lipoprotein (LDL)   Transports cholesterol from the liver to other body cells. LDL is often referred to as "bad" cholesterol because it may be taken up by muscle cells in arteries and it has been implicated in the development of atherosclerosis.

Low back pain (LBP)   Pain in the lower back often caused from weak abdominal muscles and tight lower back and hamstring muscles.

Low-impact aerobics   At least one foot is touching the floor throughout the aerobic portion.

Lumen   Inside opening of artery.

Lung diffusion   The rate at which gases diffuse from the lung air sacs to the blood in the pulmonary capillaries.

M

Mason-Likar   The 12-lead exercise EKG system.

Maximal anaerobic power   Anaerobic power is the ability to exercise for a short time period at high power levels, and is important for various sports where sprinting and power movements are common.

Maximal heart rate   The highest heart rate of which an individual is capable. A broad rule of thumb for estimating maximal heart rate is 220 (beats per minute) minus the person's age (in years).

Maximal oxygen uptake   The highest rate of oxygen consumption of which a person is capable. Usually expressed in milliliters of oxygen per kilogram of body weight per minute. Also called maximal aerobic power, maximal oxygen consumption, maximal oxygen intake.

Mean arterial pressure   Equals 1/3 (systolic blood pressure diastolic blood pressure) + diastolic blood pressure.

Mean corpuscular volume   Stage 3 iron deficient anemia is characterized by a drop in hemoglobin. The bone marrow produces an increasing number of smaller and less brightly red colored red blood cells. This is measured when the mean corpuscular volume (MCV) falls below 80 fl.

Media   Middle layer of muscle in artery wall.

Medical history   A list of a person's previous illnesses, present conditions, symptoms, medications and health risk factors. Used to help classify an individual as apparently healthy, at risk for disease, or with known disease.

Mesomorphic   An athletic, muscular body type.

Met   A measure of energy output equal to the basal metabolic rate of a resting subject. Assumed to be equal to an oxygen uptake of 3.5 milliliters per kilogram of body weight per minute, or approximately 1 kilocalorie per kilogram of body weight per hour.

Microcytic   A small red blood cell.

Mild obesity   Defined as being 20 percent to 40 percent overweight.

Mineral   Of the nearly 45 dietary nutrients known to be necessary for human life, 17 are minerals. Although mineral elements represent only a very small fraction of human body weight, they play very important roles throughout the body. They help form hard tissues such as bones and teeth, aid in normal muscle and nerve activity, act as catalysts in many enzyme systems, help control your body water levels, and are integral parts of organic compounds in the body like hemoglobin and the hormone thyroxine. Evidence is growing that certain minerals are related to prevention of disease and proper immune system function.

Minute ventilation   The volume of air that is breathed into the body each minute.

Mitochondria   The slender filament or rod inside of cells that are the source of energy. Enzymes important to producing energy from fat and carbohydrates are found inside the mitochondria.

Mode   Type of exercise.

Moderate obesity   Defined as being 40 percent to 100 percent overweight.

Monosaccharides   The simplest carbohydrate containing only one molecule of sugar. Glucose, fructose, and galactose and the primary monosaccharides.

Monounsaturated fatty acids   (See fats).

Motor neuron   A nerve cell which conducts impulses from the central nervous system to a group of muscle fibers to produce movement.

Motor unit   A motor neuron and the muscle fibers activated by it.

Muscle glycogen supercompensation   The practice of exercising tapering combined with a high carbohydrate diet that stores very high levels of glycogen in the muscles before long endurance events.

Muscle spindle Organ in a muscle that senses changes in muscle length, especially stretches. Rapid stretching of the muscle results in messages being sent to the nervous system to contract the muscle, thereby limiting the stretch.

Muscular endurance Defined as the ability of the muscles to apply a submaximal force repeatedly or to sustain a muscular contraction for a certain period of time.

Musculoskeletal fitness Is comprised of three components: flexibility, muscular strength, and muscular endurance.

Myocardial infarction A common form of heart attack, in which the blockage of a coronary artery causes the death of a part of the heart muscle.

Myofilaments Within the muscle cell, actin and myosin protein fibers are called myofilaments.

Myoglobin A muscle protein molecule that contains iron. Myoglobin carries oxygen from the blood to the muscle cell.

N

National Health and Nutrition Examination Survey (NHANES) A periodic survey administered by the National Center for Health Statistics. These surveys provide a wealth of information about dietary patterns and practices of representative samples of the U.S. population.

Net energy expenditure Equals the Calories expended during the exercise session minus the Calories expended for the resting metabolic rate and other activities that would have occupied the individual had they not been formally exercising.

Non-Insulin Dependent Diabetes Mellitus (NIDDM) See diabetes mellitus.

Nonpharmacologic approaches Use of nondrug methods to treat hypertension, hypercholesterolemia, or other health problems.

Non-weight bearing activities Activities such as bicycling, swimming, and brisk walking, that do not overstress the musculoskeletal system.

Norms Represent the achievement level of a particular group to which the measured scores can be compared.

Nutritional assessment Involves the use of a wide variety of clinical and biochemical methods to assess the state of health as characterized by body composition, tissue function, and metabolic activity.

O

Obesity Excessive accumulation of body fat.

Oligomenorrhea Scanty or infrequent menstrual flow.

Omega-3-fatty acids A type of fat found in fish oils and associated with lower blood cholesterol levels, lower blood pressure, and reduced blood dotting.

One repetition maximum, 1-RM The maximum resistance with which a person can execute one repetition of an exercise movement.

Oral glucose tolerance test (OGTT) The OGTT is a 75 gram glucose solution given after an overnight fast of 10–16 hours.

Osmolarity The concentration of a solution participating in osmosis.

Osteoarthritis A noninflammatory joint disease of older person. The cartilage in the joint wears down, and there is bone growth at the edges of the joints. Results in pain and stiffness, especially after prolonged exercise.

Osteoclasts The cells that break down hone.

Osteoblasts Bone cells that build bone.

Osteoporosis Defined as an age-related disorder, characterized by decreased bone mineral content, and increased risk of fractures.

Overload Subjecting a part of the body to efforts greater than it is accustomed to, in order to elicit a training response. Increases may be in intensity or duration.

Overuse Excessive repeated exertion or shock which results in injuries such as stress fractures of bones or inflammation of muscles and tendons.

Oxygen debt The oxygen required to restore the capacity for anaerobic work after an effort has used those reserves. Measured by the extra oxygen that is consumed during the recovery from the work.

Oxygen deficit The energy supplied anaerobically while oxygen uptake has not yet reached the steady state which matches energy output. Becomes oxygen debt at end of exercise.

Oxygen uptake The amount of oxygen used up at the cellular level during exercise. Can be measured by determining the amount of oxygen exhaled as compared to the amount inhaled, or estimated by indirect means.

Ozone Produced by the photochemical reaction of sunlight on hydrocarbons and nitrogen dioxide from car exhaust.

P

Pangamic acid   So called vitamin B_{15} which is claimed to enhance performance. Reputable nutritionists do not support this claim or even the fact that a vitamin B_{15}, exists.

Parasympathetic   The craniosacral division of the autonomic nervous system.

Parcourse   An outdoor circuit system that combines calisthenics with running.

Passive smoking   Breathing of air that has cigarette smoke in it.

Pellagra   A disease of niacin deficiency.

Percentage of total calories   Nutritionists use this concept when representing the percentage of protein, carbohydrate, and fat calories present in the diet. This is a useful skill to know, and is calculated from the fact that one gram carbohydrate, protein, and fat equals 4 Calories, 4 Calories, and 9 Calories respectively.

Percent saturation   During iron-deficient erythropoiesis (stage 2 iron deficiency) percent saturation falls (<16 percent is abnormal).

Phenylpropanolamine (PPA)   This is the active ingredient in most nonprescription weight-control products, such as Dexatrim, Appedrine, Control, Dietac, Prolamine and Adrinex. PPA is related to amphetamines and has similar side effects, such as nervousness, insomnia, headaches, nausea, tinnitus (ringing in the ears), and elevated blood pressure.

Phospholipids   Substances found in all body cells. They are similar to lipids, but contain only two fatty adds and one phosphorus containing substance.

Physical activity   Any form of muscular movement.

Physical activity readiness questionnaire (PAR-Q)   A questionnaire for screening out high risk people prior to exercise testing that has been used very successfully in Canada.

Physical fitness   A dynamic state of energy and vitality that enables one to carry out daily tasks, to engage in active leisure-time pursuits, and to meet unforeseen emergencies without undue fatigue. In addition, physically fit individuals have a decreased risk of hypokinetic diseases, and are more able to function at the peak of intellectual capacity while experiencing "joie de vivre."

Physical work capacity (PWC)   An exercise test that measures the amount of work done at a given, submaximal heart rate. The work is measured in oxygen uptake, kilopond meters per minute, or other units, and can be used to estimate maximal heart rate and oxygen uptake.

Placebo   An inactive substance given to satisfy a patient's demand for medicine.

Platelets   The clotting material in the blood.

Polarized   Charged heart cells in the resting state (negative ions inside the cell, positive outside), but when electrically stimulated, they depolarize (positive ions go inside the heart cell, negative ions go outside) and contract.

Polydipsia   Excessive thirst.

Polyphagia   Unsatisfied hunger.

Polyunsaturated fat   Dietary fat whose molecules have more than one double bond open to receive more hydrogen. Found in safflower oil, corn oil, soybeans, sesame seeds, sunflower seeds.

Polyuria   Excessive urination.

Power   Work performed per unit of time. Measured by the formula: work equals force times distance divided by time. A combination of strength and speed.

Pre-event meal   A meal 3 to 5 hours before an exercise event that emphasizes low fiber, high carbohydrate foods.

Premature ventricular contraction (PVC)   One of the most common EKG abnormalities during the exercise test where a spot on the ventricle becomes the pacemaker, superseding the SA node.

Primary air pollutants   Include carbon monoxide (CO), carbon dioxide (CO_2), sulfur dioxide (SO_2), nitrogen oxide (NO), and particulate material such as lead, graphite carbon, and fly ash.

Primary osteoporosis   May occur in two types: Type I osteoporosis (postmenopausal) which is the accelerated decrease in bone mass that occurs when estrogen levels fall after menopause; and Type II osteoporosis (age-related) which is the inevitable loss of bone mass with age that occurs in both men and women.

Progressive resistance exercise   Exercise in which the amount of resistance is increased to further stress the muscle after it has become accustomed to handling a lesser resistance.

Pronation   Assuming a face-down position. Of the hand, turning the palm backward or downward. Of the foot, lowering the inner (medial) side of the foot so as to flatten the arch. The opposite of supination.

Proprioceptive neuromuscular facilitation (PNF) stretch   Muscle stretches that use the proprioceptors (muscle spindles) to send inhibiting (relaxing) messages to the muscle that is to be stretched. Example: The contraction of an agonist muscle sends inhibiting signals that relax the antagonist muscle so that it is easier to stretch,

Protein A complex nitrogen carrying compound which occurs naturally in plants and animals and yield amino acids when broken down. The amino acids are essential for the growth and repair of living tissue. Proteins are also a source of heat and energy for the body. Protein is found widely in both animal and plant products.

Protoporphyrin A derivative of hemoglobin. Formed from heme by deletion of an atom of iron.

Prudent diet Defined in this book as the diet adhering to the 1958 Surgeon General's Report on Nutrition and Health.

Puberty The period in life when one becomes functionally capable of reproduction.

P wave Transmission of electrical impulse through the atria.

Q

QRS complex Impulse through the ventricles.

Quetelet index Body weight in kilograms divided by height in meters squared. This is the most widely accepted body mass index.

R

Racquet sports Sports like racquetball, squash, and tennis that use a racquet.

Radial pulse The pulse at the wrist.

Rating of perceived exertion (RPE) A means to quantify the subjective feeling of the intensity of an exercise. Borg scales, charts which describe a range of intensity from resting to maximal energy outputs, are used as a visual aid to exercisers in keeping their efforts in the effective training zone.

Reaction time Relates to the time elapsed between stimulation and the beginning of the reaction to it.

Recommended Dietary Allowances (RDA) The (RDA) established by the National Research Council of the National Academy of Sciences, have become the premier nutrient standard in both the U.S. and the world. The RDA are a technical standard used for nutrition policies and decision making. The RDA today are used for a wide variety of purposes ranging from development of new food products to being the standard for federal nutrition assistance programs.

Relative risk An expression of disease risk that usually compares death rates from groups varying in a certain practice.

Relative weight The body weight divided by the midpoint value of the weight range.

Relaxation therapy A treatment that involves teaching a patient to accomplish a state of both muscular and mental deactivation by the systematic use of relaxation or meditation exercises to reduce high blood pressure.

Reliability Deals with how consistently a certain element is measured by the particular test.

Residual volume The volume of air remaining in the lungs after a maximum expiration. Must be calculated in the formula for determining body composition through underwater weighing.

Respiratory exchange ratio (R) The ratio between the amount of carbon dioxide produced and the amount of oxygen consumed by the body during exercise.

Resting metabolic rate (RMR) This represents the energy expended by your body to maintain life and normal body functions, such as respiration and circulation.

R.I.C.E. Treatment of musculoskeletal pain and injury during the first 48 to 72 hours centers around rest, ice, compression, and elevation.

Risk factors Characteristics that are associated with higher risk of developing a specific health problem.

S

Sarcolemma The membrane of the muscle cell.

Sarcomere The smallest functional skeletal muscle subunit capable of contraction.

Satiety The feeling of fullness and satisfaction.

Saturated fat Dietary fat whose molecules are saturated with hydrogen. They are usually hard at room temperature and are readily converted into cholesterol in the body. Sources include animal products as well as hydrogenated vegetable oils.

Scurvy A disease of vitamin C deficiency.

Secondary air pollutants Formed by chemical action of the primary pollutants and the natural chemicals in the atmosphere. Examples include ozone (O_3), sulfuric acid (H_2SO_4), and nitric acid (HNO_3), peroxyacetyl nitrate, and a host of other inorganic and organic compounds.

Secondary osteoporosis May develop at any age as a consequence of hormonal, digestive, and metabolic disorders, as well as prolonged bedrest and weightlessness (space flight) that result in loss of bone mineral mass.

Senile dementia A form of organic brain syndrome, a mental disorder associated with impaired brain function in the elderly.

Serum erythropoietin A hormone that regulates red blood cell production.

Serum iron   During iron-deficient erythro-poiesis (stage 2 iron deficiency) serum iron levels fall.

Set   A group of repetitions of an exercise movement done consecutively, without rest, until a given number, or momentary exhaustion, is reached.

Severe obesity   Defined as more than 100 percent overweight.

Skeletal muscle   Muscle which is connected with a bone.

Skill-related fitness   Elements of fitness such as agility, balance, speed, coordination. While the elements of skill-related fitness are important for participation in various dual and team sports, they have little significance for the day-to-day tasks of Americans or their general health.

Skinfoid measurements   The most widely used method for determining obesity is based on the thickness of skinfolds. Calipers are used to measure the thickness of a double fold of skin at various sites.

Slow-twitch fibers   Muscle fiber type that contracts slowly and is used most in moderate-intensity, endurance exercises, such as distance running. Also called Type I fibers.

Smokeless tobacco   Use of smokeless tobacco takes two forms. Dipping involves placing a pinch of moist or dry powdered tobacco (snuff) between the cheek or lip and the lower gum. Chewing involves placing a golfball-sized amount of loose leaf tobacco between the cheek and lower gum where it Is sucked and chewed.

Sodium   This electrolyte is the major cation (positive ion) of fluids outside the body cells. Sodium and chloride ions tend to concentrate outside of body cell walls (extracellular), while potassium tends to concentrate inside of body cell walls (intracellular). This arrangement is essential in maintaining the balance of tissue fluids inside and outside of cells. Sodium, potassium, and chloride work with bicarbonate in regulating the acid-base balance of the body. Sodium has an important role in regulating normal muscle tone. The Food and Nutrition Board has established safe and adequate daily dietary intakes for sodium which is 1100–3300 mg.

Sodium bicarbonate   A substance used by some athletes to enhance performance in events lasting 1–3 minutes. Sodium bicarbonate ingestion increases the pH of the body, allowing greater lactic add to be produced and buffered.

Sodium to potassium ratio (Na:K)   A ratio of the dietary sodium to potassium intake which may be important as an indicator of hypertension risk.

Specificity   The principle that the body adapts very specifically to the training stimuli it is required to deal with. The body will perform best at the specific speed, type of contraction, muscle-group usage and energy-source usage it has been accustomed to in training.

Speed   Relates to the ability to perform a movement within a short period of time.

Sphygmomanometer   Consists of an inflatable, compression bag enclosed in an unyielding covering called the cuff, plus an inflating bulb, a manometer from which the pressure is read, and a controlled exhaust to deflate the system during measurement of blood pressure.

Spirulina   This is a dark green powder or pill derived from algae that has been promoted as a weight-loss product.

Spot reducing   An effort to reduce fat at one location on the body by concentrating exercise, manipulation, wraps, etc. on that location. Research indicates that any fat loss is generalized over the body, however.

Stadiometer   A vertical ruler with a horizontal headboard that can be brought into contact with the most superior or highest point on the head.

Starch   A polysaccharide made up of glucose monosaccharides.

Starch blockers   This enzyme inhibitor is supposed to block the digestion and absorption of ingested carbohydrate. Several studies have now shown these not only to be ineffective, but also a possible risk to health.

Step-care therapy   An approach with lifestyle techniques and various drugs to treat hypertension.

Sterols   A type of lipid such as cholesterol, estrogen, testosterone, and vitamin D.

Stethoscope   Made up of rubber tubing attached to a device that amplifies the sounds of blood passing through the blood vessels during measurement of blood pressure.

Strength   The amount of muscular force that can be exerted.

Stress   The general physical and psychological response of an individual to any real or perceived adverse stimulus, internal or external, that tends to disturb the individual's homeostasis.

Stretching   Lengthening a muscle to its maximum extension; moving a joint to the limits of its extension.

Stroke A form of cardiovascular disease that affects the blood vessels that supply oxygen and nutrients to the brain.

Stroke volume The volume of blood pumped out of the heart (by the ventricles) in one contraction.

ST segment depression An indication of atherosclerotic blockage in the coronary arteries.

Sugars Defined as monosaccharides (glucose, fructose, galactose) and disaccharides (lactose, mannose, sucrose).

Supermarket diets A type of diet which includes such foods as chocolate chip cookies, salami, cheese, marshmallows, milk chocolate, peanut butter, and sweetened whole milk used to produce obesity in rats.

Supplementation Use of vitamin or mineral pills to supplement the regular diet.

Systolic blood pressure The pressure of the blood upon the walls of the blood vessels when the heart is contracting. A normal systolic blood pressure ranges between 90 and 139 mm Hg. When the systolic blood pressure is measured on more than one occasion to be more than 140 mm Hg, high blood pressure is diagnosed.

Submaximal Less than maximum. Submaximal exercise requires less than one's maximum oxygen uptake, heart rate or anaerobic power. Usually refers to intensity of the exercise, but may be used to refer to duration.

Supination Assuming a horizontal position facing upward. In the case of the hand, it also means turning the palm to face forward. The opposite of pronation.

Systolic blood pressure Blood pressure during the contraction of the heart muscle.

T

Tachycardia Excessively rapid heart rate. Usually describes a pulse of more than 100 beats per minute at rest.

Target heart rate (THR) The heart rate at which one aims to exercise. For example, the American College of Sports Medicine recommends that healthy adults exercise at a THR of 60 to 90 percent of maximum heart rate reserve. Also called training heart rate.

Testosterone An androgen hormone produced by the testicles and adrenal cortex. It accelerates growth in tissues.

Thematic effect of food (TEF) The increase in energy expenditure above the resting metabolic rate that can be measured for several hours after a meal.

Thrombosis Formation or existence of a blood clot within the blood vessel system.

Tidal volume The amount of air per breath.

Total iron binding capacity (TIBC) During iron-deficient erythropoiesis (inadequate formation of red blood cells), total iron binding capacity is increased.

Total lung capacity (TLC) Represents the total amount of air in the lung.

Total peripheral resistance The sum of all the forces that oppose blood flow in the body's blood vessel system. During exercise, total peripheral resistance decreases because the blood vessels in the active muscles increase in size.

Trabecular bone Spongy, internal end bone.

Triglyceride A type of fat made of glycerol with three fatty adds. Most animal and vegetable fats are triglycerides.

T wave Electrical recovery or repolarization of the ventricles.

U

Underwater weighing The most widely used laboratory procedure for measuring body density. In this procedure, whole body density is calculated from body volume according to Archimedes' principle of displacement which states that an object submerged in water is buoyed up by the weight of the water displaced.

US-RDA These are a set of standards developed by the Food and Drug Administration (FDA) for use in regulating nutrition labeling. Although these standards were taken from the RDA, they are based on very few categories, and only 19 vitamins and minerals were chosen.

V

Validity Refers to the degree to which the test measures what it was designed to measure.

Valsalva maneuver A strong exhaling effort against a closed glottis, which builds pressure in the chest cavity that interferes with the return of blood to the heart. May deprive the brain of blood and cause fainting.

Vasoconstriction The narrowing of a blood vessel to decrease blood flow to a body part.

Vasodilation The enlarging of a blood vessel to increase blood flow to a body part.

Very-low-calorie diets (VLCD) Also called the protein-sparing modified fast. The VLCD provides 400–1700 Calories per day for people trying to lose weight. Protein is emphasized to help avoid loss of muscle tissue. Patients can use either special formula beverages or natural foods such as fish, fowl, or lean meat (along with mineral and vitamin supplements).

Very low density lipoproteins (VLDL) Transports triglycerides to body tissues.

Vital capacity The amount of air that can be expired after a maximum inspiration; the maximum total volume of the lungs, less the residual volume.

Vitamin Vitamins are nutrients which are essential for life itself. The body uses these organic substances to accomplish much of its work. Vitamins do not supply energy, but they do help release energy from carbohydrates, fats, and proteins. They also play a vital role in chemical reactions throughout the body. There are two types of vitamins—fat-soluble (A, D, E, K) and watersoluble (eight B-complex and vitamin C). Thirteen vitamins have been discovered, the most recent in 1948.

VO$_{2max}$ Maximum volume of oxygen consumed per unit of time. In scientific notation, a dot appears over the V to indicate "per unit of time."

W

Waist to hip circumference (WHR) Ratio of waist and hip circumferences. A relatively high WHR predicts increased complications from obesity.

Warm-up A gradual increase in the intensity of exercise to allow physiological processes to prepare for greater energy outputs. Changes include: rise in body temperature, cardiorespiratory changes, increase in muscle elasticity and contractility, etc.

Watt A measure of power equal to 6.12 kilogrammeters per minute.

Weight reducing clothing Special weight-reducing clothing, including heated belts, rubberized suits, and oilskins rely chiefly on dehydration and localized pressure.

Wet-bulb thermometer A thermometer whose bulb is enclosed in a wet wick, so that evaporation from the wick will lower the temperature reading more in dry air than in humid air. The comparison of wet- and dry-bulb readings can be used to calculate relative humidity.

Wet-globe temperature A temperature reading that approximates the heat stress which the environment will impose on the human body. Takes into account not only temperature and humidity, but radiant heat from the sun and cooling breezes that would speed evaporation and convection of heat away from the body. Reading is provided by an instrument that encloses a thermometer in a wetted, black copper sphere. Cf. dry-bulb thermometer, wet-bulb thermometer.

White blood cells Special immune system cells that circulate in the blood. These include monocytes, neutrophils, basophils, eosinophils, and lymphocytes.

Index